DRUG TREATMENT IN UROLOGY

DRUG
TREATMENT
IN UROLOGY

EDITED BY

Ian Eardley
Department of Urology, St James's University Hospital, Leeds

Peter Whelan
Department of Neurology, St James's University Hospital, Leeds

Roger S. Kirby
Harley Street, London

Anthony J. Schaeffer
Northwestern University Medical School, Chicago, IL

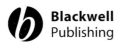
Blackwell
Publishing

© 2006 by Blackwell Publishing Ltd
Blackwell Publishing, Inc., 350 Main Street, Malden,
  Massachusetts 02148-5020, USA
Blackwell Publishing Ltd, 9600 Garsington Road,
  Oxford ox4 2DQ, UK
Blackwell Publishing Asia Pty Ltd, 550 Swanston Street,
  Carlton, Victoria 3053, Australia

First published 2006

Library of Congress Cataloging-in-Publication Data
Drug treatment in urology/edited by Ian Eardley... [et al.].
   p. ; cm.
  Includes bibliographical references.
  ISBN-13: 978-1-4051-0121-9 (alk. paper)
  ISBN-10: 1-4051-0121-0 (alk. paper)
1. Genitourinary organs –Diseases–Chemotherapy.
  [DNLM: 1. Urogenital Diseases–drug therapy. WJ 140 D794 2005] I. Eardley, Ian.

  RM375. D77 2005
  616. 6'061–dc22

                                                            2005012660

A catalogue record for this title is available from the British Library

Set in 10/13.5 Sabon by SPI Publisher Services, Pvt Ltd Pondicherry, India
Printed and bound by Replika Press PVT Ltd, Harayana, India

Commissioning Editor: Stuart Taylor
Development Editor: Julie Elliott
Production Controller: Kate Charman

For further information on Blackwell Publishing, visit our website:
http://www.blackwellpublishing.com

Contents

List of contributors, vii

Preface, x

Part 1 Functional Disorders

1 Urinary Incontinence, 3
Stephen J. Griffin & William H. Turner

2 Medical Therapy for Benign Prostatic Hyperplasia, 21
Simon R. J. Bott, Charlotte L. Foley & Roger S. Kirby

3 Drugs Used in the Treatment of Erectile Dysfunction, 39
Ian Eardley

4 Drugs Used in the Treatment of Interstitial Cystitis, 62
Mary Garthwaite & Ian Eardley

Part 2 Urinary Tract Infection

5 Treatment of Simple Urinary Tract Infection, 77
Dana Stieber & Kalpana Gupta

6 New Concepts in Antimicrobial Treatment for
Complicated Urinary Tract Infections:
Single Daily Aminoglycoside Dosing and 'Switch' Therapy, 96
Richard A. Santucci & John N. Krieger

7 Prostatitis, 120
Martin Ludwig & Wolfgang Weidner

8 Perioperative Antimicrobial Prophylaxis in
Urological Interventions of the Urinary and Male
Genital Tract, 138
Kurt G. Naber

9 Candiduria, 149
Jack D. Sobel

Part 3 Urological Oncology

10   Pharmacotherapy in the Management of Prostate Cancer, 161
     Jeetesh Bhardwa & Roger S. Kirby

11   Drugs in Superficial Bladder Cancer, 176
     Peter Whelan

12   Systemic Therapy for Bladder Cancer, 188
     J. D. Chester & M. G. Leahy

13   Testicular Cancer, 212
     Jourik A. Gietema & Dirk Th. Sleijfer

14   Renal Cancer, 234
     Naveen S. Vasudev & Poulam M. Patel

Part 4 Analgesia

15   Postoperative Analgesia, 257
     Patrick McHugh

16   Treatment of Pain in Urology, 274
     Adrian D. Joyce & William R. Cross

Index, 295

List of contributors

Jeetesh Bhardwa, MBChB, MRCS
(Eng)
Clinical Assistant in Urology
The London Clinic
20 Devonshire Place
London, UK

Simon R. J. Bott, FRCS
Specialist Registrar in Urology
South West Thames Region
London, UK

J. D. Chester
Cancer Research UK Clinical Centre
in Leeds
St James's University Hospital
Beckett Street
Leeds LS9 7TF, UK

William R. Cross, BmedSci, BMBS,
MRCS, PhD
Specialist Registrar
Pyrah Department of Urology
St James's University Hospital
Leeds LS9 7TF, UK

Ian Eardley, MB, Bchir, FRCS
Consultant Urologist
St James's University Hospital
Pyrah Department of Urology
Beckett Street
Leeds LS9 7TF, UK

Charlotte L. Foley, MRCS
Specialist Registrar in Urology
Institute of Urology and
Nephrology

The Middlesex Hospital
Mortimer street
London W1W 8AA, UK

Mary Garthwaite, MB, Bchir,
FRCS
St James's University Hospital
Pyrah Department of Urology
Beckett Street
Leeds LS9 7TF, UK

Jourik A. Gietema, MD, PhD
Department of Internal
Medicine
Division of Medical Oncology
University Hospital Groningen
9700 RB Groningen
The Netherlands

Stephen J. Griffin, MmedSc,
FRCSEd
Specialist Registrar in Urology
Department of Urology
Addenbrooke's Hospital
Hills Road
Cambridge CB2 2QQ, UK

Kalpana Gupta
Department of Medicine
University of Washington
Division of Allergy and Infectious
Diseases
Seattle, WA 98195-6523, USA

Adrian D. Joyce, MS, FRCS (Urol)
Consultant Urologist
Pyrah Department of Urology

St James's University Hospital
Leeds LS9 7TF, UK

Roger S. Kirby, MD, FRCS (Urol)
  FEBU
Consultant Urologist
149 Harley St
London W1N 1DE, UK

John N. Krieger, MD
Department of Urology
University of Washington School of
  Medicine
Seattle, WA, USA

M. G. Leahy
Cancer Research UK Clinical Centre
  in Leeds
St James's University Hospital
Beckett Street
Leeds LS9 7TF, UK

Martin Ludwig, MD
Klinik und Poliklinik für Urologie
  und Kinderurologie
Universitatsklinikum Giessen
Rudolf-Buchheim-Strasse 7
D-35385 Giessen, Germany

Patrick McHugh, FRCA,
  FFARCSI
Department of Anaesthesia
Leeds General Infirmary
Leeds LSI 3EX, UK

Kurt G. Naber, MD, PhD
Applied Professor of Urology
Urologic Clinic
Hospital St. Elisabeth
Teaching Hospital of the Medical
School of the Technical University of
  Munich,
St. Elisabethstrasse 23
D-94315 Straubing, Germany

Poulam M. Patel, MBBS, PhD,
  FRCP
Professor of Clinical Oncology
University of Nottingham
Division of Clinical Oncology
City Hospital, Nottingham, UK

Richard A. Santucci, MD
Department of Urology
Wayne State University School of
  Medicine
Detroit, MI 48201, USA

Anthony J. Schaeffer, MD
Northwestern University Medical
  School
303 East Chicago Avenue
Chicago, IL 60611, USA

Dirk Th. Sleijfer, MD, PhD
Department of Internal Medicine
Division of Medical Oncology
University Hospital Groningen
9700 RB Groningen
The Netherlands

Jack D. Sobel, MD
Professor of Medicine
Division of Infectious Diseases
Wayne State University School of
  Medicine
Detroit, MI, USA

Dana Stieber
Department of Pharmacy
University of Washington
Seattle, WA 98195-6523, USA

William H. Turner, MD, FRCS
  (Urol), Consultant Urologist
Department of Urology
Addenbrooke's Hospital
Hills Road
Cambridge CB2 2QQ, UK

Naveen S. Vasudev, MRCP, BMSc (Hons)
Specialist Registrar in Medical Oncology
St James's University Hospital
Leeds, UK

Wolfgang Weidner
Klinik und Poliklinik für Urologie und Kinderurologie
Universitatsklinikum Giessen
Rudolf-Buchheim-Strasse 7
D-35385 Giessen, Germany

Peter Whelan, MB, BS, FRCS
Consultant Urologist
Department of Neurology
St James's University Hospital
Beckett Street
Leeds LS9 7TS, UK

Preface

Urology is the most 'medical' of all the surgical specialities. Many of the conditions that present to urologists do not require surgical treatment but are best treated in other ways, including the use of drugs. While antibiotics and analgesics have been with us for many years, it is only in the past 15 years that medical therapy for urological conditions has boomed. Following the advent of effective medical therapy for benign prostatic hyperplasia, effective agents for other benign conditions including urinary incontinence and erectile dysfunction have appeared. At the same time the scientific search for an effective and safe treatment for cancer has accompanied the introduction of multiple agents for the treatment of all the urological cancers, with increasing degrees of efficacy and tolerability. It is inevitable that this progress will continue.

Given the increasing role of drugs within urology, it is perhaps surprising that there has never before been an attempt to produce a comprehensive summary of the urological drugs. This book seeks to address this deficit. The Editors, with a wide range of subspecialty interests covering the breadth of urology, have put together a series of articles that seek to provide for the reader a concise summary of the role of pharmacotherapy in urology. Each chapter deals with either a specific urological condition or with a class of drugs and seeks to outline for each respective agent, the mechanism of action, the evidence for efficacy, safety and tolerability and those practical issues relating to the use of these agents. Clearly the pharmaceutical industry is always seeking new agents either with better efficacy and tolerability than those currently marketed, or with novel mechanisms of action for new indications. Change is often rapid, and for that reason, any book such as this will only provide a snapshot of the drugs available at a particular moment in time.

At the same time as these drugs are being introduced, urology is also changing. With increasing sub-specialization of operative urology most health care systems are training significant numbers of 'office' or 'core' urologists who will inevitably become the main purveyors of medical therapy for urological conditions. It is for this group of urologists that are particularly aiming this book. We hope they will find this book useful as a guide and reference for their everyday practise.

Part 1
Functional Disorders

1: Urinary Incontinence

Stephen J. Griffin & William H. Turner

Introduction

Incontinence of urine occurs when bladder pressure exceeds urethral pressure. If bladder pressure is inappropriately high, this is detrusor overactivity with so-called urge incontinence, whereas if urethral pressure is inappropriately low, this is stress urinary incontinence (SUI). These two conditions, separately or together, cause most of the cases of urinary incontinence seen in clinical practice. A brief outline of each condition is given, together with the rationale for the use of the various types of drug treatments that have been tried for each, before an account of the details of the individual drugs that have been used.

Overactive bladder

Overactive bladder has been defined by the International Continence Society as urgency (with or without incontinence), usually with frequency and nocturia, not explained by metabolic or local pathological factors. The urodynamic manifestation of this is called detrusor overactivity and it denotes involuntary detrusor contractions during the filling phase that may be spontaneous or provoked [1]. A population-based survey in six European countries revealed a prevalence of bladder overactivity between 12% and 22% in 17000 people over 40 years old [2]. Such symptoms can have a profoundly negative influence on the quality of life, which is similar to diabetes mellitus [3], although paradoxically, many people do not seek medical advice about these symptoms. Although the physiology of the smooth muscle of the bladder is increasingly well understood [4] the pathogenesis of bladder overactivity remains to be fully elucidated, with both myogenic and neurogenic factors probably being involved [5,6].

The symptoms of bladder overactivity have been shown to respond to physical therapies. Randomized controlled trials (RCTs) investigating response rates to bladder training suggest that this is useful in the management of urge incontinence in the short term, but the data are not high quality [7]. Pelvic floor exercises appear to be an effective treatment for SUI and mixed urinary incontinence, although their efficacy with urge incontinence alone is less well documented [8]. These outcomes however, taken with the lack of side-effects of bladder training and pelvic floor exercises, emphasize their use as first-line treatment for bladder overactivity.

When behavioural techniques fail, the use of medication is appropriate, and many drugs have been used to treat bladder overactivity. Recent data suggest that the combination of bladder training and medication may offer an advantage over medication alone [9].

Drugs with a purely or largely muscarinic (M) antagonist (anticholinergic) action have been extensively used, probably on the basis that voiding contractions are mediated by release of acetylcholine (ACh) from the excitatory innervation of the detrusor, and subsequent activation of M receptors (mainly the M3 subtype) on detrusor smooth muscle cells [4]. There seem to be more M2 than M3 receptors in the detrusor, many located prejunctionally: their role is unclear at present, but stimulation may also be important in disease states [10]. It remains uncertain whether the use of anticholinergics to treat bladder overactivity actually has a rational basis, given that it is still not clear if activation of the detrusor M receptors is a critical part of the aetiology of overactive bladder contractions [11]. This might account for the generally disappointing efficacy of the anticholinergics in clinical practice [12]. Drugs that might reduce the effect of overactive bladder contractions in other ways have been used, including those that block L-type calcium channels (thereby reducing the rise in intracellular calcium necessary for detrusor cell contraction), drug with actions loosely described as smooth muscle relaxants, drugs that activate potassium channels (thereby reducing detrusor smooth muscle cell excitability), and drugs that may act on the afferent limb of the micturition reflex. The lack of high clinical efficacy of all of these drugs probably also reflects our lack of a clear understanding of the pathophysiological basis of overactive bladder contractions. Relatively few of the whole group of drugs that have been used have a level 1 evidence base [13], and although there is clear guidance on good practice for clinical trials that investigate drug therapy [14], its use in the study of drug treatment of urinary incontinence remains disappointing [15]. Only those agents in common clinical use at present (oxybutynin, propiverine, tolterodine and trospium) and those in development are discussed: other agents, now little used (e.g. dicyclomine, propantheline, flavoxate), are not considered.

Anticholinergics

Anticholinergics increase the volume to the first spontaneous detrusor contraction during filling and the bladder capacity, but decrease the amplitude of the first contraction. Currently available agents are not bladder-selective and often cause typical atropine-like side-effects (due to blockage of M receptors), including dry mouth and/or eyes, upper and lower gastrointest-inal symptoms, tachycardia and accommodation paralysis. Indeed, these agents are contraindicated in narrow angle glaucoma. Given the uncertainty about the pathophysiological basis of bladder overactivity, the wide distribution of M receptors and the lack of bladder-specific M receptors, it is not surprising that atropine-like side-effects are common. Trials report dropout rates between 12% and 63% and placebo response in up to 45% of participants [8]. The side-effect profile of presently used medication underlines the use of drug treatment as second-line therapy for bladder overactivity.

TOLTERODINE

Tolterodine is a tertiary amine that is a competitive non-selective antimuscarinic agent [16]. *In vitro*, the affinity of tolterodine for bladder muscarinic receptors is similar to that of oxybutynin, whereas its affinity for guinea-pig parotid muscarinic receptors is less than that of oxybutynin. This tissue selectivity is claimed to be preserved *in vivo* in animal models [17]. It is metabolized via cytochrome P450, yielding a 5-hydroxymethyl active metabolite [18]: both these compounds have a half-life of 2–3 h. The low lipophilicity of tolterodine and its metabolites means that they do not cross the blood–brain barrier, and this presumably accounts for a low incidence of cognitive side-effects. It is available in two preparations: immediate-release (IR) (1–2 mg twice daily) or extended-release (ER) (4 mg once daily).

Several randomized, placebo-controlled trials, over 4–12 weeks, have demonstrated benefit of IR tolterodine compared with placebo, with respect to micturition diary variables and urodynamic end points in patients with neurogenic detrusor overactivity and bladder overactivity [18,19]. Studies typically show significant improvement in the number of voids per day, urine volume per void, number of incontinent episodes and pad usage, and the volume at first detrusor contraction, volume at normal desire to void and maximum cystometric capacity are all increased. These effects are maintained with longer treatment over a 9-month period [20]. However, dry mouth is three times more likely with tolterodine than placebo [8], occurring in up to 40% of patients taking tolterodine IR [21].

ER tolterodine has become available and a large multicentre, double-blind, randomized, placebo-controlled study compared tolterodine ER 4 mg once daily with tolterodine IR 2 mg twice daily, in patients with urinary frequency, urge incontinence, and symptoms of bladder overactivity for more than 6 months [22]. More than 500 patients were enrolled into each of the three arms for the 12-week study period. Efficacy was evaluated using micturition diaries that documented the number of incontinence episodes per week, number of micturitions per 24 h, voided volume and the number of pads used per 24 h. There was a significant improvement in all micturition diary variables in both the ER and IR regimens, compared with placebo. The median reduction (from baseline) in urge incontinence episodes was 71% for tolterodine ER, 60% for tolterodine IR and 33% for placebo, and this reached statistical significance for the ER versus IR regimens ($p < 0.05$). Furthermore, dry mouth was reported significantly less often by those taking the ER preparation compared with those on tolterodine IR 2 mg twice daily. A recent secondary analysis of a placebo-controlled study showed a clinically important reduction in urgency with tolterodine ER [23]. In a follow-up study, tolterodine ER was shown to have a good side-effect profile at 12 months [24].

A number of RCTs have compared tolterodine IR 2 mg twice daily with oxybutynin IR 5 mg twice or three times daily [25–27]. There was comparable improvement in urinary frequency in all three studies and similar improvement in the number of incontinence episodes for both drugs in two studies [25,27]. Although Leung *et al.* did not show improvement with either agent with respect to incontinence episodes, improvement in urinary leakage using the urinary pad test was demonstrated with both agents [26]. However, this was statistically significantly better in the tolterodine group. Tolterodine also had a statistically significant better adverse effect profile in two out of three of these studies [25,27]. Leung *et al.* did not demonstrate significantly different adverse effect profiles between the two drugs [26].

The OBJECT study [28] prospectively compared tolterodine IR 2 mg twice daily with oxybutynin ER 10 mg once daily in patients with bladder overactivity. In this multicentre, double-blinded, parallel-group study, 378 patients were randomized and treated, and 87% completed the 12-week study. Oxybutynin ER was significantly more effective than tolterodine in each of the main outcome measures: weekly urge incontinence episodes, total incontinence episodes and urinary frequency compared with baseline values. Furthermore, there was no significant difference in dry mouth rates between the two groups. However, the study compared the ER form of oxybutynin with the standard preparation of tolterodine, and so an advantage in terms of side-effects might have been expected.

The Antimuscarinic Clinical Effectiveness Trial (ACET) addressed this issue [29]. This trial compared tolterodine ER 2 mg or 4 mg with oxybutynin ER 5 mg or 10 mg in 1289 patients with bladder overactivity. It was an open-label, multicentre trial with site selection and an 8-week treatment period. Investigators in one arm were blinded to the existence of the other arm in an attempt to limit bias. Primary efficacy variables were changes in patient perception of bladder condition and patient assessment of treatment benefit using a validated questionnaire. Severity of dry mouth was assessed using a visual analogue scale. An improved bladder condition was perceived by 70% of patients in the tolterodine ER 4 mg group, compared with 60% in the tolterodine ER 2 mg group, 59% in the oxybutynin ER 5 mg group and 60% in the oxybutynin ER 10 mg group (all $p < 0.01$ vs tolterodine ER 4 mg). In addition, patients treated with tolterodine ER 4 mg reported a significantly lower severity of dry mouth than those treated with oxybutynin ER 10 mg. However, this study lacked a placebo arm, and although open-label studies may better reflect clinical practice, the authors acknowledged that they were open to bias from both physicians and patients. The two agents in ER form were also compared in the OPERA study, and whilst oxybutynin ER had a greater impact on urinary frequency, it had a higher risk of dry mouth [30]. This study was also limited by lack of a placebo arm.

TROSPIUM CHLORIDE

Trospium chloride is a quaternary ammonium compound that blocks M1–M3 receptors non-selectively: its pharmacology has been summarized recently [31]. *In vitro*, it has higher affinity for M receptors than do flavoxate, oxybutynin or tolterodine [32]. It has a half-life of 5–15 h with low biological availability (5%), and does not cross the blood–brain barrier [16]. The standard dose is 20 mg orally, twice daily.

The efficacy of the oral regimen has been proven in a number of double-blind placebo-controlled trials in patients with neurogenic detrusor over-activity [33], detrusor overactivity and bladder overactivity [34,35]. The urodynamic effect of treatment is an increased volume at first unstable contraction, and increased maximum cystometric capacity during filling. No significant decrease in maximum detrusor pressure at first unstable contraction is observed [34,35]. Frohlich *et al.* report that 47.9% of patients treated with trospium recorded a 'cure' or 'marked improvement', compared with 19.7% receiving placebo ($p < 0.0001$) [35]. Gastrointestinal side-effects and dry mouth were experienced by 21.7% and 14%, respectively, of patients in the treatment arm, compared with 18.7% and 8.4% in the placebo arm. However, post-marketing surveillance studies in over 10 000 patients show that this drug is well tolerated [31], with dry mouth reported by 4.1% of patients and gastrointestinal upset by less than 1%, and an overall occurrence of adverse events of approximately 5%.

Twenty milligrams twice daily trospium has been compared with 5 mg oxybutynin three times daily in patients with spinal cord injury having neurogenic detrusor overactivity [36]. This randomized, double-blind, multicentre study compared the two treatment arms at 2 weeks with respect to urodynamic parameters and subjective symptoms. There were similar increases in maximum cystometric capacity, compliance and residual volume. Both regimens produced a significant decrease in maximum voiding pressure, with no statistically significant difference between the groups. However, severe dry mouth was only experienced by 4% of patients taking trospium compared with 23% in the oxybutynin arm. Furthermore, the oxybutynin group had a 16% dropout rate compared with 6% in the trospium group.

The same trospium regimen is compared with 2 mg tolterodine twice daily in patients with bladder overactivity [37]. In this placebo-controlled multicentre trial of 234 patients with bladder overactivity both treatments reduced voiding frequency, but only the decrease in the trospium-treated group reached statistical significance compared with placebo. Dry mouth was similar in both groups.

Mixed action anticholinergics

OXYBUTYNIN

Oxybutynin is a tertiary amine with antimuscarinic, muscle relaxant and local anaesthetic effects and high affinity for M1 and M3 receptors [16]. It undergoes extensive first-pass metabolism, yielding the active metabolite N-desethyl oxybutynin: the plasma half-life is around 2 h, but there is wide individual variation [38]. It is available as an IR form, (2.5–5 mg orally twice to four times daily) or ER form (5–10 mg orally once daily to a maximum of 30 mg) preparation. When taken orally, much of the pharmacodynamic effect of the drug is thought to be due to the active metabolite, N-desethyl oxybutynin, which has a higher plasma concentration than the parent compound [39]: the active metabolite may also be largely responsible for the drug's adverse effects. Oxybutynin ER yields lower plasma levels of the active metabolite compared with oxybutynin IR, suggesting decreased first-pass metabolism [40]. In addition, salivary output is higher with less dry mouth when comparing oxybutynin ER with oxybutynin IR [40–42]. Transdermal oxybutynin bypasses first-pass metabolism and is associated with less dry mouth than the IR preparation [43].

Several controlled studies have demonstrated the efficacy of oxybutynin in the treatment of bladder overactivity and detrusor hyperreflexia. Thüroff *et al.* [44] reviewed 15 RCTs that included nearly 500 patients treated with oxybutynin. The mean decreases in incontinence and frequency were 52% and 33%, respectively. The mean overall subjective improvement rate was 74%, with adverse effects reported by 70% of patients. Side-effects are typically systemic antimuscarinic effects – dry mouth, constipation, blurred vision – and are generally dose-related. However, oxybutynin can also cross the blood–brain barrier, causing cognitive impairment that can be particularly problematic with the elderly and with children treated with intravesical oxybutynin.

Oxybutynin ER uses an osmotic drug delivery system to release the drug in a controlled fashion over 24 h [45]. This reduces the variations in plasma levels that occur with the IR preparation. Studies comparing the ER with the IR preparation have failed to show any improvement in efficacy with respect to symptom control of the ER compared with the IR preparation [40–42]. However, the side-effect profile is better with the ER preparation.

Transdermal oxybutynin has demonstrable efficacy for the treatment of bladder overactivity compared with placebo [46]. The incidence of dry mouth was comparable with the placebo arm. However, the most common adverse event was site pruritis (noted in up to 16.8% of patients). Davila *et al.* [43] further demonstrated that transdermal oxybutynin had similar efficacy in the treatment of urge urinary incontinence, with less dry mouth. Transdermal oxybutynin was shown to have efficacy similar to tolterodine ER, but a lower anticholinergic side-effect profile, at the expense of more skin irritation [47].

Intravesical oxybutynin has been used successfully for the treatment of neurogenic detrusor overactivity and detrusor overactivity in both children and adults [16]. The efficacy of oxybutynin is well documented and the International Consultation on Incontinence recommended it and tolterodine as the drugs of choice for bladder overactivity [16].

PROPIVERINE

Propiverine is a benzilic acid derivative with anticholinergic and calcium antagonistic actions [48]. It has a bioavailability of 40% and undergoes extensive first-pass metabolism. There are three metabolites that seem to be active; however, the pharmacological characteristics of this drug remain to be elucidated [16]. It is administered orally 15 mg three times daily, increased to four times daily if necessary.

Nine randomized studies using propiverine for the treatment of bladder overactivity were collated by Thüroff *et al.* [44]. Subjective improvement was reported by 77%, and objective improvement in bladder capacity and urinary frequency was noted. Bladder capacity increased by 64 ml and there was a reduction in urinary frequency by 30%. Madersbacher *et al.* [48] report similar efficacy between propiverine 15 mg three times daily and oxybutynin IR 5 mg twice daily in a multicentre, randomized, double-blind placebo-controlled trial using urodynamic parameters to assess efficacy. However, the incidence and severity of dry mouth was less in the patients treated with propiverine.

Propiverine is also effective in the treatment of neurogenic detrusor overactivity in patients with spinal cord injury [33]. In a prospective, double-blind, randomized, multicentre trial, bladder capacity at first contraction increased by 72 ml, maximal cystometric capacity increased by 104 ml and maximum detrusor pressure decreased by $27 +/- 32$ cm H_2O [33]. Dry mouth was reported by 37% of patients on propiverine and 28% on placebo, with accommodation disturbance in 8% and 2%, respectively [33].

NEWER AGENTS

Darifenacin is a selective M3 receptor antagonist that is currently being evaluated in phase III studies. Initial work in patients with detrusor overactivity suggests urodynamic effects comparable with oxybutynin, with less effect on salivary flow.

Solifenacin is a long-acting antimuscarinic agent. Enhanced bladder selectivity has been claimed [49], and the preliminary results of a study comparing solifenacin with tolterodine and placebo show a significant improvement in symptoms of bladder overactivity [50], but more detail on the efficacy compared with existing anticholinergics is required.

Activation of detrusor muscle through M receptors requires influx of calcium to the detrusor muscle cell and mobilization of calcium from the sarcoplasmic reticulum [4]. The calcium channel blocker, verapamil, used intravesically can increase bladder capacity and decrease leakage in patients with detrusor overactivity [51].

Potassium channel openers (KCOs) reduce smooth muscle cell excitability, and may therefore be useful in bladder overactivity by addressing the myogenic component of its aetiology [11]. Recent *in vivo* data support this use [52]. There are KCOs currently in phase II/III studies in patients with bladder overactivity symptoms.

Stress urinary incontinence

The anatomical factors that relate to SUI have been reviewed recently [53]: they cannot be treated pharmacologically. However, it is postulated that women with SUI have reduced maximum urethral closure pressures (MUCP), as they have lower resting urethral pressures than age-matched continent women. Various agents have been used, without much success, in an attempt to improve urethral pressure. Urethral pressure is substantially mediated by activation of α-adrenoceptors in urethral smooth muscle [4,54], and so drugs that might augment the activation of these receptors have been used over some years to attempt to treat SUI. The role of the vascular plexus of the lamina propria of the female urethra remains to be agreed upon [55,56], but it seems likely that it may contribute significantly. Both the vasculature and smooth muscle within the lamina propria and the smooth muscle of the urethra may be sensitive to oestrogen, and this has been used to try to treat SUI [16].

Several α-adrenoceptor agonists have been used to treat SUI: they share the anticipated side-effects that include anxiety, tremor, headache, palpitations and hypertension, and so should be used with caution in those with cardiovascular disease. Indeed, the Food and Drug Administration (FDA) in the USA has asked for norephedrine (phenylpropanolamine) to be withdrawn from the market because of concerns about hypertension. In a placebo-controlled study, 27 of 38 patients with SUI responded to ephedrine, but those with severe symptoms did less well [57]. By contrast, in a placebo-controlled study of norephedrine, only a moderate response was seen in 25 women with SUI [58]. In a placebo-controlled study of methoxamine in women with SUI, there was no significant rise in MUCP, but systolic hypertension and symptomatic side-effects did occur [59]. The β_2-adrenoceptor agonist clenbuterol has been used to treat SUI, although the rationale is hard to see. A randomized study compared clenbuterol with pelvic floor exercises, and found that either drug or drug and pelvic floor exercises were better than pelvic floor exercises alone [60]. Currently good evidence is lacking for the use of adrenoceptor agonists or antagonists of any sub-type for the treatment of SUI.

Duloxetine inhibits re-uptake of noradrenaline and 5-HT. It has been used in a placebo-controlled study in 683 women with SUI and with mixed incontinence and produced around 50% reductions in incontinence episodes compared with around 25% reductions by placebo, in all women, and in those with more severe symptoms [61]. A recently published placebo-controlled trial compared duloxetine 40 mg bd with placebo in 494 women with SUI [62]. There were demonstrable and statistically significant reductions in the frequency of incontinent episodes (median decrease 50% vs 29%), and there was an improvement in disease-specific quality of life. Discontinuations with duloxetine were significantly higher (22% vs 5% for placebo), with nausea being the most common reason for discontinuation. There is a suggestion in the clinical trials that the nausea diminishes with time.

Vaginally administered oestrogens have been used in the treatment of SUI. Meta-analyses [63,64] of controlled trials using oestrogens to treat SUI found improvement in MUCPs and subjective symptomatic improvement. However, there was no objective improvement in the amount of urinary leakage. Oestrogens, therefore, may be helpful with the associated symptoms of frequency and urgency, but are not an effective treatment alone for SUI.

Nocturnal enuresis

Bedwetting results in low self-esteem and may affect personal relationships and career development, but self-esteem in enuretic children returns to normal after adequate treatment [65]. It has, therefore, been suggested that active treatment should be started early when a patient presents with nocturnal enuresis. Some studies have shown that one of the factors contributing to nocturnal enuresis in children is absence of a normal nocturnal increase in ADH [66].

DESMOPRESSIN

Desmopressin (1-desamino-8-D-arginine vasopressin; DDAVP) is a synthetic analogue of arginine vasopressin. It has pronounced antidiuretic effect and is practically devoid of vasopressor actions [16]. It was available initially as an intranasal spray and is now also available in oral tablet form. It has been used for the treatment of nocturnal enuresis for some years, generally at a dose of 0.02 mg intranasal spray at bedtime. Night-time administration of desmopressin increases water reabsorption in the collecting ducts of the kidneys, causing a reduction in nocturnal urine volume [67].

Studies report that treatment with desmopressin for nocturnal enuresis over a period of 6 months or more results in a halving in the number of wet nights in 50–85% whilst 40–70% report being completely dry [65]. Furthermore, patients do not develop tolerance to the drug over time. Cure rates upon cessation of therapy are difficult to interpret, as there is an annual spontaneous recovery rate of approximately 15% [65]. However, data suggest that treatment with desmopressin further improves the cure rate. In addition, tapered dose cessation is associated with better cure rates than immediate cessation of the drug.

Long-term treatment with desmopressin for nocturnal enuresis has no significant side-effects. Van Kerrebroeck [65] reviewed 1083 patients treated with desmopressin spray or tablets and found only 53 (5%) patients experienced adverse effects that could be related to treatment. The most frequent adverse effects were headache (2% of all patients) and abdominal pain (1% of all patients). Furthermore, desmopressin does not influence endogenous ADH secretion.

Neurogenic incontinence

Neurogenic lower urinary tract dysfunction can be broadly divided into two categories: bladders that fail to empty successfully and those that fail to store urine adequately. Failure to empty results from either detrusor hypocontractility or increased outlet resistance caused by detrusor sphincter dyssynergia

(DSD), whilst failure to store is neurogenic detrusor overactivity. The underlying aetiology of neurogenic lower urinary tract dysfunction can be complex and problems with storage and bladder emptying can coexist.

Failure to empty

Clean intermittent catheterization (CIC) is the main therapeutic measure used to provide adequate bladder emptying in patients with neurogenic bladder where manual dexterity is adequately preserved. Patients for whom this is not a viable option may be considered for therapy to decrease outlet resistance.

Botulinum toxin blocks the release of ACh from nerve terminals reversibly over a prolonged period of time. Insertion of toxin to selected muscular tissues has been used to treat various conditions including achalasia, anal fissure, strabismus and torticollis. Dykstra *et al.* first evaluated injection of botulinum A toxin into the rhabdosphincter of men with spinal cord injury for the treatment of DSD [68]. In this small study ($n = 11$), patients had cystoscopic injection of toxin into the rhabdosphincter via a needle electrode attached to an electromyography machine to confirm correct needle position. There was a decrease in urethral pressure profile and post-void residual urine after treatment. A similar study in patients with spinal cord injury with DSD found 21 of 24 patients were significantly improved with a significant decrease in post-void residual urine [69]. The response lasted 3–9 months, making re-injection necessary. The authors claim this is safe, although expensive, alternative management in patients with DSD who cannot perform CIC and do not want permanent surgical sphincterotomy.

Failure to store

Neurogenic detrusor overactivity is often treated with anticholinergic therapy initially, along standard lines, although this is not always effective. Recent work has turned attention to modulation of the afferent side of the innervation of the lower urinary tract, because of experimental data suggesting that unmyelinated C fibres may mediate the afferent limb of the micturition reflex in certain circumstances, such as spinal lesions [6]. This C fibre activity may also be involved in the genesis of detrusor overactivity in patients with neuropathic lower urinary tract dysfunction [6].

CAPSAICIN

Vanilloids are agents that activate vanilloid receptors, and these are expressed almost exclusively by primary sensory neurons involved in nociception and neurogenic inflammation [70,71]. Vanilloid receptors are activated by drugs like capsaicin, the active ingredient in hot peppers of the genus Capsicum. This causes initial excitation, then desensitization of the neuron. Capsaicin has been shown to prevent rhythmic bladder contractions induced by bladder distension in the spinal cat [72], and was therefore used clinically in patients with neurogenic detrusor overactivity unresponsive to conservative treatment. Capsaicin is lipid-soluble and has to be dissolved in 30% ethanol in saline in order to be suitable for intravesical instillation. It also produces profound excitation of the vanilloid receptors before desensitization, causing intense pain on instillation, sometimes requiring anaesthesia [73]. De Ridder *et al.* have reported on 79 patients with refractory neurogenic detrusor overactivity treated with intravesical capsaicin [74]. Most patients in this study had multiple sclerosis and suffered from detrusor overactivity refractory to anticholinergic medications and CIC. They report that 80% showed some degree of clinical or urodynamic response. Patients without spinal cord disease did not do well, suggesting unmyelinated C fibre afferents are important in spinal man. Greater disability was also associated with poorer outcome. However, investigations and populations in different centres were not standardized. In one centre, the policy for pretreatment instillation of lignocaine changed midstudy. In addition, there was no standardized follow-up protocol. There was no placebo arm to this study, as the authors claimed that this would be difficult due to pungency of capsaicin.

RESINIFERATOXIN

Resiniferatoxin is a natural vanilloid derived from a cactus-like plant, *Euphorbia resinifera*, commonly found in Morocco. It is 1000 times more potent than capsaicin and is therefore pharmacologically active at much lower concentrations than capsaicin. This limits excitatory effects whilst still producing rapid desensitization. Cruz *et al.* initially performed a pilot study in seven neurologically impaired patients with detrusor overactivity [75]. There was no early deterioration in symptoms as with capsaicin, and itching or mild discomfort only lasted a few minutes. Improvement in urinary frequency and increased bladder capacity was noted in approximately half the patients and was sustained for approximately 3 months. Lazzeri *et al.* found no burning sensation on instillation, and immediate significant increase in bladder capacity with intravesical resiniferatoxin (which was not sustained at 4 weeks), without significant change in bladder pressure in patients with an unstable detrusor [76]. However, the limitations of this study include the solubility of resiniferatoxin in saline without alcohol. Lazzeri *et al.* have also shown a significant increase in bladder capacity with high-dose resiniferatoxin in spinal man in whom capsaicin has failed [77]. High-dose resiniferatoxin can also induce detrusor areflexia in these patients.

BOTULINUM TOXIN

A new approach to neurogenic detrusor overactivity has been pioneered by Schurch *et al.*, who have used cystoscopic injection of botulinum A toxin [78]. The drug is injected at 20–30 sites within the bladder, excluding the trigone. At 6 weeks, 89% of patients with traumatic spinal cord injury having severe neurogenic detrusor overactivity and incontinence had restoration of continence [78]. Furthermore, significant increases in mean reflex volume, cystometric capacity, post-void residual volume and decrease in detrusor voiding pressure were recorded. The requirement for anticholinergic medication was markedly decreased or withdrawn, and improvement was sustained at 9 months after treatment, without side-effects. Recently, a retrospective European multicentre study in 200 patients with spinal cord injury/disease, neurogenic detrusor overactivity or neurogenic incontinence confirmed these findings [79]. Furthermore, there have been preliminary reports of successful use of this agent for treatment of bladder overactivity [80].

Conclusions

Urinary incontinence is a debilitating condition. Therapeutics has an important role in the treatment of incontinence. Some success has also been achieved with the treatment of SUI pharmacologically. Desmopressin has a well-accepted role in the treatment of nocturnal enuresis in children. Anticholinergic medications result in statistically significant improvement in patients with detrusor overactivity and neurogenic detrusor overactivity, with response rates of 50–70% reported. However, randomized, placebo-controlled trials have shown placebo responses up to 45% and atropine-like side-effects are common. In patients with neurogenic detrusor overactivity, intravesical botulinum A toxin can help patients who have failed to respond to anticholinergics, and it may have a role for other patient groups. Newer anticholinergic agents acting through novel pathways and drugs targeting bladder afferents may help further in the therapeutic battle against detrusor overactivity, but this remains to be seen.

References

1 Abrams P, Cardozo L, Fall M *et al.* The standardisation of terminology of lower urinary tract function: report from the Standardisation Sub-committee of the International Continence Society. *Neurourol Urodyn* 2002; **21**(2): 167–78.

2 Milsom I, Abrams P, Cardozo L, Roberts RG, Thuroff J, Wein AJ. How widespread are the symptoms of an overactive bladder and how are they managed? A population-based prevalence study. *BJU Int* 2001; **87**(9): 760–66.

3 Jackson S. The patient with an overactive bladder – symptoms and quality-of-life issues. *Urology* 1997; **50** (Suppl. 6A): 18–22; discussion 23–4.

4 Turner WH. Physiology of the smooth muscles of the bladder and urethra. In: Schick E, Corcos J, eds. *The Urinary Sphincter.* New York: Marcel Decker, 2001: 43–70.

5 Brading AF. A myogenic basis for the overactive bladder. *Urology* 1997; **50**(Suppl. 6A): 57–67.

6 de Groat WC. A neurologic basis for the overactive bladder. *Urology* 1997; **50**(Suppl. 6A): 36–52.

7 Roe B, Williams K, Palmer M. Bladder training for urinary incontinence in adults. *Cochrane Database Syst Rev* 2000; (2): CD001308.

8 Hay-Smith J, Herbison P, Ellis G, Moore K. Anticholinergic drugs versus placebo for overactive bladder syndrome in adults. *Cochrane Database Syst Rev* 2002; (3): CD003781.

9 Mattiasson A, Blaakaer J, Hoye K, Wein AJ. Simplified bladder training augments the effectiveness of tolterodine in patients with an overactive bladder. *BJU Int* 2003; **91**(1): 54–60.

10 Yamanishi T, Chapple CR, Chess-Williams R. Which muscarinic receptor is important in the bladder? *World J Urol* 2001; **19**(5): 299–306.

11 Brading AF, Turner WH. The unstable bladder: towards a common mechanism. *Br J Urol* 1994; **73**(1): 3–8.

12 Herbison P, Hay-Smith J, Ellis G, Moore K. Effectiveness of anticholinergic drugs compared with placebo in the treatment of overactive bladder: systematic review. *BMJ* 2003; **326**(7394): 841–4.

13 Abrams P *et al.* Levels of Evidence and Grades of Recommendation. In: Abrams P, Cardozo, Khoury S, Wein A, eds. *Incontinence*, 2nd edn. Plymouth: Health Publication, 2002: 10.

14 Moher D, Schulz KF, Altman DG. The CONSORT statement: revised recommendations for improving the quality of reports of parallel-group randomised trials. *Lancet* 2001; **357**(9263): 1191–4.

15 Herbison GP. The reporting quality of abstracts of randomised controlled trials submitted to the ICS meeting in Heidelberg. *Neurourol Urodyn* 2003; **22**(5): 365–6.

16 Andersson KE, Appell R, Awad S *et al.* Pharmacological treatment of incontinence. In: Abrams P, Cardozo L, Khoury S, Wein A, eds. *Incontinence*, 2nd edn. Plymouth: Health Publication, 2002: 479–511.

17 Nilvebrant L. Tolterodine and its active 5-hydroxymethyl metabolite: pure muscarinic receptor antagonists. *Pharmacol Toxicol* 2002; **90**(5): 260–67.

18 Abrams P. Evidence for the efficacy and safety of tolterodine in the treatment of overactive bladder. *Expert Opin Pharmacother* 2001; **2**(10): 1685–701.

19 Crandall C. Tolterodine: a clinical review. *J Womens Health Gend Based Med* 2001; **10**(8): 735–43.

20 Appell RA, Abrams P, Drutz HP, Van Kerrebroeck PE, Millard R, Wein A. Treatment of overactive bladder: long-term tolerability and efficacy of tolterodine. *World J Urol* 2001; **19**(2): 141–7.

21 Guay DR. Tolterodine, a new antimuscarinic drug for treatment of bladder overactivity. *Pharmacotherapy* 1999; **19**(3): 267–80.

22 Van Kerrebroeck P, Kreder K, Jonas U, Zinner N, Wein A. Tolterodine once-daily: superior efficacy and tolerability in the treatment of the overactive bladder. *Urology* 2001; **57**(3): 414–21.

23 Freeman R, Hill S, Millard R, Slack M, Sutherst J. Reduced perception of urgency in treatment of overactive bladder with extended-release tolterodine. *Obstet Gynecol* 2003; 102(3): 605–11.

24 Kreder K, Mayne C, Jonas U. Long-term safety, tolerability and efficacy of extended-release tolterodine in the treatment of overactive bladder. *Eur Urol* 2002; **41**(6): 588–95.

25 Abrams P, Freeman R, Anderstrom C, Mattiasson A. Tolterodine, a new antimuscarinic agent: as effective but better tolerated than oxybutynin in patients with an overactive bladder. *Br J Urol* 1998; **81**(6): 801–810.

26 Leung HY, Yip SK, Cheon C *et al*. A randomized controlled trial of tolterodine and oxybutynin on tolerability and clinical efficacy for treating Chinese women with an overactive bladder. *BJU Int* 2002; **90**(4): 375–80.

27 Malone-Lee J, Shaffu B, Anand C, Powell C. Tolterodine: superior tolerability than and comparable efficacy to oxybutynin in individuals 50 years old or older with overactive bladder: a randomized controlled trial. *J Urol* 2001; **165**(5): 1452–6.

28 Appell RA, Sand P, Dmochowski R *et al*. Prospective randomized controlled trial of extended-release oxybutynin chloride and tolterodine tartrate in the treatment of overactive bladder: results of the OBJECT Study. *Mayo Clin Proc* 2001; **76**(4): 358–63.

29 Sussman D, Garely A. Treatment of overactive bladder with once-daily extended-release tolterodine or oxybutynin: the antimuscarinic clinical effectiveness trial (ACET). *Curr Med Res Opin* 2002; **18**(4): 177–84.

30 Diokno AC, Appell RA, Sand PK *et al*. Prospective, randomized, double-blind study of the efficacy and tolerability of the extended-release formulations of oxybutynin and tolterodine for overactive bladder: results of the OPERA trial. *Mayo Clin Proc* 2003; **78**(6): 687–95.

31 Hofner K, Oelke M, Machtens S, Grunewald V. Trospium chloride – an effective drug in the treatment of overactive bladder and detrusor hyperreflexia. *World J Urol* 2001; **19**(5): 336–43.

32 Uckert S, Stief CG, Odenthal KP, Becker AJ, Truss MC, Jonas U. Comparison of the effects of various spasmolytic drugs on isolated human and porcine detrusor smooth muscle. *Arzneimittelforschung* 1998; **48**(8): 836–9.

33 Stohrer M, Madersbacher H, Richter R, Wehnert J, Dreikorn K. Efficacy and safety of propiverine in SCI-patients suffering from detrusor hyperreflexia – a double-blind, placebo-controlled clinical trial. *Spinal Cord* 1999; **37**(3): 196–200.

34 Cardozo L, Chapple CR, Toozs-Hobson P *et al*. Efficacy of trospium chloride in patients with detrusor instability: a placebo-controlled, randomized, double-blind, multicentre clinical trial. *BJU Int* 2000; **85**(6): 659–64.

35 Frohlich G, Bulitta M, Strosser W. Trospium chloride in patients with detrusor overactivity: meta-analysis of placebo-controlled, randomized, double-blind, multi-center clinical trials on the efficacy and safety of 20 mg trospium chloride twice daily. *Int J Clin Pharmacol Ther* 2002; **40**(7): 295–303.

36 Madersbacher H, Stohrer M, Richter R, Burgdorfer H, Hachen HJ, Murtz G. Trospium chloride versus oxybutynin: a randomized, double-blind, multicentre trial in the treatment of detrusor hyper-reflexia. *Br J Urol* 1995; **75**(4): 452–6.

37 Jünemann KP, Al-Shukri S. Efficacy and tolerability of trsopium chloride and tolterodine in 234 patients with urge-syndrome: a double-blind, placebo-controlled multicentre clinical trial. *Neurourol Urodyn* 2000; **19**: 488.

38 Douchamps J, Derenne F, Stockis A, Gangji D, Juvent M, Herchuelz A. The pharmacokinetics of oxybutynin in man. *Eur J Clin Pharmacol* 1988; **35**(5): 515–20.

39 Waldeck K, Larsson B, Andersson KE. Comparison of oxybutynin and its active metabolite, N-desethyl-oxybutynin, in the human detrusor and parotid gland. *J Urol* 1997; **157**(3): 1093–7.

40   Sathyan G, Chancellor MB, Gupta SK. Effect of OROS controlled-release delivery on the pharmacokinetics and pharmacodynamics of oxybutynin chloride. *Br J Clin Pharmacol* 2001; **52**(4): 409–17.

41   Birns J, Lukkari E, Malone-Lee JG. A randomized controlled trial comparing the efficacy of controlled-release oxybutynin tablets (10 mg once daily) with conventional oxybutynin tablets (5 mg twice daily) in patients whose symptoms were stabilized on 5 mg twice daily of oxybutynin. *BJU Int* 2000; **85**(7): 793–8.

42   Versi E, Appell R, Mobley D, Patton W, Saltzstein D. Dry mouth with conventional and controlled-release oxybutynin in urinary incontinence. The Ditropan XL Study Group. *Obstet Gynecol* 2000; **95**(5): 718–21.

43   Davila GW, Daugherty CA, Sanders SW. A short-term, multicenter, randomized double-blind dose titration study of the efficacy and anticholinergic side effects of transdermal compared to immediate release oral oxybutynin treatment of patients with urge urinary incontinence. *J Urol* 2001; **166**(1): 140–45.

44   Thuroff JW, Chartier-Kastler E, Corcus J *et al.* Medical treatment and medical side effects in urinary incontinence in the elderly. *World J Urol* 1998; **16**(Suppl 1): S48–61.

45   Dmochowski R, Kell S, Staskin D. Oxybutynin chloride: alterations in drug delivery and improved therapeutic index. *Expert Opin Pharmacother* 2002; **3**(4): 443–54.

46   Dmochowski RR, Davila GW, Zinner NR *et al.* Efficacy and safety of transdermal oxybutynin in patients with urge and mixed urinary incontinence. *J Urol* 2002; **168**(2): 580–6.

47   Dmochowski RR, Sand PK, Zinner NR, Gittelman MC, Davila GW, Sanders SW. Comparative efficacy and safety of transdermal oxybutynin and oral tolterodine versus placebo in previously treated patients with urge and mixed urinary incontinence. *Urology* 2003; **62**(2): 237–42.

48   Madersbacher H, Halaska M, Voigt R, Alloussi S, Hofner K. A placebo-controlled, multicentre study comparing the tolerability and efficacy of propiverine and oxybutynin in patients with urgency and urge incontinence. *BJU Int* 1999; **84**(6): 646–51.

49   Ikeda K, Kobayashi S, Suzuki M *et al.* M(3) receptor antagonism by the novel antimuscarinic agent solifenacin in the urinary bladder and salivary gland. *Naunyn Schmiedebergs Arch Pharmacol* 2002; **366**(2): 97–103.

50   Chapple C, Rechberger T, Al-Shukri S, Meffan P, Everaert K, Ridder A. Results of a randomized phase 3 study comparing solifenacin succinate with tolterodine and placebo in patients with symptomatic overactive bladder. *Neurourol Urodyn* 2003; **22**(5): 534–5.

51   Mattiasson A, Ekström B, Andersson KE. Effects of intravesical instillation of verapamil in patients with detrusor hyperactivity. *J Urol* 1989; **141**(1): 174–7.

52   Fey TA, Gopalakrishnan M, Strake JG *et al.* Effects of ATP-sensitive K+ channel openers and tolterodine on involuntary bladder contractions in a pig model of partial bladder outlet obstruction. *Neurourol Urodyn* 2003; **22**(2): 147–55.

53   Blander DS, Zimmern PE. Urinary incontinence and prolapse. In: Stanton SL, Zimmern PE, eds. *Female Pelvic Reconstructive Surgery.* London: Springer, 2003: 13–20.

54   Donker PJ, Ivanovici F, Noach EL. Analyses of the urethral pressure profile by means of electromyography and the administration of drugs. *Br J Urol* 1972; **44**(2): 180–93.

55   Turner WH. An experimental urodynamic model of lower urinary tract function and dysfunction. MD, University of Cambridge, 1998.

56   Bump RC, Friedman CI, Copeland WJ. Non-neuromuscular determinants of intraluminal urethral pressure in the female baboon: relative importance of vascular and nonvascular factors. *J Urol* 1988; **139**(1): 162–4.

57   Diokno AC, Taub M. Ephedrine in treatment of urinary incontinence. *Urology* 1975; **5**(5): 624–5.

58 Ek A, Andersson KE, Gullberg B, Ulmsten U. The effects of long-term treatment with norephedrine on stress incontinence and urethral closure pressure profile. *Scand J Urol Nephrol* 1978; **12**(2): 105–110.

59 Radley SC, Chapple CR, Bryan NP, Clarke DE, Craig DA. Effect of methoxamine on maximum urethral closure pressure in women with genuine stress incontinence: a placebo-controlled, double-blind crossover study. *Neurourol Urodyn* 2001; **20**(1): 43–52.

60 Ishiko O, Ushiroyama T, Saji F *et al.* Beta(2)-adrenergic agonists and pelvic floor exercises for female stress incontinence. *Int J Gynaecol Obstet* 2000; **71**(1): 39–44.

61 Zinner N, Dmochowski R, Miklos J, Norton P, Yalcin I, Bump R. Duloxetine versus placebo in the treatment of stress urinary incontinence (SUI). *Neurourol Urodyn* 2002; **21**(4): 383–4.

62 van Kerrebroeck P, Abrams P, Lange R, Slack R, Wyndaele JJ, Yalcin I, Bump RC. Duloxetine versus placebo in the treatment of European and Canadian women with stress urinary incontinence. *Int J Obstet Gynaecol*, 2004; **111**: 249–57.

63 Sultana CJ, Walters MD. Estrogen and urinary incontinence in women. *Maturitas* 1994; **20**(2–3): 129–38.

64 Fantl JA, Cardozo L, McClish DK. Estrogen therapy in the management of urinary incontinence in postmenopausal women: a meta-analysis. First report of the Hormones and Urogenital Therapy Committee. *Obstet Gynecol* 1994; **83**(1): 12–18.

65 van Kerrebroeck PE. Experience with the long-term use of desmopressin for nocturnal enuresis in children and adolescents. *BJU Int* 2002; **89**(4): 420–5.

66 Hjalmas K. Desmopressin treatment: current status. *Scand J Urol Nephrol Suppl* 1999; **202**: 70–72.

67 Robertson GL, Norgaard JP. Renal regulation of urine volume: potential implications for nocturia. *BJU Int* 2002; **90**(Suppl. 3): 7–10.

68 Dykstra DD, Sidi AA, Scott AB, Pagel JM, Goldish GD. Effects of botulinum A toxin on detrusor-sphincter dyssynergia in spinal cord injury patients. *J Urol* 1988; **139**(5): 919–22.

69 Schurch B, Hauri D, Rodic B, Curt A, Meyer M, Rossier AB. Botulinum-A toxin as a treatment of detrusor-sphincter dyssynergia: a prospective study in 24 spinal cord injury patients. *J Urol* 1996; **155**(3): 1023–9.

70 De Ridder D, Baert L. Vanilloids and the overactive bladder. *BJU Int* 2000; **86**(2): 172–80.

71 Szallasi A, Fowler CJ. After a decade of intravesical vanilloid therapy: still more questions than answers. *Lancet Neurol* 2002; **1**(3): 167–72.

72 de Groat WC, Kawatani M, Hisamitsu T *et al.* Mechanisms underlying the recovery of urinary bladder function following spinal cord injury. *J Auton Nerv Syst* 1990; **30**(Suppl.): S71–7.

73 Fowler CJ, Beck RO, Gerrard S, Betts CD, Fowler CG. Intravesical capsaicin for treatment of detrusor hyperreflexia. *J Neurol Neurosurg Psychiatry* 1994; **57**(2): 169–73.

74 De Ridder D, Chandiramani V, Dasgupta P, Van Poppel H, Baert L, Fowler CJ. Intravesical capsaicin as a treatment for refractory detrusor hyperreflexia: a dual center study with long-term followup. *J Urol* 1997; **158**(6): 2087–92.

75 Cruz F, Guimaraes M, Silva C, Reis M. Suppression of bladder hyperreflexia by intravesical resiniferatoxin. *Lancet* 1997; **350**(9078): 640–1.

76 Lazzeri M, Beneforti P, Turini D. Urodynamic effects of intravesical resiniferatoxin in humans: preliminary results in stable and unstable detrusor. *J Urol* 1997; **158**(6): 2093–6.

77 Lazzeri M, Spinelli M, Beneforti P, Zanollo A, Turini D. Intravesical resiniferatoxin for the treatment of detrusor hyperreflexia refractory to capsaicin in patients with chronic spinal cord diseases. *Scand J Urol Nephrol* 1998; **32**(5): 331–4.

78 Schurch B, Stöhrer M, Kramer G, Schmid DM, Gaul G, Hauri D. Botulinum-A toxin for treating detrusor hyperreflexia in spinal cord injured patients: a new alternative to anticholinergic drugs? Preliminary results. *J Urol* 2000; **164**(3 Pt 1): 692–7.

79 Reitz A, Stöhrer M, Kramer G *et al*. European experience of 200 cases treated with Botulinum-A toxin injections into the detrusor muscle for neurogenic incontinence. *Eur Urol Suppl* 2003; **2**(1): 140.

80 Loch A, Loch T, Osterhage J, Alloussi S, Stöckle M. Botulinum-A toxin detrusor injections in the treatment of non-neurologic and neurologic cases of urge incontinence. *Eur Urol Suppl* 2003; **2**(1): 172.

2: Medical Therapy for Benign Prostatic Hyperplasia

Simon R. J. Bott, Charlotte L. Foley & Roger S. Kirby

Introduction

Lower urinary tract symptoms (LUTS) resulting from benign prostatic hyperplasia (BPH) have now been treated medically for over 2 decades. Although surgery by transurethral resection of prostate (TURP) was the therapy of choice for most patients up to the mid-1990s, medical therapy is now widely used as first-line treatment, except in cases of complicated bladder outflow obstruction (BOO) where surgery is more usually performed or in very mild cases where watchful waiting is the norm. The number of patients undergoing TURP in the USA has halved over the last decade and Europe is gradually mirroring this decline [1]. This phenomenon is occurring despite the progressive ageing of the male population, which has been accompanied by an increased prevalence of BPH. We are likely to see further increases in the prevalence of BPH given that currently about 15% of the total population in the USA is over 65 years old. By 2025 this figure is expected to rise to 22% [2].

The epidemiology of BPH has been extensively studied, but the terminology that has been used to describe BPH, its symptoms and effects, has sometimes been inconsistent and this has resulted in varying incidence figures. Overall, it seems likely that the prevalence of BPH is uniform across the developed world. The American Agency for Health Care Policy and Research (AHCPR) estimates that of the 22.5 million white men aged between 50 and 79 years in the USA, 5.6 million (25%) will have symptoms of sufficient severity to warrant a discussion of treatment options. The criteria used by the AHCPR were an International Prostate Symptom Score (IPSS) of > 7 and a maximum flow rate of < 15 ml/s. Community-based studies in Europe show similar results. For example, in Austria the proportion of men with an IPSS > 7 was 27.1% in men aged 50–59 years and 36% in those aged 70–79 [3]. In the UK between 29% and 51% of men aged 50 or over had an IPSS $\geqslant$ 8, depending on the age group studied [4].

Although the incidence of symptomatic BPH is similar, the management strategies vary significantly from country to country. For example in France and the UK the number of elderly men is approximately equal at around 4 millions; however, while France spends in the order of 180 million Euros in ex-factory sales of medical therapies for BPH the value of similar sales in the

UK is less than 50% of this figure [5]. This is probably due to a variety of reasons. Men in the UK tend to accept their LUTS as a natural feature of ageing and it may be that they are also relatively unaware of the risk of prostate cancer and so do not seek medical help for their symptoms. Other possible causes include the relatively tight financial constraints of the UK's National Health Service (NHS) where doctors may be more willing to advise a 'watch and wait' policy in men with mild or moderate LUTS. A further difference between France and the UK is that patients in France are more likely to receive phytotherapeutic agents, which make up nearly 40% of the medicinal market share. As these are widely perceived as being more 'natural' and 'holistic' there may be a lower threshold for initiating one of these agents than for a standard pharmaceutical product.

It is perhaps surprising that despite a large body of evidence describing the effects of medical therapies there is not a greater consensus on their role in the management of men with BPH. More data are required on the efficacy and safety of phytotherapies, and a management strategy along the lines proposed in the AHCPR guidelines [6] or the International Consultation on BPH [7] would appear to offer a more rational approach to BPH management.

The natural history of BPH

The likely outcome of a watch-and wait-policy is being addressed by the ongoing longitudinal community trial in Olmsted County, USA. Encompassing over 2000 untreated men and with follow-up of up to 11 years, this represents one of the largest and longest observational studies of its kind. From a randomly selected subset of 25% of patients aged 40–79 years, the IPSS, peak flow and prostate volume have been measured every 18–24 months [8] [29]. This study has shown a prostate growth rate of 2.4% per year by volume, with greater rates in men with higher baseline prostate volumes (> 30 ml) and also those with higher baseline prostate-specific antigen (PSA) values. Prostate growth rate was only mildly related to the symptom score and not related to the baseline peak urinary flow rate. Prostatic enlargement, PSA and age were all associated with an increased risk of developing acute urinary retention (AUR) and requiring BPH-related treatment [9]. The Olmsted county study therefore provides a rationale for targeted preventative therapy for men with either a prostate volume > 30 ml or an elevated PSA (> 1.6 ng/ml) since these men are more likely to have faster-growing BPH and are, as a result, more likely to progress and require intervention in the future.

The impact of LUTS on sexual function was addressed in a large study by Rosen *et al.* [10]. They reported on 14 000 European and American men aged 50–79 years who completed the IPSS, the Danish Prostate Symptom Score for Sexual function (DAN-PSS-sex) and the International Index for Erectile function (IIEF) questionnaires. The study group found that across Europe and the USA the mean frequency of sexual intercourse/activity was 5.8 times per month. In men with no LUTS this varied from a mean of 8.6 times per month for a man aged 50–59 years down to 4.0 times per month for a man aged 70–79 years. Notably, men who had moderate or severe LUTS had sexual frequency, erectile function and sexual desire equivalent to a man without significant urinary symptoms a decade their senior. This large study exposes the extent and the effect of LUTS upon men's sexual function.

Alpha-adrenergic antagonists

Alpha-adrenergic blockers constitute the most widely used medical therapy for symptomatic BPH, reflecting both their efficacy and safety in men with symptomatic BPH. While the lower urinary tract contains both α_1- and α_2-adrenoceptors, prostatic smooth muscle contains predominantly α_1-adrenoceptors, the three subtypes identified being α_{1A}, α_{1B} and α_{1D}. Lower urinary tract smooth muscle contraction is mediated through the α_{1A} subtype and α-blockers act by blocking these receptors, thereby interrupting the motor sympathetic adrenergic nerve supply, which in turn results in relaxation of the smooth muscle of the prostatic stroma, capsule and the bladder neck. The first α-blocker used in the treatment of symptomatic BPH was phenoxybenzamine, a non-selective α_1 and α_2 inhibitor [11]. Phenoxybenzamine is now obsolete since α_2 receptor blockade resulted in excessive cardiovascular side-effects and there were also concerns about possible carcinogenic side-effects. Subsequently, prazosin, a selective α_1-blocker that had been originally used as an antihypertensive agent, was developed for the treatment of BPH. A second generation of α-blockers followed including doxazosin, alfuzosin, terazosin and indoramin, and these drugs were marketed as having fewer side-effects than the earlier drugs. With the discovery of the three receptor subtypes a third generation α_{1A}/α_{1D}-selective blocker, tamsulosin, has been developed more recently.

Interestingly, α-blockers are particularly effective at treating the irritative symptoms associated with BPH and only provide fairly modest improvements in urinary flow rates. Surgery, on the other hand, is very effective at relieving obstructive symptoms and improving flow rates, but is not as immediately efficient at relieving irritative symptoms. These findings may point to another role of α-blockers besides simple smooth muscle relaxation in and around the prostate [12]. Alpha-1 receptors are found in the human bladder and the spinal cord and in contrast to the prostate these have been shown to be predominantly α_{1D}-adrenoceptors. The possible role of

α_{1D}-adrenoceptor inhibition in the symptomatic improvement seen with α-blockers is further suggested by rat studies that show that α_{1D}-adreno-ceptor antagonists inhibit detrusor overactivity, possibly via inhibition at the levels of the bladder and the spinal cord [13].

While our understanding of exactly how α-blockers exert their effect on the prostate and lower urinary tract is incomplete, this should not detract from the large body of evidence supporting their efficacy and safety. Data from large multicentre placebo-controlled trials of all the main α-blockers have been available for a number of years and several meta-analyses have recently pooled these data. In one such meta-analysis of 92 phase II and III trials involving 44 000 patients, α-blockers were shown to provide superior efficacy when compared with placebo [14]. The efficacy of the different α-blockers appeared to be similar. Symptom scores improved with treat-ment by an average of 35% and the maximum flow rate increased by between 1.8 and 2.5 ml/s. The authors concluded however, that selective α_1-blockers significantly reduced the incidence of side-effects compared with the unselective drugs.

In a separate review, Chapple [15] specifically examined the more specific α-blockers with respect to their efficacy and safety. Pooling together four studies involving nearly 3000 patients he reported that alfuzosin, terazosin, doxazosin and tamsulosin significantly improved symptom scores by 17–38% and flow rates by 1.4–2.4 ml/s.

As all α-blockers seem to be broadly similar in their efficacy, their side-effect profile may dictate which agent is used in a particular patient. In a further meta-analysis Djavan reported that the discontinuation rates due to unwanted side-effects such as orthostatic hypertension and dizziness were higher in trials involving prazosin, terazosin and doxazosin [16]. In fact, these cardiovascular 'side-effects' may actually be beneficial in some patients. For example, doxazosin has been shown to reduce the blood pressure of hypertensive but not normotensive individuals [17] and this has suggested a role in the treatment of men with both BPH and hypertension.

The other main side-effects of α-blockers are their adverse effects upon sexual function and these effects are summarized in Table 2.1.

5-α reductase inhibitors (5ARIs)

Finasteride, a 5-α reductase type 2 inhibitor, has been available for over 10 years and although prescribing patterns vary, it commands up to a third of the market share in many European countries [5]. Finasteride was one of the first 'designer drugs' with a structure akin to that of testosterone, so that it competitively inhibits 5-α reductase type 2, without directly inhibiting the

Table 2.1 The effects of alpha blockers on sexual function

	Impotence (%)		Ejaculation failure (%)		Reduced libido (%)	
	Drug	Placebo	Drug	Placebo	Drug	Placebo
Alfuzosin ($n = 358$)	2.2	—	0	—	0.6	—
Terazosin ($n = 305$)	6	5	0.3	1	3	1
Tamsulosin ($n = 381$)	0.8	1.6	4.5[*]	1	1	0
($n = 381$)						

$*p < 0.05$. Adapted from *FMJ Debruyne Urol* 2000; 56(Suppl. 5A): 20.

testosterone receptor. By blocking the enzyme that produces the more potent testosterone metabolite, dihydrotestosterone (DHT), finasteride reduces prostate gland size and reverses the disease process of BPH.

Finasteride does not have immediate efficacy, but does produce objective improvement over a matter of several months. Long-term, randomized studies have confirmed its efficacy in reducing LUTS, improving flow rates and reducing the incidence of AUR and the need for surgical intervention [18–20]. Prostate volumes are typically reduced by 25–30%. There is evidence that men with larger prostates respond better to finasteride than men with smaller prostates. In a meta-analysis of 2600 patients, Boyle *et al.* noted that differences in prostate size accounted for about 85% of the variation in outcome seen between the six randomized trials in this study. Significant benefits over placebo were only seen in men with prostate glands of volume greater than 40 ml and these benefits increased with prostate size [21].

Finasteride inhibits only 5-α reductase type 2, which is the isoform found predominantly within the prostate. Inhibition of both the type 1 (which is found within the skin and liver) and the type 2 isoforms should reduce the circulating levels of DHT still further and dutasteride is a drug that achieves this [22]. To be included in the phase III dutasteride trials, men had to be at least 50 years old, with prostate volumes of 30 ml or more, an IPSS score of 12 points or more and a maximum flow rate of 15 ml/s or less. Men with a PSA value less that 1.5 ng/ml or greater than 10 ng/ml were excluded. The minimum prostate volume and PSA levels were set in these studies as a consequence of the finasteride trials, which demonstrated greater efficacy in men with glands of 30 ml or more and a serum PSA in excess of 1.4 ng/ml. A total of 4325 patients were randomized in three parallel placebo-controlled trials lasting 24 months. Dutasteride was shown to rapidly lower serum DHT measurements in the majority of men by 90% or more and prostate volume measurements showed a significant decline from as early as the first month of the trial. Although the AUA symptom index scores improved in one of the three studies within 3 months, when pooled together significant improvement was not seen until 6 months. At 24 months the treated group experienced a mean improvement of 4.5 points compared with an improvement of 2.3 for the placebo controls ($p < 0.001$) (Table 2.2). Flow rate improvements were significantly better from 1 month and thereafter in the treatment arm, up to 2.2 ml/s compared with 0.6 ml/s in the placebo group. Interestingly, serum PSA levels fell by just over half in the dutasteride group, a reduction similar to that seen with finasteride. There was a relative risk reduction of 57% for developing AUR and 48% for BPH-related surgical intervention. Dutasteride was well tolerated although impotence, decreased libido, ejaculation disorders and gynaecomastia were significantly greater in the active treatment arm during the first year of the study. In addition, the incidence of newly diagnosed prostate cancer was 1.9% in the placebo arm and 1.1% in the dutasteride group. While this represents only a small absolute risk reduction, the relative risk reduction of over 40% has prompted a larger trial to look at its possible role in prostate cancer prevention.

Dutasteride is clearly very effective at rapidly lowering serum DHT and shrinking the prostate in general and the transition zone of the gland in particular. Despite its dual action its efficacy and side-effect profile is similar to finasteride [18]. Currently it remains unclear whether the additional effect of antagonizing both isoenzymes is better than type 2 alone. Until a comparative study is performed, this agent appears to be comparable to finasteride.

Combination therapy

The concept of combining an α-blocker, which relaxes the smooth muscle in the bladder neck and prostate, with a 5ARI, which by acting on the epithelial component reverses the natural progression of BPH, seems sound. Yet, until recently large randomized placebo-controlled studies failed to show a significant difference when finasteride was added to either the α-blocker terazosin [23] or doxazosin [24]. Perhaps this was not surprising since the mean prostate

Table 2.2 Results of placebo-controlled clinical trials on dutasteride [22]

	Dutasteride	Placebo	p value
Median change in serum DHT	−90.2%	+9.6%	$p < 0.001$
Change in prostate volume (ml)	−14.6	+0.8	$p < 0.001$
Change in symptom score	−4.5	−2.3	$p < 0.001$
Change in Qmax (ml/s)	+2.2	+0.6	$p < 0.001$
Patients with AUR	39 (1.8%)	90 (4.2%)	$p < 0.001$, relative risk reduction 57%
Patients requiring BPH-related surgery	47 (2.2%)	89 (4.1%)	$p < 0.001$, relative risk reduction 48%

size in these two studies was below the 40-ml volume cut-off at which finasteride has been shown to provide a significant improvement. Furthermore, the follow-up period in each of these two trials was for 1 year only.

Recently however, the Medical Therapy of Prostate Symptoms (MTOPS) trial has been reported (Figs 2.1–2.3) [25]. The aim of this study was to determine whether medical therapy prevents or delays the clinical progression of BPH. This multicentre, randomized, placebo-controlled, double-blind study assigned 3047 men to receive doxazosin monotherapy (4–8 mg), finasteride monotherapy (5 mg), combined doxazosin and finasteride or placebo. The primary outcome was the time to clinical progression after a minimum follow-up of 4 years and a mean follow-up of 5 years. Mean baseline patient characteristics were IPSS 17.0 (range 12.0–21.0), Qmax 10.6 ml/s (range 8.5–12.3) and prostate size 36 ml (+/ − 20 ml).

A total of 350 men progressed to at least one of the predefined clinical end points; 78% had an IPSS rise greater than 4 points, while 12 % developed AUR, 9% developed incontinence and 1% developed recurrent urinary infection. None developed renal insufficiency secondary to BPH.

In comparing the different arms of the trial, monotherapy with either doxazosin or finasteride produced an equivalent but significant reduction in the incidence of BPH progression compared with placebo while combination therapy was substantially more effective when compared with monotherapy (Table 2.3). Interestingly, finasteride alone was equally effective at preventing AUR as combination therapy, with an overall risk reduction of

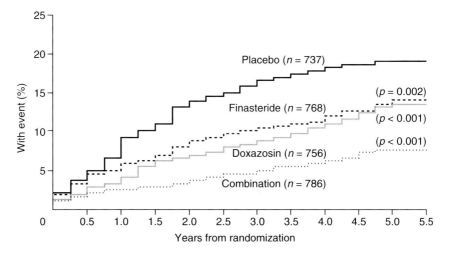

Figure 2.1 Impact of Medical Therapy of Prostate Symptoms (MTOPS) study: effect of finasteride, doxazosin, combination therapy or placebo on benign prostatic hyperplasia (BPH) progression. Combination vs placebo 66% risk reduction. Risk reduction with finasteride and doxazosin was significantly greater than with either drugs alone. Finasteride alone vs placebo 34% risk reduction. Doxazosin alone vs placebo 39% risk reduction.

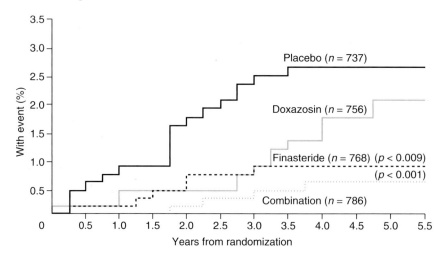

Figure 2.2 Medical Therapy of Prostate Symptoms (MTOPS) study: effect of finasteride, doxazosin, combination therapy or placebo on the risk of acute urinary retention (AUR). Combination vs placebo 81% risk reduction. Finasteride alone reduced the risk of AUR by 68% vs placebo. Doxazosin alone did not significantly reduce the risk of AUR vs placebo.

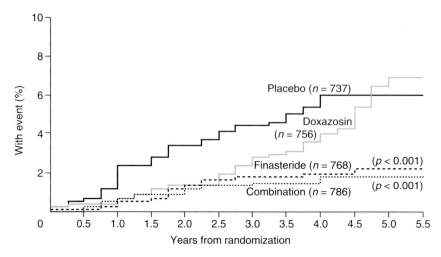

Figure 2.3 Medical Therapy of Prostate Symptoms (MTOPS) study: effect of finasteride, doxazosin, combination therapy or placebo on the risk of surgical intervention. Combination vs placebo 67% risk reduction. Finasteride and doxazosin significantly reduced the incidence of BPH-related surgery vs placebo. Finasteride alone significantly reduced the incidence of BPH-related surgery vs placebo. Doxazosin alone did not significantly reduce the incidence of BPH-related surgery.

70–80%. The α-blockers postponed the time to occurrence of AUR, although over the whole course of the trial there was no reduction in risk of AUR in the doxazosin monotherapy arm. Likewise, finasteride monotherapy and combination therapy significantly reduced the incidence of an

Table 2.3 Summary of the results of the MTOPS trial

	Placebo	Doxazosin	Finasteride	Combination
Reduction in median AUA symptom score	4.0	6.0	5.0	7.0
Increase in median maximum flow rate (ml/s)	1.4	2.5	2.2	3.7
Disease progression (per 100 patient years) (%)	4.5	2.7	2.9	1.5
Risk reduction of progression compared to placebo	—	39%	34%	67%
AUR rate (per 100 patient years) (%)	0.6	0.4	0.2	0.1
Rate of invasive therapy for BPH (per 100 patient years) (%)	1.3	1.2	0.5	0.4

invasive procedure while doxazosin monotherapy delayed the occurrence but not the overall rate of invasive procedures.

McConnell *et al.* [25] emphasized that combination therapy was particularly beneficial with respect to symptom score and flow rate improvements over the longer term. The prostate volume increased in both the placebo and the doxazosin monotherapy arms by an average 4.5% per annum, while in the finasteride monotherapy and combination therapy arms a mean reduction of 13% and 16%, respectively, was reported.

The incidence of adverse events was similar to what might have been predicted from previous studies. It was concluded that combination therapy in selected patients might be the most effective way of improving symptom score and flow rate while at the same time reducing the risk of clinical progression with its associated sequelae.

Other approaches to combination therapy have also been reported; α-blockers provide rapid relief of symptomatic BPH while 5ARIs, on the other hand, take longer to achieve symptomatic relief, but sustain this relief over a period of many years by modifying the disease process. Diamond *et al.* [26] therefore took the logical step of randomizing 120 patients to receive an α-blocker in combination with a 5ARI and then, after a period of time withdrawing the α-blocker from the patients in the test arm. This double-blind trial used tamsulosin and finasteride in group 1 and tamsulosin and placebo in a second parallel control group. In both groups tamsulosin was stopped at 6, 9 and 12 months and patients were re-evaluated 1 month after discontinuation of treatment. All 120 patients in this trial had prostates greater than 40 g in size, and IPSS > 17 and a Qmax < 15 ml/s and hence reflect the moderate to severe end of the BPH spectrum.

At 6 months, 55% of patients from the first group reported no change in symptom scores after discontinuing tamsulosin compared with 20% of men in the control arm. The study group had an increase in Qmax of 2.5 ml/s over

baseline. By 9 months 80% of group 1 men successfully discontinued tamsulosin compared with 25% in the control group and at 12 months 85% of
group 1 were successfully discontinued compared with 20% in group 2. This
study concluded that finasteride maintains the subjective and objective effects of combination therapy after 9–12 months in patients with enlarged
prostate and LUTS. A similar study by Baldwin *et al.* [27] used the α-blocker
doxazosin rather than tamsulosin. They reported no worsening of symptom
scores in 13–15% of men who discontinued doxazosin at 3 months, 40–48%
at 6 months, 73–84% at 9 months and 84–87% at 12 months.

The Symptom Management after Reducing Therapy (SMART) trial randomized 327 men with IPSS $\geqslant$ 12 and prostate volumes $\geqslant$ 30 ml in a
prospective, multicentre, double-blind study involving combination therapy
followed by withdrawal [28]. Initially, all patients received dutasteride in
combination with tamsulosin for a period of 24 weeks. In the study arm, the
tamsulosin was then withdrawn and replaced by placebo and the trial continued for a further 12 weeks. In the men in whom the α-blocker was discontinued 77% felt their symptoms were the same or better 6 weeks after stopping
tamsulosin and this was maintained in 93% of patients at the end of the study
period. In a subsidiary part of the trial a close correlation was noted between
IPSS scores and an assessment of how the patient felt generally.

The role of combination therapy in the management of symptomatic
BPH has yet to be defined. Adding two therapies together not only increases
the cost of treatment but also raises the incidence of side-effects. Moreover,
both finasteride and dutasteride are only effective in men with prostates of
more than 40 ml, so the value of combination therapy in men with glands
smaller than this is questionable. Nevertheless, in men with larger glands,
combination therapy may be the best option, particularly in patients where
surgery would best be avoided. It offers rapid and lasting symptom relief,
enhanced quality of life and a reduced risk of complications secondary to
BPH. While MTOPS suggested an additive effect with regard to efficacy in
combination therapy, most other studies have not confirmed this. It may be
possible to maintain symptom and quality of life improvements by using
combination therapy at least for 6–12 months and then discontinuing the
α-blocker without seeing a worsening in symptoms. Recently guidelines
have been developed for primary care physicians in the UK that are aimed
at helping them make more rational prescribing decisions for their patients
with symptomatic BPH (Fig. 2.4).

Phytotherapy

Men have used phytotherapy for centuries for the treatment of a variety of
ailments, including symptomatic BPH. Although not a new medical therapy,

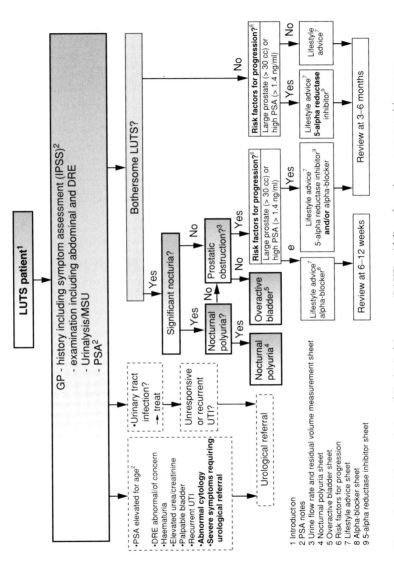

Figure 2.4 British Association of Urological Surgeons (BAUS) guidelines for primary care practitioners on pharmacotherapy for BPH. (Reproduced with permission from *BJU Int* 2004.)

the rapid expansion of this market in recent years has focused our attention on these products. Currently over 90% of men in the USA referred with LUTS have tried or are using complimentary therapy [29]. The market for these treatments has increased dramatically, rising in the USA from $500 000 in 1996 to over $1 billion today [29]. In Europe, the use of phytotherapy is more variable. It is the first-line therapy of choice in Germany, Austria, France and Spain and over 90% of all drugs prescribed for BPH in Austria and Germany are phytotherapeutic agents. In contrast, in the UK, Italy and Poland their share of the BPH medicines market is less than 10% [5].

Phytotherapeutic agents are typically derived from roots, seeds, bark, fruits, flowers and leaves. They are sold either as monopreparations or as mixtures of a number of agents. Several manufacturers supply a combination of different plant extracts to create their own 'prostate health pill' that can then be registered while single-plant monopreparations have no patent protection. Furthermore, there is a suggestion that combinations may have enhanced marketability by having a 'unique formula' or 'enhanced efficacy'.

The problem with performing studies to investigate these compounds is not only the variability of the combinations, but also the varying dose of active ingredients within any mixture. The same plant species may produce different amounts of active products depending on the conditions in which it grows as well as the techniques used in the extraction process. Since the 'active' compound is frequently unknown, quantifying the optimal dosing may be little more than guesswork. Indeed, when the National Consumer Laboratory in the USA analysed the free fatty acid content (which is the presumed active ingredient) in 27 different saw palmetto products [30], they found this to vary by up to 95%, with only 17 of the products containing the 'standard' 85% dose.

Studies aimed at investigating the mechanism of action of phytotherapies are almost all performed *in vitro* on tissue cultures and with supraphysiological doses, which are unlikely to reflect the *in vivo* effects accurately [31]. The mechanisms of action most commonly suggested include anti-inflammatory actions, 5α-reductase inhibition or growth factor alteration. Until recently, very little reliable safety or efficacy data were available on these compounds. Even now, properly performed placebo-controlled studies are rare and the complexity and uncertain constituents of these preparations must limit any conclusions that are reached.

Despite these reservations, these products do appear to have stood the test of time and the fact that so many men go out and buy them is perhaps testimony to their effects even if they have not passed through the rigorous scrutiny of conventional pharmacological agents. However, although they are perceived as natural and therefore presumed safe, it remains to be demonstrated objectively in large-scale trials.

Serenoa repens

Serenoa repens is the most popular and most studied of the phytotherapeutic agents used in BPH. It is also known as Saw palmetto, American dwarf palm, *Sabal serrulatum* (its botanical name) and Permixon (its trade name). The mechanism of action probably involves inhibition of the enzyme 5α-reductase [32] although there may be other mechanisms, such as an anti-inflammatory effect via inhibition of cyclo-oxgenase synthesis [32], inhibition of the growth factors β-FGF and EGF [33] or some possible anti-estrogenic effects [34]. Significantly, *S. repens* does not reduce serum PSA levels, unlike finasteride, and therefore its mechanism of action, although antiandrogenic, may differ from the highly competitive 5ARIs [35,36]. There have been a large number of trials assessing the efficacy of *S. repens* but the vast majority are uncontrolled open-label studies. Of those that are placebo-controlled, none meet the accepted criteria for assessing treatment in men with LUTS developed by the International Consultation on BPH [37] either because there are only small patient numbers, limited follow-up or lack of a standardized symptom scoring system.

Two large meta-analyses have been performed in an attempt to combine the results of these trials and to derive the best possible information. The first by Wilt *et al.* [38] combined 21 randomized trials involving 3139 men receiving *S. repens* either as monotherapy or in combination. They concluded that *S. repens* provided a mild to moderate improvement in urinary symptoms (weighted mean difference -1.41 points, 95% CI $= -2.52, -0.30$) and urinary flow (weighted mean difference 1.86 ml/s, 95% CI $= 0.60, 3.12$). In two studies that compared *S. repens* with finasteride there were similar improvements with both agents. Side-effects were mild and infrequent, occurring in 9% of men compared with 11% in the two studies involving finasteride. In the second meta-analysis performed by Boyle [39], 13 trials were combined incorporating 2859 men receiving Permixon only. Only 2 of the 13 trials used the standard IPSS questionnaire, so the only common end points were nocturia and peak flow rates, with the latter of these not reported in two studies. Although some heterogeneity existed between trials, Permixon significantly reduced the mean number of episodes of nocturia by an additional $0.50 +/- 0.012$ episodes per night and the flow rate by an additional $2.20 +/- 0.51$ ml/s over and above the placebo effect. No valuable data were accrued by either meta-analysis with regard to the effects of *S. repens* on the incidence of AUR or the need for surgical intervention.

Unfortunately, meta-analyses are by design inherently flawed due to the heterogeneity of studies incorporated, each with their different aims, different designs and different outcome measures. These findings may not reflect the results of future long-term, randomized, placebo-controlled trials, although they do suggest that *S. repens* is probably safe and effective at least to some extent. The results of two ongoing large placebo-controlled trials sponsored and coordinated by the National Institute of Health and the United States National Institute of Diabetes and Diseases of the Kidney should provide a more objective assessment of *S. repens*.

Published more recently and therefore not included in these meta-analyses was a study over a period of 12 months comparing Permixon with the α-blocker, tamsulosin [35]. This double-blind, multicentre European trial involved 811 men with IPSS scores ⩾ 10. Both drugs produced very similar improvements in the IPSS scores (decreased by 4.4 in both groups) and maximum flow rates (increased by 1.8 ml/s with Permixon and by 1.9 ml/s with tamsulosin). Both compounds were well tolerated. This is the first valid comparison of *S. repens* with an α-blocker, although further studies and longer follow-up is required before these two products can be considered equally efficacious.

The use of *S. repens* in combination with tamsulosin was addressed in a study reported by Glemain [40]. Over 300 patients with IPSS scores ⩾ 13 were randomized to receive either 0.4 mg tamsulosin monotherapy or tamsulosin in combination with 160 mg *S. repens*. While tamsulosin monotherapy reduced IPSS scores by a mean 5.2 units (S.D. 6.4), combination with *S. repens* provided no additional benefit.

Pygeum africanum

Pygeum africanum or the African plum is believed to act by modulating growth factor–induced cell growth and proliferation [32]. Its effects on the bladder were elegantly demonstrated by Levine *et al.* [41], who showed in a rabbit model that the increases in the bladder wall mass and decreases in compliance caused by partial outflow obstruction could be reduced by treatment with *P. africanum*.

Clinical trials, although numerous, are largely inadequate and none have met the criteria of the International Consultation on BPH for assessing treatment in men with LUTS [37]. Studies currently underway include the Tadenam–IPSS study and the sponsored trials by the United States National Institute of Diabetes and Diseases of the Kidney. The results of these trials are awaited before meaningful efficacy and safety conclusions can be drawn about this product.

Hypoxis rooperi

Also known as South African star grass, *Hypoxis rooperi* contains beta-sitosterol and other sterols, which, *in vitro*, elevate levels of transforming growth factor-β_1 and induce apoptosis [42]. Although these effects have not been demonstrated *in vivo* the results of some of the clinical trials are dramatic. In a double-blind, placebo-controlled trial of 200 patients [43], later extended to an open-label study [44], *H. rooperi* improved symptom score and maximum urinary flow rates very significantly. The IPSS improved by 7.4 points in the test arm compared with 2.3 points in the control arm and the maximum flow rate by 5.2 ml/s in the test compared with 1.1 ml/s in the placebo group [43]. In the follow-up open-label study, men who continued on *H. rooperi* maintained their symptom and flow rate improvements, but interestingly the 14 men who stopped all BPH therapy maintained similar improvements over the following 12 months, suggesting a possible use of *H. rooperi* in intermittent therapy [44].

Another compound, Azuprostat, containing beta-sitosterol, derived from *H. rooperi* as well as *Pinus* (pine) and *Picea* (spruce), was evaluated in a 6-month randomized placebo-controlled trial involving 177 men [45]. The IPSS improvements were 8.2 units in the treated arm and 2.8 units in the placebo arm. The urinary flow rate improved by 8.9 ml/s in the treatment arm and by 4.4 ml/s in the control group. The magnitude of these improvements is far greater than any other medical treatment and if reproducible would produce figures similar to those achieved by surgical intervention. However, this study raised several issues. The placebo group achieved a mean flow rate improvement of 4.4 ml/s – greater than the reported flow rate improvements seen in the *treatment* arm of most published trials of medical therapy, let alone the placebo arm. Furthermore, although the patients had a mean age of 65 years the mean flow rate in the treatment group was 19.4 ml/s, a value well in excess of the norm for this age.

These studies, together with results from other trials, led Wilt *et al.* [46] in a recent meta-analysis to conclude that beta-sitosterol does improve the symptom score and flow rate of men with BPH. However, the long-term effectiveness, safety and ability to prevent the complications of BPH remain to be established.

While there are over 30 phytotherapeutic treatments for symptomatic BPH the remainder have been evaluated even less rigorously than those described above. While there is undoubtedly a role for these agents in the medicinal armamentarium, too little is known about their efficacy and safety at the present time.

Conclusions

Current medical agents are not as immediately effective at treating BPH as surgery, although patients usually perceive them as being safer. This, together with the demands of the ageing population, seems likely to drive both an increased usage of medical therapy as well as further research to find newer, more effective medical and minimally invasive treatments. Our understanding of the safety and efficacy of α-blockers and 5ARIs is becoming established, and important questions, like the place of combination therapy, have recently been addressed by the landmark MTOPS study [25]. These data provide good evidence that while α-blockers have an almost immediate beneficial effect on symptoms and flow, they have no significant impact on the risk of disease progression. By contrast, 5ARIs, when used in men with larger prostates, are capable of both arresting disease progression and reducing the incidence of AUR or the need for BPH-related surgery. The use of both an α-blocker and a 5ARI in combination seems appropriate in older men with larger glands and an elevated PSA. High-quality, long-term placebo-controlled data are required before plant extracts can be recommended for the treatment of men with this most prevalent of conditions.

References

1   Holtgrewe HL, Bay-Nielsen H, Carlesson P, Coast J, Echtle D, Fitzpatrick F *et al.* Proceedings of the 4th International Consultation on Benign Prostatic Hyperplasia (BPH). Plymouth: Plymbridge Distributors, 1998.

2   US Bureau of the Census. www.census.gov. 5-10-2000.

3   Madersbacher S, Haidinger G, Temml C, Schmidbauer CP. Prevalence of lower urinary tract symptoms in Austria as assessed by an open survey of 2096 men. *Eur Urol* 1998; 34(2): 136–41.

4   Trueman P, Hood SC, Nayak US, Mrazek MF. Prevalence of lower urinary tract symptoms and self-reported diagnosed 'benign prostatic hyperplasia', and their effect on quality of life in a community-based survey of men in the UK. *BJU Int* 1999; 83(4): 410–15.

5   McNicholas TA. Lower urinary tract symptoms suggestive of benign prostatic obstruction: what are the current practice patterns? *Eur Urol 1 A.D* 39 (Suppl. 3): 26–30.

6   McConnell JD, Barry MJ, Bruskewitz R. Clinical practice guideline for benign prostatic hyperplasia: Diagnosis and treatment. 1994. Department of Health and Human Services. AHCPR publication no. 94-0582.

7   Denis L, McConnell JD, Yoshida O, Khoury S, Abrams P, Barry M *et al.* Proceedings of the 4th International Consultation on Benign Prostatic Hyperplasia (BPH). Plymouth: Health Publication, 1997: 669–83.

8   Rhodes T, Jacobson DJ, Jacobson SJ, Girman CJ, Roberts RO, Lieber MM. Longitudinal prostate volume in a community-based sample: long-term followup in the Olmsted county study of urinary symptoms and health status among men. American Urological Association Annual meeting, 1059. 2002.

9   Anderson JB, Roehrborn CG, Schalken JA, Emberton M. The progression of benign prostatic hyperplasia: examining the evidence and determining the risk. *Eur Urol* 2001; 39(4): 390–99.

10 Rosen R, Altwein J, Boyle P, Kirby RS, Lukacs B, Mueleman, O'Leary M, Puppo P, Robertsom C, Giuliano F. Lower urinary tract symptoms and male sexual dysfunction: the multinational study of the aging male (MSAM-7) *Eur Urol* 2003; 44: 637–49.

11 Caine M, Perlberg S, Meretyk S. A placebo-controlled double-blind study of the effect of phenoxybenzamine in benign prostatic obstruction. *Br J Urol* 1978; 50(7): 551–4.

12 Michel MC, Schafers RF, Goepel M. Alpha-blockers and lower urinary tract function: more than smooth muscle relaxation? *BJU Int* 2000; **86**(Suppl. 2): 23–8.

13 Broten T, Scott A, Siegl PKS, Forray C. Alpha-1adrenoceptor blockade inhibits detrusor instability in rats with bladder outlet obstruction. *FASEB J* 1998; **12**: A445.

14 Heimbach D, Muller SC. Treatment of benign prostatic hyperplasia with alpha 1-adrenoreceptor antagonists. *Urologe A* 1997; **36**(1): 18–34.

15 Chapple CR. Pharmacotherapy for benign prostatic hyperplasia – the potential for alpha 1-adrenoceptor subtype-specific blockade. *Br J Urol* 1998; **81**(Suppl. 1): 34–47.

16 Djavan B, Marberger M. A meta-analysis on the efficacy and tolerability of alpha 1-adrenoceptor antagonists in patients with lower urinary tract symptoms suggestive of benign prostatic obstruction. *Eur Urol* 1999; **36**(1): 1–13.

17 Kirby RS. Doxazosin in benign prostatic hyperplasia: effects on blood pressure and urinary flow in normotensive and hypertensive men. *Urology* 1995; **46**(2): 182–6.

18 McConnell JD, Bruskewitz R, Walsh P, Andriole G, Lieber M, Holtgrewe HL *et al.* The effect of finasteride on the risk of acute urinary retention and the need for surgical treatment among men with benign prostatic hyperplasia. Finasteride Long-Term Efficacy and Safety Study Group. *N Engl J Med* 1998; **338**(9): 557–63.

19 Nickel JC, Fradet Y, Boake RC, Pommerville PJ, Perreault JP, Afridi SK *et al.* Efficacy and safety of finasteride therapy for benign prostatic hyperplasia: results of a 2-year randomized controlled trial (the PROSPECT study). PROscar Safety Plus Efficacy Canadian Two year Study. *CMAJ* 1996; **155**(9): 1251–9.

20 Andersen JT, Ekman P, Wolf H, Beisland HO, Johansson JE, Kontturi M *et al.* Can finasteride reverse the progress of benign prostatic hyperplasia? A two-year placebo-controlled study. The Scandinavian BPH Study Group. *Urology* 1995; **46**(5): 631–7.

21 Boyle P, Gould AL, Roehrborn CG. Prostate volume predicts outcome of treatment of benign prostatic hyperplasia with finasteride: meta-analysis of randomized clinical trials. *Urology* 1996; **48**(3): 398–405.

22 Roehrborn CG, Boyle P, Nickel JC, Hoefner K, Andriole G. Efficacy and safety of a dual inhibitor of 5-alpha-reductase types 1 and 2 (Dutasteride) in men with benign prostatic hyperplasia. *Urology* 2002; **60**(3): 434–41.

23 Lepor H, Williford WO, Barry MJ, Brawer MK, Dixon CM, Gormley G *et al.* The efficacy of terazosin, finasteride, or both in benign prostatic hyperplasia. Veterans Affairs Cooperative Studies Benign Prostatic Hyperplasia Study Group. *N Engl J Med* 1996; **335**(8): 533–9.

24 Kirby RS, Roehrborn CG, Boyle P, for the PREDICT Study Investigators. Efficacy and tolerability of doxazosin and finasteride, alone or in combination, in treatment of symptomatic benign prostatic hyperplasia: the Prospective European Doxazosin and Combination Therapy (PREDICT) trial. *Urology* 2003; **61**: 119–26.

25 McConnell JD, Roehborn CG, Bautista OM, The long-term effect of doxazosin, finasteride, and combination therapy on the clinical progression of benign prostatic hyperplasia. *N Engl J Med* 2003; **349**: 2387–98.

26 Diamond SM, Ismail M, Hubosky S, El-Gabry E. Placebo controlled trial of alpha blockers and finasteride in men with enlarged prostates and LUTS: subjective and objective results after discontinuation of alpha blockers. American Urological Association. 2002.

27 Baldwin KC, Ginsberg PC, Roehrborn CG, Harkaway RC. Discontinuation of alphablockade after initial treatment with finasteride and doxazosin in men with lower urinary tract symptoms and clinical evidence of benign prostatic hyperplasia. *Urology* 2001; **58**(2): 203–209.

28 Barkin J, Guimaraes M, Do Castelo V, Jacobi G, Pushkar D, Taylor S *et al.* Dutasteride provides sustained symptom relief following short term combination treatment with tamsulosin. American Urological Association. 2002.

29 Lowe FC, Fagelman E. Phytotherapy in the treatment of benign prostatic hyperplasia: an update. *Urology* 1999; **53**(4): 671–8.

30 ConsumaLab.com. Independent Tests of Herbal, Vitamin and Mineral Supplements. http://www.ConsumerLab.com. 2000.

31 Lowe FC. Phytotherapy in the management of benign prostatic hyperplasia. *Urology* 2001; **58**(6 Suppl. 1): 71–6.

32 Plosker GL, Brogden RN. Serenoa repens (Permixon). A review of its pharmacology and therapeutic efficacy in benign prostatic hyperplasia. *Drugs Aging* 1996; **9**(5): 379–95.

33 Paubert-Braquet M, Momboisse JC, Boichot-Lagente JC. *Pygeum africanum* extract inhibits bFGF and EFG induced proliferation of 3T3 fibroblasts. *Biomed Pharmacother* 1994; **48**: 43–7.

34 Marwick C. Growing use of medicinal botanicals forces assessment by drug regulators. *JAMA* 1995; **273**(8): 607–609.

35 Debruyne F, Koch G, Boyle P, Da Silva FC, Gillenwater JG, Hamdy FC *et al.* Comparison of a phytotherapeutic agent (Permixon) with an alpha-blocker (Tamsulosin) in the treatment of benign prostatic hyperplasia: a 1-year randomized international study. *Eur Urol* 2002; **41**(5): 497–506.

36 Carraro JC, Raynaud JP, Koch G, Chisholm GD, Di Silverio F, Teillac P *et al.* Comparison of phytotherapy (Permixon) with finasteride in the treatment of benign prostate hyperplasia: a randomized international study of 1,098 patients. *Prostate* 1996; **29**(4): 231–40.

37 Roehrborn CG. BPH clinical research criteria. In: Denis L, Griffiths K, Khoury S, eds. Proceedings of the 4th International Consultation on BPH. Plymouth: Health Publications, 1997: 437–514.

38 Wilt T, Ishani A, MacDonald R. Serenoa repens for benign prostatic hyperplasia (Cochrane Review). The Cochrane Library Issue 3. 2002. Oxford: Update Software.

39 Boyle P, Robertson C, Lowe F, Roehrborn C. Meta-analysis of clinical trials of permixon in the treatment of symptomatic benign prostatic hyperplasia. *Urology* 2000; **55**(4): 533–9.

40 Glemain P, Coulange C, Grapin FN, Muszynski RC. No benefit in combining tamsulosin with Serenoa repens versus tamsulosin alone on storage/filling and voiding lower urinary tract symptoms. American Urological Association Annual meeting. 2002.

41 Levin RM, Riffaud JP, Bellamy F, Rohrmann D, Krasnopolsky L, Haugaard N *et al.* Effects of tadenan pretreatment on bladder physiology and biochemistry following partial outlet obstruction. *J Urol* 1996; **156**(6): 2084–8.

42 Kassen A, Berges R, Senge T. Effect of beta-sitosterol (Harzol®) on the expression and secretion of growth factors in primary human prostate stromal cell cultures in vitro (abstract 31). Fourth International Consultation on BPH. 1997.

43 Berges RR, Windeler J, Trampisch HJ, Senge T. Randomised, placebo-controlled, double-blind clinical trial of beta-sitosterol in patients with benign prostatic hyperplasia. Beta-sitosterol Study Group. *Lancet* 1995; **345**(8964): 1529–32.

44 Berges RR, Kassen A, Senge T. Treatment of symptomatic benign prostatic hyperplasia with beta-sitosterol: an 18-month follow-up. *BJU Int* 2000; **85**(7): 842–6.

45 Klippel KF, Hiltl DM, Schipp B. A multicentric, placebo-controlled, double-blind clinical trial of beta-sitosterol (phytosterol) for the treatment of benign prostatic hyperplasia. German BPH-Phyto Study group. *Br J Urol* 1997; **80**(3): 427–32.

46 Wilt TJ, MacDonald R, Ishani A. Beta-sitosterol for the treatment of benign prostatic hyperplasia: a systematic review. *BJU Int* 1999; **83**(9): 976–83.

3: Drugs Used in the Treatment of Erectile Dysfunction

Ian Eardley

Physiology of erection

Sexual stimuli that may be visual, auditory, imaginative or even olfactory stimulate descending neural pathways that probably originate within the hypothalamus. From there, fibres descend within the spinal cord to the sacral segments S2, S3 and S4. Parasympathetic nerves pass across the pelvis, around the rectum to the base of the bladder, and then along the postero-lateral aspect of the prostate, before exiting the pelvis just lateral to the urethra. The fibres penetrate the corpora cavernosa, innervating the penile arteries and the smooth muscle that lies within the cavernosal sinusoids. The parasympathetic nerves can also be activated via reflex pathways, with the sensory limb initiated by tactile stimulation of the penis, and with impulses travelling proximally in the dorsal nerve of the penis. The parasympathetic nerves release a cocktail of neurotransmitters, including acetylcholine and vasoactive intestinal polypeptide (VIP), but the most important is nitric oxide (Fig. 3.1). Acetylcholine also stimulates the release of nitric oxide by the vascular endothelium that lines the sinusoidal spaces and it is the nitric oxide derived both from the parasympathetic nerves and the vascular endothelium that results in the smooth muscle relaxation that is crucial for an erection to occur.

Nitric oxide is able to pass through the smooth muscle cell membrane, where it stimulates the enzyme guanylate cyclase to convert guanylate triphosphate (GTP) to cyclic guanylate monophosphate (cGMP), the active intracellular second messenger, and via a sequence of events characterized by phosphorylation, smooth muscle relaxation ensues. The action of the cGMP is terminated by the enzyme phosphodiesterase type 5 (PDE5) (Fig. 3.1).

While the parasympathetic nerves are particularly active during sexual stimulation, at other times there is tonic activity of the sympathetic nervous system that results in release of noradrenaline, which in turn causes smooth muscle contraction. The balance between the opposing sympathetic (contractile) and parasympathetic (relaxant) systems determines the state of contraction of the penile smooth muscle; when the smooth muscle is relaxed the penis is erect, and when it is contracted, the penis is flaccid.

Smooth muscle relaxation results in arterial dilatation with increased blood flow into the penis. This is accompanied by relaxation of the sinus-

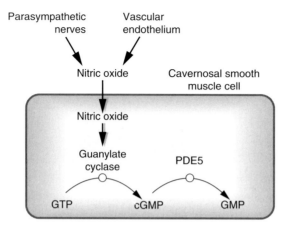

Figure 3.1 Physiology of the cavernosal smooth muscle cell. Nitric oxide, released from both parasympathetic nerve endings and from the vascular endothelium, stimulates guanylate cyclase to convert guanylate triphosphate (GTP) to its active second messenger, cyclic guanylate monophosphate (cGMP). Phosphodiesterase type 5 (PDE5) breaks down cGMP.

oidal tissue and pooling of blood in the vascular spaces, which in turn leads to swelling of the cavernosal tissue. As the swelling occurs within the tough outer layer of the corpora (known as the tunica albuginea), the penis becomes more rigid and efferent veins that penetrate the tunica are compressed against it. This results in reduced venous outflow from the penis, increasing the penile swelling and rigidity. When sexual activity is over, the sympathetic nerves become dominant, the smooth muscle contracts and the vascular changes reverse, leading to penile flaccidity.

Causes of erectile dysfunction

The complex neurovascular process outlined briefly above is susceptible to interference at multiple levels (Table 3.1). Psychological and psychiatric disease can interfere with normal erection, while neurological disease affecting the basal ganglia, the brainstem and the spinal cord can also have deleterious effects. The parasympathetic nerves are susceptible to surgical damage as they traverse the pelvis, and vascular disease can also impair the normal vascular response to neural stimulation. A large number of drugs used in the therapy of hypertension, prostate cancer, psychiatric disease and depression can also precipitate erectile dysfunction (ED). Metabolic disease such as diabetes and renal failure can result in endothelial and smooth muscle dysfunction with associated impairment of normal erections. Finally, the whole system is modulated by testosterone and conditions that result in low serum testosterone can also induce ED.

Table 3.1 Some of the causes of erectile dysfunction: varying types of pathology can interfere with normal penile erection (although the list is by no means exhaustive)

Type	Examples
Psychological	Anxiety
	Depression
Neurological	Multiple sclerosis
	Spinal cord injury
	Parkinson's disease
Vascular	Atherosclerosis
Endocrine	Hypogonadism
	Hyperprolactinaemia
Metabolic	Diabetes
	Renal failure
Iatrogenic	Surgery that damages the pelvic nerves, e.g. radical retropubic prostatectomy
	Pelvic radiotherapy
Drugs	Antihypertensives (especially beta-blockers, thiazide diuretics)
	Antipsychotics
	Antiandrogens
	Antidepressant

Principles of therapy

At the current time, there are three principal mechanisms that drugs employ to improve erectile function. The first (and most widely utilized) involves facilitation of penile smooth muscle relaxation. The second involves stimulation of central neural pathways, and the third involves testosterone replacement in those men who have the specific problem of low serum testosterone.

Historically, the first drug to be widely used was papaverine. It was administered by intracavernosal injection, and for 15 years or so, a variety of smooth muscle relaxants were used as injectables for the treatment of ED. Currently, the only drug that is widely licensed for use in this way is prostaglandin E1 (also called alprostadil). Both alprostadil and papaverine produce smooth muscle relaxation directly while other drugs that have also been used such as phentolamine and moxisylate are adrenoceptor-blocking agents that block sympathetic nervous activity. All these drugs have to be administered locally (usually by intracavernosal injection), first, because the concentrations required for efficacy are too high to allow systemic administration and, second, because systemic administration would cause unacceptable side-effects.

The first licensed orally active smooth muscle relaxant was sildenafil, an inhibitor of PDE5, while more recently two new drugs of this class, tadalafil and vardenafil, have also been licensed (Table 3.2). Phentolamine is an

Method of administration		Drugs
Locally administered drugs	Intraurethral	Prostaglandin E1
	Intracavernosal	Prostaglandin E1 VIP/Phentolamine Papaverine Moxisylate
Systemically administered drugs	Oral	PDE5 inhibitors, e.g. sildenafil, vardenafil, tadalafil Adrenoceptor antagonists, e.g. phentolamine

Table 3.2 Drugs that facilitate smooth muscle relaxation

adrenoceptor-blocking agent that has been licensed for use in some parts of the world (although not in Europe or the USA).

Animal experiments have suggested that dopaminergic neurotransmission within the hypothalamus is important in penile erection and the first licensed centrally acting drug, apomorphine, used this purported mechanism for its mode of action. Active when administered sublingually, apomorphine is a dopaminergic agonist that appears to improve penile erections. Other drugs with a possible central mechanism of action that have been used for the treatment of ED include yohimbine (an α-2-adrenoceptor antagonist) and trazadone (which has some α-adrenergic antagonist properties and some inhibition of serotonin reuptake actions). At this time a number of other centrally acting drugs (including the melanocortin analogues) are under development.

Orally active agents

Phosphodiesterase type 5 inhibitors

There are many similarities between the three licensed PDE5 inhibitors. All are highly potent drugs that inhibit the target enzyme with considerable but slightly incomplete selectivity (see below). All are orally active, and all require sexual stimulation to be effective. The reason for this is that without the nitric oxide release that is induced by sexual stimulation, the PDE5 inhibitor will have no effect. This functional selectivity actually has considerable therapeutic benefit for the patient. First, although the enzyme PDE5 is present in other tissues of the body, it is the release of nitric oxide within the penis, in response to a sexual stimulus, that allows very low levels of these drugs to improve erections without undue side-effects. Second, it simulates normal erectile function in that when the man is sexually aroused, nitric oxide is released and the drug has its effect, and when the sexual act is complete, the nitric oxide release diminishes and the effect of the drug ceases. Subsequent sexual arousal will allow the drug to become 'active' again, until such time as the tissues levels fall below that needed for efficacy.

As was alluded to above, the enzyme PDE5 is found in other parts of the body, particularly the vasculature, the nasopharynx and the gastrointestinal tract. Side-effects can occur due to inhibition of this enzyme in these loci, and these side-effects of headache, flushing, indigestion and nasal congestion are common to all the PDE5 inhibitors.

Despite their similarities, there are differences between the three PDE5 inhibitors. Biochemically, the main areas of variation are their selectivity and their pharmacokinetics. There are in fact 11 classes of phosphodiesterase within the body, and they are differentially distributed in different tissues. The ideal PDE5 inhibitor would not produce significant inhibition of any of these other enzymes, but in fact all of them have some inhibitory activity against specific isoenzymes. This can be ascertained by calculation of selectivity ratios for the three drugs, and although different laboratories produce slightly differing results for these ratios, it is generally accepted that at high doses, tadalafil inhibits PDE type 11 (PDE11), while sildenafil (at high doses) inhibits PDE type 6 (PDE6). Vardenafil probably also has some clinically significant activity against PDE6, although less so than sildenafil. Tadalafil has no significant activity against PDE6 while neither sildenafil nor vardenafil has any significant activity against PDE11.

PDE6 is found only in the retina and is involved in phototransduction. At high doses, sildenafil can induce reversible visual changes such as blue vision or bright vision. Research has demonstrated a transient change in the electroretinogram, but no permanent deleterious effects [1]. PDE11 is found widely in the body, although its function is currently unclear. It is certainly found within the testis, but studies have not demonstrated any deleterious effects upon testicular function, either in terms of endocrine function or spermatogenesis [2].

The second area of difference is in the pharmacokinetic properties of the drugs. In clinical studies there are differences in the time to maximal plasma concentration following oral administration (T_{max}) and in the half-life of the drugs ($T_{1/2}$) (Table 3.3) [3–5]. Such values are important for the speed of

Table 3.3 Time to maximal plasma concentration (T_{max}) and half-life ($T_{1/2}$) of the PDE5 inhibitors [3,4,5]	T_{max} (h)	$T_{1/2}$ (h)
Sildenafil	1.16	3.82
Tadalafil	2.0	17.5
Vardenafil	0.66	3.94

onset of action of the drug and for the duration of action, issues that are pertinent to the use of drugs that are used 'as required'.

All the PDE5 inhibitors are licensed for use across the range of aetiologies of men with ED, and in the absence of head-to-head comparative trials they appear to have broadly similar efficacy. Details of the individual drugs are outlined below. They share a number of contraindications, of which the most important is a contraindication to use in men who take nitrates or nitric oxide donor medication. This not only applies to prescription drugs used for the treatment of ischaemic heart disease, but also applies to recreational drugs such as amyl nitrate (poppers).

SILDENAFIL

Sildenafil was first licensed in 1998 as an oral therapy for the treatment of men with ED. It is rapidly absorbed with peak plasma concentrations being achieved in around 1 h [3]. Absorption is slightly delayed by food and this may be of importance to some men. It is metabolized primarily in the liver, with a half-life of around 4 h. The usual starting dose is 50 mg, with titration up to 100 mg or down to 25 mg according to efficacy and side-effects. In elderly patients, patients with moderate to severe renal impairment, those with significant liver disease and those using cytochrome P450 enzyme CYP3A2 inhibitors, a starting dose of 25 mg is advisable.

Sildenafil has proven efficacy and safety in a wide range of patient populations. Following reports of efficacy and safety in broad populations of men with ED [6], several subsequent large, placebo-controlled trials demonstrated efficacy in men with diabetes [7–9], spinal cord injury [10], depression [11], coronary artery disease [12,13] and in men using antidepressants [14] and antihypertensives [15]. Multiple efficacy end points were used in these studies. In the broad population study, the successful intercourse rate was 69% in men taking sildenafil compared with 19% in men taking placebo [6]. The erectile function (EF) domain of the International Index for Erectile Function (IIEF) [16] at the end of the study was 22.1 in those taking sildenafil and 12.2 in those taking placebo, while 74% of men taking sildenafil had improved erections compared with 19% of those taking placebo. This success rate varied by the aetiology of the ED and representative results are shown in Table 3.4. As can be seen, the efficacy is less impressive in men with diabetes.

Patients who use sildenafil can expect to obtain a clinical effect within 1 h and in some patients the onset may be much faster, as shown in small laboratory-based studies [18] or in 'at home' studies [19]. These studies were performed, however, in men who had not eaten for variable periods of time, and given the known delay in absorption caused by food [3], patients should be

Table 3.4 Efficacy of sildenafil in phase III and phase IV clinical trials

Senior author	Year	Population	Results at end of treatment					
			EFD placebo	EFD sildenafil	Intercourse success with placebo (%)	Intercourse success with sildenafil (%)	Improved erections with placebo (%)	Improved erections with sildenafil (%)
Goldstein [6]	1998	Broad	12.2	22.1	22	69	19	74
Chen [17]	2001	Broad	18.1	24.3	30	62	38.4	88.2
Rendell [7]	1999	Diabetes	10.4	17.5	12	48	10	56
Boulton [8]	2001	Diabetes type 2	11.5	20.4	14.4	58.8	11	65
Seidman [11]	2001	Depression	12.4	23.4	NR	NR	11	91
Giuliano [10]	1999	Spinal cord injury	NR	NR	NR	NR	4	76
Olsson [12]	2001	Cardiovascular disease	NR	NR	NR	NR	24	71
Debusk [13]	2004	Coronary artery disease	15	19.8	25	51	28	59

NR, not recorded.

advised to wait longer for efficacy following a meal. The other end of the window of efficacy has not been studied as extensively, but laboratory-based studies certainly demonstrate some efficacy out to 8 and even 12 h [20].

The side-effects most commonly seen with sildenafil include headache, flushing, indigestion and nasal congestion [21]. These side-effects are all dose-dependent and are thought to reflect inhibition of PDE5 in tissues other than the penis, such as vascular smooth muscle, the nasopharyngeal mucosa and smooth muscle of the urinary tract. At high doses, sildenafil also inhibits PDE6, which is found only within the retina. This inhibition results in visual side-effects, such as bluish vision or bright vision. Careful studies have demonstrated a transient and reversible effect upon the electroretinogram, but no permanent effect upon other aspects of visual function [1].

The effect of sildenafil upon vascular smooth muscle, alluded to above, can be seen in the modest falls in blood pressure seen following administration [22]. In fact, the clinical consequences of this hypotensive effect are minor. There are however interactions with other drugs affecting the cardiovascular system. Co-administration with nitrates such as glyceryl trinitrate or nitroprusside leads to significant falls in both systolic and diastolic blood pressure [23]. In clinical practice, sildenafil is contraindicated in all patients taking nitrates. Another interaction is occasionally seen in men taking α-adrenoceptor-blocking agents, where again, there may be transient falls in blood pressure. Co-administration of sildenafil with α-blocking agents should only be entertained with caution and should only be considered at least 4 h after ingestion of the α-blocker. The exact regulatory labelling details vary between countries.

The safety of sildenafil in men with cardiovascular disease has been extensively investigated, following on from early press reports suggesting an increased risk of myocardial infarction. In fact, all the available data suggest that sildenafil has no increased cardiac risk. Analysis of the placebo-controlled trials shows no excess incidence either of myocardial infarction or of death [1] and post-marketing studies also show no excess risk [24]. Studies of cardiac function in men with coronary artery disease also demonstrate no deleterious effects [25,26].

TADALAFIL

Tadalafil was licensed in 2002 in Europe and in 2003 in the USA. It is absorbed following oral administration, with achievement of peak plasma levels in around 2 h [4]. Its absorption is minimally affected by prior food. It is metabolized primarily within the liver by the cytochrome P450 enzyme system and it has a half-life of around 17.5 h [4]. The licensed starting dose varies by country. In Europe and the USA, the licensed starting dose is 10 mg with titration up to 20 mg if required. In some other countries, a starting dose of 20 mg has been approved. No dosing alterations are needed in the elderly, but in men with impaired renal or hepatic function titration up to 20 mg is not advised.

Tadalafil has proven efficacy in large trials of both the broad population of men with ED and men with a specific aetiological cause for their ED, such as men with diabetes and men who have undergone radical retropubic prostatectomy. As with sildenafil, multiple efficacy end points were used in the trials. In the primary publication, reporting pooled data from five large placebo-controlled trials, the successful intercourse rate for tadalafil 20 mg was 75% compared with 32% for placebo, the end of trial EF domain score was 23.9 for tadalafil 20 mg compared with 15.1 for placebo and tadalafil 20 mg improved erections in 81% of men compared with 35% of men who took placebo [27]. As with sildenafil, the efficacy in diabetics was reduced [28] (Table 3.5).

The onset of action of tadalafil (as with the other PDE5 inhibitors) is in advance of its maximum plasma concentration, with at-home studies suggesting that many patients have successful intercourse in less than 1 h [29]. This study was performed with no restriction on food intake. The duration of activity of tadalafil has been extensively studied. One large study clearly demonstrated efficacy at 36 h after administration [30], and pooled data from large placebo-controlled trials have confirmed this [27].

The side-effect profile is similar to that seen with sildenafil, with headache, flushing, indigestion and nasal congestion occurring in a dose-dependent fashion [27]. These side-effects are thought to reflect PDE5 inhibition in tissues other than the penis. However, there are two important differences

Table 3.5 Efficacy of tadalafil in phase III clinical trials

Senior author	Year	Population	Results at end of treatment					
			EFD placebo	EFD tadalafil	Intercourse success with placebo %	Intercourse success with tadalafil %	Improved erections with placebo %	Improved erections with tadalafil %
Brock [27]	2002	Broad	15.1	23.9 (20-mg dose)	32%	75% (20-mg dose)	35%	81% (20-mg dose)
Saenz de Tejada [28]	2002	Diabetes	12.2	18.8 (20-mg dose)	NR	NR	25%	64% (20-mg dose)

NR, not recorded.

in the side-effect profile from sildenafil. First, visual side-effects are not seen, reflecting a lack of significant inhibition of PDE6. Second, a small proportion of men get backache, proximal girdle pain or limb pain. The exact cause is unclear, but is thought to reflect prolonged PDE5 inhibition (since it was occasionally seen in early sildenafil trials, when sildenafil was being taken three times per day).

In healthy subjects, tadalafil has a mild hypotensive effect. As with sildenafil, co-administration with nitrates results in marked hypotensive effects in some patients [31] and accordingly tadalafil is contraindicated in all men taking such drugs. As with sildenafil, occasional interactions are seen with α-blockers such as doxazosin, although there was no significant interaction seen in an interaction study with tamsulosin [32]. Clinically, there should be caution in prescribing tadalafil to men using α-blockers: indeed, until recently in the USA co-administration with all α-blockers other than tamsulosin is contraindicated, although the exact labelling restrictions vary between countries.

The cardiac safety of tadalafil has been demonstrated in a number of ways. Pooled data from the pivotal placebo-controlled trials have revealed no excess incidence of either myocardial infarction or death [33] while treadmill studies of men with cardiovascular disease who have been administered tadalafil have also shown no deleterious effects [34].

VARDENAFIL

Vardenafil was licensed in 2003 for use in men with ED. It is absorbed following oral administration, with achievement of peak plasma levels in around 0.7 h [5]. It is metabolized primarily within the liver by the cytochrome P450 enzyme system and it has a half-life of approximately 4 h [5]. The licensed starting dose is 10 mg with titration up to 20 mg or down to

5 mg if indicated by efficacy or tolerability. In elderly patients, patients with impaired hepatic or renal function, and patients using inhibitors of the CYP3A4 system, a starting dose of 5 mg is recommended. While the dose can be increased to 10 mg or 20 mg in the elderly and in those with hepatic or renal impairment, in patients using inhibitors of the CYP3A4 system the maximum advisable dose is 5 mg.

Placebo-controlled trials with vardenafil have demonstrated efficacy both in the broad population of men with ED [35] and in men with diabetes [36] and men who have undergone radical retropubic prostatectomy [37] (Table 3.6). As with sildenafil, multiple efficacy end points were used in the trials. In the North American pivotal trial, the successful intercourse rate for vardenafil 20 mg was 64.5% at 12 weeks compared with 32.2% for placebo, the 12-week EF domain score was 21.4 for vardenafil 20 mg compared with 15 for placebo, and vardenafil 20 mg improved erections in 80.9% of men compared with 38.6% of men who took placebo. As with the other two drugs the efficacy in diabetics was reduced.

At-home placebo-controlled studies have confirmed a rapid onset of action for vardenafil [39], with many men responding in less than 1 h, and sometimes much faster. While a high-fat meal delays absorption of vardenafil, less fatty meals do not [40]. The duration of clinical effectiveness has been studied less extensively, although common sense suggests efficacy for at least 1.5–2 half-lives (i.e. 6–8 h).

The dose-related PDE5 side-effects of headache, flushing, indigestion and nasal congestion are seen as they are with the other PDE5 inhibitors [38].

Table 3.6 Efficacy of vardenafil in phase III trials

Senior author	Year	Population	Results at end of treatment					
			EFD placebo	EFD vardenafil	Intercourse success with placebo	Intercourse success with vardenafil	Improved erections with placebo	Improved erections with vardenafil
Hellstrom (at 12 weeks) [35]	2002	Broad	15	21.4 (20-mg dose)	32.2%	64.5% (20-mg dose)	38.6%	80.9% (20-mg dose)
Hatzichristou [38]	2004	Broad	14.5	23.3 (flexible dose)	30%	69% (flexible dose)	33%	84% (flexible dose)
Goldstein [36]	2003	Diabetes	12.6	19 (20-mg dose)	23%	54% (20-mg dose)	13%	72% (20-mg dose)
Brock [37]	2003	Radical retropubic prostatectomy	9.2	15.3 (20-mg dose)	10%	34% (20-mg dose)	9%	60% (20-mg dose)

However, neither back pain nor visual side-effects are commonly encountered. Biochemically, there is a minor degree of inhibition of PDE6, but the absence of visual side-effects in the clinical trials suggest that it is insignificant.

As with the other PDE5 inhibitors, vardenafil has mild hypotensive effects. When combined with organic nitrates the fall in blood pressure can be significant, and co-administration is contraindicated. Similarly until recently co-administration with α-blockers is contraindicated in the USA because of occasional falls in blood pressure. In Europe, the co-administration of α-blockers is a caution to the use of vardenafil, but as with the other drugs in this class, the exact labelling restrictions vary between countries. Currently there are no interaction data relating to the co-administration of vardenafil with so-called uroselective α-blockers such as tamsulosin. The cardiac safety of tadalafil has been demonstrated in treadmill studies of men with cardiovascular disease who have been administered tadalafil but have shown no deleterious effects [41]. Pooled data from the clinical trials also appear to show no excess incidence of cardiac complications in men taking vardenafil compared with men taking placebo [42].

COMPARISON OF THE PHOSPHODIESTERASE TYPE 5 INHIBITORS

In terms of efficacy (at the time of writing) there seems little to choose between the three drugs. Given the lack of true comparative trials, and given the different populations studied in the pivotal trials, the efficacy of the PDE5 inhibitors seems to be similar, with approximately 70% of men from the 'broad' population having successful intercourse. All drugs show reduced efficacy rates in diabetics. In terms of the window of efficacy, the lack of comparative trials makes it impossible to judge whether one drug is appreciably faster than the others. All drugs have been tested in at-home stopwatch studies, but the different populations studied do not facilitate comparison (Table 3.7). The duration of action of tadalafil is clearly much greater than sildenafil and vardenafil. The latter two have efficacy for perhaps 6–8 h or so, (i.e. 2 half-lives) while tadalafil has proven efficacy for at least 36 h.

Table 3.7 Comparison of the onset of action studies of the PDE5 inhibitors

Drug	Patient population with respect to response to PDE5 inhibitors	Response rate
Sildenafil [19]	Prior sildenafil responders only	67.8% at 30 min
Tadalafil [29]	No restrictions	52% at 30 min
Vardenafil [39]	No restrictions	53% at 25 min with 20 mg vardenafil

In terms of side-effects, all three drugs have similar profiles (with the minor exceptions noted above), all have minor hypotensive effects and all have significant interactions with nitrates leading to a contraindication for all of the PDE5 inhibitors in men using organic nitrates. There appear to be no detrimental effects upon cardiac function, and the most obvious difference between the drugs is the degree of interaction with α-blockers. Even here, the apparent differences probably only reflect the different trials, and we might expect to see the labelling restrictions in this respect move towards conformity.

Comparative trials have been performed to attempt to identify patient's preference [43,44,45]. At the time of writing, none of these trials has had an ideal design leading to possibly incorrect conclusions. Whether true comparative trials will demonstrate differences in efficacy, safety or preference remains to be seen.

Centrally acting agents

APOMORPHINE

Apomorphine is a dopaminergic agonist that activates D1 and D2 receptors. As an injectable agent it has been available for over 30 years, and early research demonstrated its ability to produce an erection following injection into both normal men and men with ED. In the 1990s an oral formulation of the drug was developed which was active when taken sublingually. It is thought to work centrally by stimulation of dopaminergic neurones within the hypothalamus, thus initiating sexual activity, although in humans sexual arousal is necessary. It was licensed in Europe in 2001, and at the time of writing remains under regulatory review in the USA.

Apomorphine is administered sublingually and reaches peak plasma concentrations within 40–60 min [46]. Given the mode of administration, there is no food interaction. It is primarily metabolized within the liver with an elimination half-life of 3 h. The starting dose is 2 mg, with patients usually titrated up to 3 mg. This appears to minimize the risk of unwanted side-effects. No dosing adjustments are needed in the elderly, but in those with either renal or hepatic impairment, the upper dosing limit should be 2 mg. There are few interactions with other drugs, although apomorphine should not be combined with other centrally acting dopaminergic agonists or antagonists. Caution should be exercised when administering apomorphine to men taking nitrates or other antihypertensive agents, because of the possibility of hypotension. Alcohol does appear to increase the risk of side-effects.

Apomorphine has proven efficacy in the treatment of the broad population of men with ED, although no specific studies have been performed in men with specific aetiologies. In pooled data from 3 pivotal phase III trials the end of treatment EF domain of the IIEF score was 13.29 for placebo compared with

16.64 for apomorphine [47]. Post hoc subgroup analysis demonstrated that maximal efficacy was achieved in men with mild to moderate ED, where the end of treatment successful intercourse rate was 60% for apomorphine (compared to 43% for placebo). The sublingual mode of administration facilitates a rapid onset of action with a median onset of action at 18.8 min in the clinical trials [46]. Duration of activity has not formally been studied.

Apomorphine is well tolerated at licensed doses, with the most common side-effects being nausea, headache and dizziness. The most serious adverse event seen at higher doses is syncope, but in the pooled trial database, syncope was rarely seen at therapeutic lower doses. There is clear evidence that dose titration minimizes adverse events [48]. The trial data showed evidence that neither concomitant medication nor moderate alcohol consumption increased the risk of adverse events. Formal studies were not performed with respect to cardiovascular issues, but the pooled trial data did not show any evidence of cardiac risk.

COMPARISON OF PDE5 INHIBITORS AND APORMORPHINE

Only one trial has been published comparing the efficacy and safety of sildenafil and apomorphine [49]. This was a randomized open-label crossover trial with full-dose titration being possible in patients who were naive to therapy. The trial showed clear superiority for sildenafil over apomorphine in all measurable end points (including intercourse success rate, EF domain of the IIEF and global assessment questions). The vast majority of patients expressed a preference for sildenafil. No trials have been published comparing either tadalafil or vardenafil and apomorphine.

Other occasionally used oral agents

PHENTOLAMINE

Phentolamine is a non-selective α-adrenoceptor antagonist that had been used with papaverine as an intracavernosal agent in the 1980s and early 1990s. An oral preparation underwent clinical trials in the 1990s, and was subsequently licensed in some parts of the world. It was not licensed for use however in western Europe or North America, where trials were stopped in 1999 because of safety concerns. It probably works by inhibition of the sympathetic tone that normally results in smooth muscle contraction within the penis, although there may also be some additional central effects. It had been noted that when injected on its own as an intracavernosal agent, phentolamine was not particularly effective and it was thus theorized that there may be an additional mechanism of action analogous to that of yohimbine, a centrally acting α-2-adrenoceptor antagonist.

As an oral formulation it had modest efficacy in placebo-controlled clinical trials at doses of 40 mg and 80 mg [50]. For the 80-mg dose, the EF domain improved by 3.6 points compared with a placebo change of − 0.98. Side-effects included headache, dizziness and nasal congestion, although generally the drug was well tolerated. For a 40-mg dose taken orally, the maximum plasma concentration is achieved in around 0.69 h and the half-life is 2.14 h. Toxicology trials suggested an increased incidence of brown fat tumours in rats, and trials in the USA were stopped in 1999 [51].

Although the relative efficacy with PDE5 inhibitors has not been formally tested in clinical trials, the magnitude of change in the IIEF EF domain appears to be much less than in those seen with PDE5 inhibitors and in those countries where it is licensed, phentolamine currently has a secondary role in the modern management of men with ED.

YOHIMBINE

Yohimbine is a drug that has long been reputed to have useful efficacy in men with ED. It is an alkaloid, derived from the bark of the yohimbe tree. Pharmacologically it has α-2-adrenoceptor–blocking actions, and this is thought to represent its mechanism of action in ED either at a central or at a peripheral site of action, with the former thought to be more likely. Dosing regimes have been variable, ranging from 15 to 30 mg per day in divided doses. A meta-analysis of randomized placebo-controlled trials in 1998 [52] identified seven studies that were of sufficient quality to justify inclusion, and although two of these trials showed no significant difference between placebo and yohimbine, the overall meta-analysis demonstrated an odds ratio of 3.85 (95% CI 2.22–6.67) in favour of yohimbine. It is important to remember that the end points used in these trials were generally not as rigorous as those used in the modern studies of PDE5 inhibitors. The commonest side-effects were anxiety, agitation, headache, tachycardia and gastrointestinal disturbances, although in general yohimbine was well tolerated.

In comparison with the PDE5 inhibitors, yohimbine appears to have lower efficacy. However, recent interest has centred upon possible combination therapy involving yohimbine [53], and it continues to have a small role in the therapy of men with ED, usually as a second-line agent.

TRAZODONE

Trazodone hydrochloride is an oral antidepressant that has anxiolytic and sedative properties. There have been occasional reports of its efficacy in the treatment of men with ED. Trazodone has several pharmacological actions including inhibition of serotonin re-uptake and α-2-adrenoceptor antagonism. The latter is thought to represent the most likely mechanism of action for this drug in the treatment of ED, although it is unclear whether this is a central or a peripheral effect. The usual dose that has been used in men with ED is 150 mg per day, taken either singly or in divided doses. A systematic review of placebo-controlled trials [54] suggested, in a pooled analysis of six controlled trials, that men taking trazodone were more likely to have a positive response to therapy than men receiving placebo. However, the magnitude of this effect was variable, and most importantly the improvement did not reach statistical significance (Table 3.8). The group of patients with the most marked response were those with psychogenic ED, although even here there was no statistically significant improvement. The commonest adverse events in this meta-analysis were dry mouth, sedation, dizziness and fatigue. Given the efficacy of the PDE5 inhibitors, trazodone has little role in the modern management of men with ED.

Licensed locally active agents

INTRACAVERNOSAL ALPROSTADIL

Prostaglandin E1 (alprostadil) is a potent relaxant of cavernosal smooth muscle. It directly activates cell surface receptors on the smooth muscle of the cavernosal trabeculae and the penile arteries to activate the enzyme adenylate cyclase, thereby increasing intracellular concentrations of cyclic AMP, which in turn acts as second messenger causing smooth muscle relaxation in an entirely analogous way to the action of cGMP.

As an intracavernosal injection, alprostadil was licensed in 1992 and is available in doses up to 40 μg. The usual starting dose is around 10 μg, with titration up to an effective dose. If a patient is thought to have psychogenic or neurogenic ED, then a low starting dose of perhaps 2.5 μg should be used, because these patients can be especially sensitive to alprostadil. Unlike the oral PDE5 inhibitors, it does not require a sexual stimulus to be effective, and the

Table 3.8 Efficacy of trazodone in pooled analysis of placebo-controlled trials (from Fink et al. [54])	Number of patients with positive response to therapy (%)		
	Trazodone	Placebo	Efficacy ratio for trazodone: placebo (95% CI)
All patients	38/104 (37%)	21/105 (20%)	1.6 (0.8–3.3)
Patients with psychogenic ED	29/46 (63%)	10/43 (23%)	2.7 (0.9–8)

erection typically develops within 10–15 min, persisting for around 30–120 min. Several trials have demonstrated efficacy in the broad population of men with ED [55] and in those with ED that is resistant to oral therapy [56]. The commonest complications are penile pain at the time of injection (seen in around 30% of men), a prolonged erection lasting more than 4 h (which is a medical emergency requiring urgent treatment, but which only occurs in around 1% of men at the initial injection) and penile scarring, probably secondary to the repeated intracavernosal injection [57].

Currently the primary indication for the use of intracavernosal injection therapy is in men who have failed to respond to oral therapy, or in men who are unsuitable for oral therapy. Practical issues involves tuition in the injection technique, which should take place into the side of the corpora, thereby missing the dorsal neurovascular complex. Intracavernosal therapy is contraindicated in a small group of patients. For example, patients who are at risk of developing priapism, such as patients with sickle cell anaemia, multiple myeloma or leukaemia, should not be treated by this method. Use of anticoagulants is not a contraindication to treatment, although extra care must be taken to avoid excessive bruising. Patients with Peyronie's disease can probably also be treated safely by injection therapy. Patients who have previously had a prolonged erection following intracavernosal injection are often reluctant to continue with self-injection and require careful evaluation before instituting therapy.

INTRAURETHRAL ALPROSTADIL

Prostaglandin E1 can also be applied within the urethra with benefit. The urethra close to the external urethral orifice is lined with stratified squamous epithelium while more proximally the lining acquires a more complex stratified and pseudostratified columnar structure. It seems likely that from the urethra alprostadil traverses the epithelium to gain access to spongiosal veins that communicate with veins of the corpus cavernosum. Retrograde flow through these veins would allow drugs introduced into the urethra to reach the cavernosal smooth muscle, although larger doses of drug will inevitably need to be applied in order for a therapeutic dose to reach its target tissue.

Using a specially designed device (the MUSE® device) doses of between 125 and 1000 μg alprostadil can be applied to achieve an erection [58] and the MUSE system was licensed for the treatment of men with ED in 1997. Clinical trials have demonstrated efficacy in men with ED, although these trials were performed before the introduction of sildenafil [58]. Side-effects include penile pain.

Trials comparing intraurethral alprostadil with intracavernosal injections, and with sildenafil, appear to show that the MUSE device is an inferior therapy for men with ED [59,60]. Accordingly it has only a minor role in the modern treatment of men with ED.

Testosterone therapy

In the pharmacological treatment of men with ED, testosterone therapy has a unique position. Unlike the other drugs described above, which can often be used regardless of the cause of the ED, testosterone has a role under specific circumstances, i.e. when there is a proven deficiency in the levels of serum testosterone. However, beyond this statement, a number of controversies and uncertainties lie. Firstly, hypogonadism does not always result in ED. There is usually a reduction in the frequency of sexual thoughts, in the frequency, volume and quality of the ejaculate, but visual evoked erections are often possible in men taking antiandrogens. Current thinking suggests that nocturnal erections are androgen-dependent while erections arising from erotic stimuli have only partial androgen dependence [61]. A further area of controversy surrounds the biochemical diagnosis of hypogonadism. This is a complex issue that lies beyond the scope of this review but recent guidelines have begun to clarify the area for the clinician [62].

Testosterone can be administered in a number of ways (Table 3.9) and the method of administration has a significant bearing upon both efficacy and side-effects. Depot preparations (the intramuscular injections and implants) do not replicate the normal diurnal changes in plasma testosterone concentrations, which are best replicated by the topical preparations and potentially by the oral preparations. However, the oral preparations are prone to significant hepatic metabolism, and the alkylated androgen preparations (such as methyl testosterone) can result in significant hepatotoxicity, such that their use is not now advised. Oral testosterone undecanoate is however licensed in many countries around the world and appears to be safe. The topical patches can occasionally cause skin irritation, which is a problem that is less commonly seen with the gel preparations. The absorption of these preparations is variable, and careful monitoring of serum levels is required to achieve the appropriate dose.

The efficacy of testosterone replacement in men with ED has only limited evidence to support it. One meta-analysis only identified five studies where appropriate placebo responses had been measured, and the total number of patients studied was only 109 men [63]. The response rate (with varying methods of therapy) to testosterone was 65.4% compared with a response-rate to placebo of 16.7%.

Adverse events that can occur with testosterone preparations are either dependent upon the mode of administration (see above) or are more generalizable. There is a tendency for the haematocrit to rise slightly and for there

Table 3.9 Common testosterone preparations

Route of administration	Compound	Trade name (where available)	Dosing regime
Intramuscular pellet	Testosterone	Non-proprietary	200–800 mg/3 months
Oral	Methyl testosterone	—	10–40 mg daily
—	Testosterone undecanoate	Restandol®	120–160 mg daily
		Andriole®	(maintenance 40–120 mg)
Intramuscular injection	Testosterone propionate	Virormone® (also present in Sustanon 100® and Sustanon 250®)	As per instructions
—	Testosterone enanthate	Non-proprietary	200–400 mg every 2–3 weeks
—	Testosterone cypionate	Non-proprietary	200–400 mg every 2–3 weeks
Topical	Testosterone patch	Andropatch® Androderm®	2.5–7.5 mg/day
—	Testosterone patch (scrotal skin only)	Testoderm®	4–6 mg daily
—	Testosterone gel	Testogel® Androgel®	5–10 grams of gel per day (equivalent to 50–100 mg testosterone per day)
—	Testosterone gel	Testim®	50–100 g/day

to be a degree of fluid retention. There are anabolic effects with increased muscle mass, and there may be reversal of osteoporosis. The effects upon serum lipids and cardiovascular function are complex, although not necessarily detrimental. Finally, the effect upon the prostate is poorly understood at this time. Whether testosterone can promote either prostatic growth or the development of prostate cancer is unknown, and at present it seems prudent to monitor testosterone therapy with regular assessment of the haematocrit, the serum lipids and prostate-specific antigen (PSA).

One potential future area of use is in combination with other oral therapies for the treatment of ED. There is limited evidence that some men who are initially poor responders to the PDE5 inhibitors can be converted to being a responder by combination with testosterone [64].

Agents under development

MELANOCORTIN ANALOGUES

Animal studies have implicated α-melanocyte-stimulating hormone (α-MSH) and ACTH in the control of penile erection and sexual behaviour.

The action is mediated via so-called melanocortin (MC) receptors, probably within the hypothalamus, of which there are several types. A number of synthetic analogues of α-MSH have been developed of which one, Melanotan II, has entered clinical trials for the treatment of male ED. Early studies demonstrated erectogenic activity in men with both psychogenic and organic ED following subcutaneous injection of Melanotan II [65], and recently an intranasal formulation of the compound has been developed. Side-effects include stretching and yawning and it has also been reported to provoke an increased level of sexual desire [66]. At the time of writing, its role remains under investigation.

PHENTOLAMINE AND VASOACTIVE INTESTINAL POLYPEPTIDE COMBINATIONS

A combination of phentolamine and VIP underwent clinical trials in the late 1990s as a potential agent for intracavernosal injection. VIP 25 μg was combined with phentolamine 1 mg or 2 mg for intracavernosal injection. As with intracavernosal alprostadil, no sexual stimulation was required for efficacy, with erections typically appearing within 10–15 min. Clinical trials produced promising results [67], with efficacy that appeared to be at least equivalent to intracavernosal alprostadil. The principal side-effect was facial flushing, while priapism was rare and intracavernosal pain was absent. At the time of writing, the combination therapy is still awaiting licensing and launch.

TOPICAL ALPROSTADIL

Prostaglandin E1 gel can also be effective when applied onto the skin of the penis, and a topical preparation is currently under trial to assess its efficacy and safety. It is combined with a soft enhancer of percutaneous absorption (SEPA), an amphiphilic molecule that reversibly alters the lipid structure of the epidermis, thus allowing improved absorption of small molecules. The SEPA enhances absorption of the alprostadil and modest efficacy has been reported [68]. Side-effects are mild but include penile erythema. Phase III trials of this preparation are underway at the time of writing and the place of such an agent is unclear.

Conclusion

At the present time, the PDE5 inhibitors remain first-line therapy for most men with ED. While testosterone has a specific indication, other oral therapies are very much second-line treatments. Injectables are indicated following failure of initial oral therapy. The place of topical therapy is not yet apparent. There is developing interest in pharmacological management of other aspects of sexual function such as desire and ejaculatory dysfunction, but no drugs are yet licensed for these indications. One possible future area of interest is combination of drugs that work centrally with drugs that work peripherally, although it is important to remember that while different agents may have synergistic benefits, adverse events may also be increased.

References

1 Padma-Nathan H, Eardley I, Kloner R, Laties AM, Montorsi F. A 4 year update on the safety of sildenafil citrate. *Urology* 2002; **60**(Suppl. 2B): 67–90.
2 Hellstrom WJG, Overstreet JW, Yu A *et al*. Tadalafil has no detrimental effect on human spermatogenesis or reproductive hormones. *J Urol* 2003; **170**: 887–1.
3 Nichols DJ, Muirhead GJ, Harness JA. Pharmacokinetics of sildenafil citrate after single oral doses in healthy male subjects: absolute bioavailability, food effects and dose proportionality. *Br J Clin Pharm* 2002; **53**(Suppl. 1): 5S–12S.
4 Patterson B, Bedding A, Jewell H, Payne C, Mitchell M. Dose normalised pharmacokinetics of tadalafil (IC351) administered as a single dose to healthy volunteers. *Int J Impot Res* **13**(Suppl. 4), Abstract 120.
5 Klotz T, Sachse R, Heidrich A, Jockenhovel F, Rohde G, Wensing G, Horstmann R, Engelmann R. Vardenafil increases penile rigidity and tumescence in erectile dysfunction patients: a rigiscan and pharmacokinetic study. *World J Urol* 2001; **19**: 32–9.
6 Goldstein I, Lue T, Padma-Nathan H, Rosen R, Steers W, Wicker P, for the Sildenafil Study Group. Oral sildenafil in the treatment of erectile dysfunction. *N Engl J Med* 1998; **338**: 1397–404.
7 Rendell M, Rajfer J, Wicker P, Smith M, Sildenafil Diabetes Study Group. Sildenafil for treatment of erectile dysfunction in men with diabetes: a randomized control trial. *JAMA* 1999; **281**: 421–6.
8 Boulton AJM, Selam JL, Sweeney M, Ziegler D. Sildenafil for the treatment of erectile dysfunction in men with type II diabetes mellitus. *Diabetologia* 2001; **44**: 1296–301.
9 Stuckey B, Jadzinsky MN, Murphy L, Montorsi F, Kadioglu A, Fraige F, Manzano P, Deerochanawong C. Sildenafil citrate for treatment of erectile dysfunction in men with type 1 diabetes: results of a randomized controlled trial. *Diabetes Care* 2003; **26**: 279–84.
10 Giuliano F, Hultling C, El Masry WS, Smith M, Osterloh I, Orr M, Maytom M, for the Sildenafil Study Group. Randomized trial of sildenafil for the treatment of erectile dysfunction in spinal cord injury. *Ann Neurol* 1999; **46**: 15–21.
11 Seidman SN, Roose SP, Menza MA, Shabsigh R, Rosen RC. Treatment of erectile dysfunction in men with depressive symptoms: results of a placebo-controlled trial with sildenafil citrate. *Am J Psychiatry* 2001; **158**: 1623–30.
12 Olsson AM, Persson C-A. Efficacy and safety of sildenafil citrate for the treatment of erectile dysfunction in men with cardiovascular disease. *Int J Clin Prac* 2001; **55**: 171–6.
13 DeBusk RF, Pepine CJ, Glasser DB, Shpilsky A, De Riesthal H, Sweeney M. Efficacy and safety of sildenafil citrate in men with erectile dysfunction and stable coronary artery disease. *Am J Cardiol* 2004; **93**: 147–53.
14 Nurnberg HG, Hensley PL, Gelenberg AJ, Fava M, Lauriello J, Paine S. Treatment of antidepressant-associated sexual dysfunction with sildenafil: a randomized controlled trial. *JAMA* 2003; **289**: 56–64.
15 Kloner R, Brown M, Prisant LM, Collins M, for the Sildenafil Study Group. Effect of sildenafil in patients with erectile dysfunction taking antihypertensive therapy. *Am J Hypertens* 2001; **14**: 70–3.

16   Rosen RC, Cappelleri JC, Gendrano III, N. The International Index of Erectile Function (IIEF): a state-of-the-science review. *Int J Impot Res* 2002; **14**: 226–44.

17   Chen KK, Hsieh JT, Huang ST, Jiaan DBP, Lin JSN, Wang CJ, for the Assess 3 Study Group. ASSESS-3: a randomised, double-blind, flexible-dose clinical trial of the efficacy and safety of oral sildenafil in the treatment of men with erectile dysfunction in Taiwan. *Int J Impot Res* 2001; **13**: 221–9.

18   Eardley I, Ellis P, Boolell, Wulff M. Onset and duration of action of sildenafil citrate for the treatment of erectile dysfunction. *Br J Clin Pharm* 2002; **53**(Suppl. 1): 61S–65S.

19   Padma-Nathan H, Stecher VJ, Sweeney M, Orazem J, Tseng L-J, deRiesthal H. Minimal time to successful intercourse after sildenafil citrate: results of a randomized, double-blind, placebo-controlled trial. *Urology* 2003; **62**: 400–403.

20   Gepi-Atee S, Sultana SR, Hodgson G, Wulff MB, Gingell C. Duration of action of sildenafil citrate among men with erectile dysfunction of no known organic cause. *Int J Impot Res* 2001; **13**(Suppl. 1): 26.

21   Morales A, Gingell C, Collins M, Wicker PA, Osterloh IH. Clinical safety of oral sildenafil citrate (VIAGRA®) in the treatment of erectile dysfunction. *Int J Impot Res* 1998; **10**(2): 69–74.

22   Zusman RM, Prisant LM, Brown MJ. Effect of sildenafil citrate on blood pressure and heart rate in men with erectile dysfunction taking concomitant antihypertensive medication. *J Hypertens* 2000; **18**: 1865–9.

23   Webb DJ, Muirhead GJ, Wulff M *et al.* Sildenafil citrate potentiates the hypotensive effects of nitric oxide donor drugs in male patients with stable angina. *J Am Coll Cardiol* 2000; **36**: 25–31.

24   Shakir SA, Wilton LV, Boshier A *et al.* Cardiovascular events in users of sildenafil: results from first phase of prescription event monitoring in England. *BMJ* 2001; **322**: 651–2.

25   Hermann HC, Chang G, Klugherz BD *et al.* Hemodynamic effects of sildenafil in men with severe coronary artery disease. *N Engl J Med* 2000; **342**: 1622–6.

26   Arruda-Olson AM, Mahoney DW, Nehra A *et al.* Cardiovascular effects of sildenafil during exercise in men with known or probable coronary artery disease. *JAMA* 2002; **287**: 719–25.

27   Brock, GB, McMahon, CG, Chen, KK *et al.* Efficacy and safety of tadalafil for the treatment of erectile dysfunction: results of integrated analyses. *J Urol* 2002; **168**: 1332–6.

28   Saenz de Tejada I, Knight JR, Anglin G, Emmick JT. Effects of tadalafil on erectile function in men with diabetes. *Diabetes Care* 2002; **25**: 2159–64.

29   Padma-Nathan H, Rosen RC, Shabsigh R, Saikali K, Watkins V, Pullman B. Cialis (IC351) provides prompt response and extended period of responsiveness for the treatment of men with erectile dysfunction (ED). American Urological Association. 2001; Abstract 923: Anaheim, California, p. 224.

30   Porst H, Padma-Nathan H, Giuiano F, Anglin G, Varnese L, Rosen RC. Efficacy of tadalafil for the treatment of erectile dysfunction at 24 and 36 hours after dosing: a randomized controlled trial. *Urology* 2003; **62**: 1–5.

31   Emmick JT, Stuewe SR, Mitchell M. Overview of the cardiovascular effects of tadalafil. *Eur Heart J* 2002; Vol 4 (Suppl. H): 32–47.

32   Jackson G, Kloner RA, Emmick JT, Mitchell MI, Bedding A, Pereira A. Interaction between tadalafil and two alpha blockers: Doxazosin and Tamsulosin. *Int J Impot Res* 2003; **15**(Suppl. 6). Abstract P-037: p. S60

33   Kloner RA, Mitchell M, Emmick JT. Cardiovascular effects of tadalafil. *Am J Cardiol* 2003; **92**(Suppl.): 37–46.

34   Patterson D, McDonald TM, Effron MB, Emmick JT, Mitchell M, Bedding A, Kloner RA. Tadalafil does not affect time to ischaemia during exercise stress testing in patients with coronary artery disease. *Int J Impot Res* 2002; **14**(Suppl. 3): S102.

35 Hellstrom WJ, Gittelman M, Karlin G, Segerson T, Thibonnier M, Taylor T, Padma-Nathan H. Vardenafil for treatment of men with erectile dysfunction: efficacy and safety in a randomized, double-blind, placebo-controlled trial. *J Androl* 2002; **23**: 763–71.

36 Goldstein I, Young JM, Fischer J, Bangerter K, Segerson T, Taylor T, Vardenafil Diabetes Study Group. Vardenafil, a new phosphodiesterase type 5 inhibitor, in the treatment of erectile dysfunction in men with diabetes: a multicenter double-blind placebo-controlled fixed-dose study. *Diabetes Care* 2003; **26**: 777–83.

37 Brock G, Nehra A, Lipshultz LI, Karlin GS, Gleave M, Seger M, Padma-Nathan H. Safety and efficacy of vardenafil for the treatment of men with erectile dysfunction after radical retropubic prostatectomy. *J Urol* 2003; **170** (Pt 1): 1278–83.

38 Hatzichristou D, Montorisi F, Taylor T. Efficacy of vardenafil in a flexible dose regimen: a placebo controlled trial. *Eur Urol* 2004; Vol 45. p. 634–41.

39 Montorsi F, Padma-Nathan H, Buvat J, Beneke M, Ulbrich E, Bandel T, Porst H. Time to onset of action leading to successful sexual intercourse by vardenafil in men with erectile dysfunction. *Sex Relationship Ther* 2004; **19**(Suppl. 1): S66.

40 Rajagopalan P, Mazzu A, Xia C, Dawkins R, Sundaresan P. Effect of high-fat breakfast and moderate-fat evening meal on the pharmacokinetics of vardenafil, an oral phospho-diesterase-5 inhibitor for the treatment of erectile dysfunction. *J Clin Pharmacol* 2003; **43**(3): 260–67.

41 Thadani U, Smith W, Nash S, Bittar N, Glasser S, Narayan P, Stein RA, Larkin S, Mazzu A, Tota R, Pomerantz K, Sundaresan P. The effect of vardenafil, a potent and highly selective phosphodiesterase-5 inhibitor for the treatment of erectile dysfunction, on the cardiovas-cular response to exercise in patients with coronary artery disease. *J Am Coll Cardiol* 2002; **40**(11): 2006–12.

42 Kloner R, Mohan P, Norenberg C *et al*. Cardiovascular safety of vardenafil a potent highly selective PDE5 inhibitor in patients with erectile dysfunction: an analysis of 5 placebo controlled trials. *Pharmacotherapy* 2002; **22**: 1371.

43 Ströberg-P, Murphy-A, Costigan-T. Switching patients with erectile dysfunction from sildenafil citrate to tadalafil: results of a European multicenter, open-label study of patient preference. *Clin Ther* 2003; **25**(11): 2724–37.

44 Grovier-F, Potempa-A, Kaufman-J, Denne-J, Kovalenko-P, Ahuja-S. A multicenter, ran-domized, double-blind, crossover study of patient preference for tadalafil 20 mg or silde-nafil citrate 50 mg during initiation of treatment for erectile dysfunction. *Clin Ther* 2003; **25**: 2709–23.

45 Von Keitz A, Rajfer J, Segal S, Murphy A, Denne J, Costigan T, Lockhart D, Beasley J, Emmick J. A multicenter, randomized, double-blind, crossover study to evaluate patient preference between tadalafil and sildenafil. *Eur Urol* 2004; **45**: 499–509.

46 Heaton JP. Apomorphine: an update of clinical trial results. *Int J Impot Res* 2000; **12** (Suppl. 4): S67–73.

47 Stief C, Padley RJ, Perdok RJ, Sleep DJ. Cross-study review of the clinical efficacy of Apomorphine SL 2 mg and 3 mg: pooled data from three placebo-controlled fixed-dose crossover studies. *Eur Urol Suppl* 2002; **1**: 12–20.

48 Ralph DJ, Sleep DJ, Perdok RJ, Padley RJ. Adverse events and patient tolerability of apomorphine SL 2 mg and 3 mg: a cross data analysis of phase II and III studies. *Eur Urol Suppl* 2002; **1** (21–7).

49 Eardley I, Wright P, MacDonagh R, Hole J, Edwards A. An open label, randomised, flexible dose, crossover study to assess the comparative efficacy and safety of sildenafil citrate and apomorphine hydrochloride in men with erectile dysfunction. *BJU Int* 2004; **93**: 1271–5.

50 Goldstein I. Oral phentolamine: an alpha-1, alpha-2 adrenergic antagonist for the treat-ment of erectile dysfunction. *Int J Impot Res* 2000; **12**(Suppl. 1): S75–80.

51 Hopps CV, Mulhall JP. Novel agents for sexual dysfunction. *Br J Urol Int* 2003; **92**: 534–8.

52 Ernst E, Pittler MH. Yohimbine for erectile dysfunction: a systematic review and meta-analysis of randomised clinical trials. *J Urol* 1998; **159**: 433–6.

53 Lebret T, Herve JM, Gorny P, Worcel M, Botto H. Efficacy and safety of a novel combination of L-arginine glutamate and yohimbine hydrochloride: a new oral therapy for erectile dysfunction. *Eur Urol* 2002; **41**: 608–13.

54 Fink HA, MacDonald R, Rutks IR, Wilt TJ. Trazodone for erectile dysfunction: a systematic review and meta-analysis. *Br J Urol Int* 2003; **92**: 441–6.

55 Linet OI, Ogrinc FG. Efficacy and safety of intracavernosal alprostadil in men with erectile dysfunction. *N Engl J Med* 1996; **334**: 873–7.

56 Shabsigh R, Padma-Nathan H, Gittleman M, McMurray J, Kaufman J, Goldstein I. Intracavernous alprostadil alfadex (Edex/Viridal) is effective and safe in patients with erectile dysfunction after failing sildenafil (Viagra). *Urology* 200; **55**: 477–80.

57 Juenemann KP, Manning M, Krautschick A, Alken P. 15 years of injection therapy in erectile dysfunction – a review. *Int J Impot Res* 1996; **8**: A60.

58 Padma-Nathan H, Hellstrom W, Kaiser FE *et al.* Treatment of men with erectile dysfunction with transurethral alprostadil. *N Engl J Med* 1997; **336**: 1–7.

59 Shabsigh R, Padma-Nathan H, Gittleman M, McMurray J, Kaufman J, Goldstein I. Intracavernous alprostadil alfadex is more efficacious, better tolerated, and preferred over intraurethral alprostadil plus optional actis: a comparative, randomised, crossover multicentre study. *Urology* 2000; **55**: 109–13.

60 Gauthier A, Rutchik DS, Winters CJ, Fuselier AH, Woo H, Prats JL, Bardot S. Relative efficacy of sildenafil compared to other treatment options for erectile dysfunction. *South Med J* 2000; **93**: 962–5.

61 Morales A, Heaton JPW. Hypogonadism and erectile dysfunction: pathophysiological observations and therapeutic outcomes. *Br J Urol Int* 2003; **92**: 896–9.

62 Morales A, Lunenfeld B. Investigation, treatment and monitoring of late-onset hypogonadism in males. Official recommendations of the International Society for the Study of the Aging Male. *Aging Male* 2002; **5**: 74–86.

63 Jain P, Redemaker AW, McVary KT. Testosterone supplementation for erectile dysfunction: a meta-analysis. *J Urol* 2000; **164**: 371–5.

64 Shabsigh R, Kaufman JM, Steidle C, Padma-Nathan H. Testosterone converts sildenafil non-responders to responders in men with hypogonadism and erectile dysfunction who failed prior sildenafil therapy. *J Urol* 2003; **169**: 247 (Abstract).

65 Wessells H, Levine N, Hadley ME, Dorr R, Hruby V. Melanocortin receptor agonists, penile erection and sexual motivation: human studies with Melanotan II. *Int J Impot Res* 2000; **12**(Suppl. 4): S74–9.

66 Wessells H, Padma-Nathan H, Rajfer J, Feldman R, Rosen R, Molinoff P, Diamond L, Earle D, Powers B. At-home efficacy of an intranasally administered melanocortin receptor agonist, PT-141 in men with erectile dysfunction. *J Urol* 2004; **171**(Suppl. 1): Abstract 1197.

67 Dinsmore WW, Gingell C, Hackett G, Kell P, Savage D, Oakes R, Frentz GD. Treating men with predominantly nonpsychogenic erectile dysfunction with vasoactive intestinal polypeptide and phentolamine mesylate in a novel auto-injector system: a multicentre double-blind placebo controlled study. *BJU Int* 1999; **83**: 274–9.

68 Goldstein I, Payton TR, Schecter PJ. A double blind, placebo controlled, efficacy and safety study of topical gel formulation of 1% alprostadil (Topiglan™) for the in-office treatment of erectile dysfunction. *Urology* 2001; **57**: 301–304.

4: Drugs Used in the Treatment of Interstitial Cystitis

Mary Garthwaite & Ian Eardley

Introduction

Interstitial cystitis (IC) is a chronic, debilitating condition that is character-ized by urinary frequency and urgency, together with chronic pelvic or perineal pain. It is a condition that affects mainly Caucasian women, with a female-to-male ratio of approximately 10:1. The available epidemi-ological data are based on the rigid diagnostic criteria formulated in 1987 by the National Institute of Diabetes, Digestive and Kidney Diseases (NIDDK) [1] although many clinicians feel that strict adherence to these criteria has led to underdiagnosis of the condition [2]. In fact, recent data suggest that IC or painful bladder syndrome might affect more men than was previously thought and that it also might affect children [3]. Worldwide estimates of prevalence range between 8 and 510 cases per 100 000 [4] and the average age at diagnosis is reported to be around 42–48 years (although this may not reflect the actual age at onset of symptoms) [5]. It has been reported that approximately 25% of patients are under 30 years of age at the time of diagnosis [6].

At this time, IC is primarily a clinical diagnosis that is based upon the patient's history of irritative voiding symptoms and chronic, often episodic, urinary tract-related pain in conjunction with physical examination and cystoscopic examination. Findings at cystoscopy include inflammation, scarring, glomerulations and Hunner's ulcers.

Unfortunately, IC remains a diagnosis of exclusion and as yet there is no specific diagnostic test [7]. In 1987 the NIDDK produced a set of criteria for the diagnosis of IC, which were revised in 1988 [1]. These criteria were originally intended to aid clinical research into this condition but they were also widely adopted by urologists around the world due to a lack of other clinical guidelines. It has become clear that there are some problems with the criteria; for instance one particular issue is that the cardinal sign of pain and its severity are missing from the criteria. As a consequence it has been reported that only 36% of patients with IC actually fulfil all the criteria [8], and many patients with probable IC have been omitted from treatment trials on this basis. Current thinking is that while the criteria will identify patients with established IC, patients in the early stages of the disease may be missed as there may be no decrease in the bladder capacity, while glomerulations or Hunner's ulcers may also be absent at cystoscopy [10]. It is felt by many that a further revision of the criteria is required in order to include the whole spectrum of IC and provide a useful clinical tool in the diagnosis of both early and advanced cases [10,11].

IC can have a devastating impact on an individual's quality of life. As well as the social and physical difficulties caused by the severe urinary frequency and urgency associated with the condition, there are also emotional and psychological sequelae. The patient-driven support groups, such as the Interstitial Cystitis Support Group (ICSG) in the UK and its American counterpart, the Interstitial Cystitis Association (ICA), are working to raise awareness of the condition within both the medical and patient communities [7]. One of the benefits of this increased public awareness has been a dramatic increase in IC-centred research within the last few years.

Principles of therapy

The precise aetiology of IC remains unclear and is likely to be multifactorial. The pathophysiology of IC is the focus of intense research efforts but the study of this disease is complex and the development of targeted treatments therefore remains an extremely difficult task. Postulated aetiologies (either primary or contributory) include:

1 infection;
2 epithelial dysfunction (e.g. glycosaminoglycan (GAG) layer defect);
3 autoimmune response;
4 allergic reaction (e.g. mast cell disorders);
5 neurogenic inflammation;
6 toxic urogenous substrates;
7 inherited susceptibility;
8 lymphatic or vascular obstruction.

As the clinical features of IC are so variable it is possible that a variety of aetiological factors and pathophysiological processes underlie the development and progression of the disorder in individual patients. It may well be possible that the term 'interstitial cystitis' actually represents a number of different pathological processes and disease states, and this is partly the rationale for the recent tendency to call this condition the 'painful bladder syndrome'.

Given the different theories of aetiology and pathogenesis, there have been a number of different approaches to therapy, and these can be conveniently divided into five types of therapy: urothelial protection, mast cell inhibition, immune response modulation, neurogenic inflammation modulation and modulation of nociception.

Urothelial protection

Therapeutic agents used to maintain or enhance the barrier properties of the urothelial lining of the bladder work on the rationale that IC results from injury to the bladder epithelium, resulting in urothelial dysfunction and increased permeability. The increased permeability allows the passage of irritative or toxic substances in the urine through into the underlying tissues of the bladder wall, leading to the development of inflammation and pain. Pentosan polysulphate (PPS, Elmiron®), heparin, chondroitin sulphate, hyaluronic acid and its derivative sodium hyaluronate (Cystistat®) all act by maintaining or enhancing the protective mucopolysaccharide layer over-lying the urothelium [4].

Mast cell/histamine release inhibition

It has been shown that there is often proliferation and activation of mast cells within the bladder wall of patients with IC. It has been postulated that the release of histamine from activated mucosal mast cells is the underlying cause of the chronic pain experienced by these patients. Therapeutic agents that inhibit mast cell activation and histamine release potentially reduce or eliminate pain in IC. Agents that have been used include cromolyn (mast cell stabilizer), hydroxyzine (H_1-receptor antagonist) and cimetidine (H_2-receptor antagonist). Mast cell inhibition is also thought to be involved in the mechanism of action of dimethyl sulphoxide (DMSO) (Rimso 50®) although this agent is also known to have anti-inflammatory, analgesic and muscle-relaxant properties.

Immunogenic response modulation

One theory regarding the aetiology of IC is that an autoimmune process is involved. Interestingly, it has been reported that many patients with IC have other concomitant allergic or autoimmune disorders [12]. The mechanism of action of bacille Calmette–Guérin (BCG) therapy in the treatment of IC remains unclear but is thought to involve local immune modulation within the bladder. Cyclosporin is an immunosuppressive agent that inhibits T cell activation and cytokine release. Its use as an immune modulator is well established in the field of organ transplantation and its use as an experimental drug in the treatment of IC is based on the premise that the condition has an autoimmune aetiology.

Modulation of neurogenic inflammation

High levels of nitric oxide (NO) have been detected in the bladders of IC patients but importantly its activity appears reduced [13]. NO is a vasodilator and a neurotransmitter and is known to play a role in pain processing within the spinal cord. Inhibitors of NO are associated with increased mast cell degranulation and inflammation [14] while within the bladder NO has been shown to promote smooth muscle relaxation [15]. L-arginine, a substrate for NO production, has been used with the intention of potentiating some of these effects in patients with IC, particularly the beneficial inflammatory effects. Misoprostol is an oral prostaglandin E_1 analogue that regulates a number of immunological cascades [16]. Its use in IC is based on the rationale that prostaglandins may be cytoprotective in the bladder. Montelukast, a leukotriene D receptor antagonist that has been used in the treatment of asthma because of its anti-inflammatory properties, has also been proposed as a treatment of IC [17].

Modulation of nociception

Antidepressants are known to have analgesic properties. The mechanism of action underlying their analgesic effect is unclear but it has been postulated that they act via the inhibition of serotonin or norepinephrine re-uptake at the neural synapse and thereby inhibit nociception at central sites. They are also thought to act directly on the urinary system via anticholinergic and sedative effects and may even increase bladder capacity and inhibit histamine secretion from mucosal mast cells [18]. Amitriptyline, a commonly used tricyclic antidepressant, has been employed in the treatment of IC. Gabapentin (Neurontin®), an anticonvulsant with proven effectiveness in neuropathic pain syndromes, has been used to treat the neuropathic pain elements of IC. It acts by mimicking $GABA_B$-receptor activation, thereby benefiting pain and enhancing sleep. Opioid and non-steroidal anti-inflammatory drugs (NSAIDs) are frequently utilized in the management of the chronic pain associated with IC.

Drugs used in the treatment of interstitial cystitis

Given the problems with diagnosis, and given the relative rarity of this condition (or conditions), there is a paucity of clinical trial data for agents used to treat this condition. In particular there are few placebo-controlled randomized clinical trials and for many of the agents listed below there is little supportive data for their use. The agents listed under 'Clinical trial data' are those that tend to be used more commonly, where licensing regulations permit. The basics of dosing, side-effects, cautions and contraindications are listed in Table 4.1.

Table 4.1 Drugs commonly used in interstitial cystitis

Drug	Regimen	Side-effects	Cautions	Contraindications
Pentosan polysulphate (PPS, Elmiron®) Low molecular weight, heparin-like compound. First oral drug approved in USA specifically for the treatment of IC.	100 mg tds per oral	Bleeding complications: (gums, epistaxis, retinal haemorrhage), alopecia, diarrhoea, nausea and vomiting, rash, liver function abnormalities, gastritis, leukopenia, thrombocytopenia	Heparin insufficiency, pregnancy, lactation	Known sensitivity to related compounds
Sodium hyaluronate (Cystistat®) Hyaluronic acid derivative.	Bladder instillations 40 mg weekly for 4 weeks then monthly	Few adverse effects but localized irritation reported		
Dimethyl sulphoxide (DMSO®, Rimso-50®) FDA approved treatment for IC in USA.	Bladder instillation 50 ml 0f 50% solution every 1–2 weeks-For 6–8 weeks depending on response	Urethral burning during voiding, garlic-like taste or odour for 1–2 days following treatment (solvent excreted via the lungs)		
Hydroxyzine (Atarax®, Vistiril®) H_1-receptor antagonist.	25–75 mg orally nocte	Drowsiness, dry mouth, gastric disturbances, dizziness, headache, rash, sedative effects (may be beneficial at reducing nocturia if taken at night)	Pregnancy, BPH, urinary retention, glaucoma, hepatic disease, renal impairment, epilepsy	
Cimetidine (Tagamet®) H_2-receptor antagonist.	200 mg tds orally	Dry mouth, gastric disturbances, drowsiness, dizziness, headache, rash, pancreatitis (rare)	Pregnancy, lactation, hepatic disease, renal impairment	Warfarin Phenytoin Theophylline
Amitriptyline Tricyclic antidepressant.	25–75 mg orally at night	Dry mouth, sedation, blurred vision, constipation, tachycardia,	Cardiac disease, epilepsy, pregnancy, lactation,	Recent myocardial infarction, arrhythmias,

Continued

Table 4.1 (*Continued*)

Drug	Regimen	Side-effects	Cautions	Contraindications
		postural hypotension, arrhythmias sweating, tremor	elderly, hepatic impairment, thyroid disease, glaucoma	severe liver disease
Gabapentin (Neurontin®) Anticonvulsant.	100 mg orally at night	Drowsiness, dizziness, ataxia, fatigue, nystagmus, tremor, weight gain, arthralgia, urinary incontinence	Elderly, history of psychotic illness, renal impairment, ;diabetes, pregnancy, lactation	
L-arginine Amino acid available over the counter.	500 mg tds orally (for minimum of 6 months)			

Clinical trial data

Agents licensed for this indication

PENTOSAN POLYSULPHATE (ELMIRON®)

PPS is the most widely used drug in the treatment of IC. It was the first drug approved specifically for the treatment of IC by the Food and Drug Administration (FDA) in the USA. One randomized, double-blind, placebo-controlled, multicentre, prospective study [19] looked at 148 patients with IC and compared PPS (100 mg tds) with placebo. The treatment duration was 3 months. They reported significant overall improvements compared with baseline, with reduced pain and a reduced pressure to urinate. A further long-term study of PPS showed that improvements were sustained for 1–2 years [20]. The largest, prospective, randomized trial, looking at the safety and efficacy of up to 900 mg per day of PPS in patients with IC, found that the higher doses may increase the degree of symptomatic improvement gained but also could increase the incidence of gastrointestinal side-effects [21]. A more recent study comparing PPS, hydroxyzine, combination therapy and placebo showed little difference between PPS and placebo [22].

HYALURONIC ACID/SODIUM HYALURONATE (CYSTISTAT®)

There are no reported published placebo-controlled studies demonstrating efficacy for intravesical sodium hyaluronate in IC. In a small study of ten patients with IC, intravesical hyaluronic acid was used at a dose of 40 mg weekly for 6 weeks, and monthly thereafter, for 6 months [23]. Response rates were low, with satisfactory improvement reported in only 30% of the patients. Few adverse effects were reported but included localized irritation. A further study used 40 mg administered intravesically weekly for 3 weeks then monthly, for 3 months, in 19 patients [24]. Patients were followed up for 3 years and results suggested a beneficial long-term effect with decreased pain and frequency.

DIMETHYL SULPHOXIDE (DMSO®, RIMSO-50®)

Studies comparing DMSO with placebo have shown 50–70% improvement rates, with reported relapse rates of between 35% and 40% [25]. Patients who did relapse were often responsive to repeated treatment. In a small, randomized trial of 20 IC patients intravesical DMSO was shown to be more effective than intravesical BCG therapy [26]. This was an open-label study reflecting the garlic-like odour of the DMSO.

Agents without a license for this indication

HYDROXYZINE (ATARAX®, VISTIRIL®)

In one case series of IC patients a 40% reduction in symptom scores was reported in two-thirds of patients [27]. However, the randomized trial exploring the efficacy of PPS and hydroxyzine mentioned earlier [22] showed no significant difference from placebo.

CIMETIDINE (TAGAMET®)

One randomized trial of cimetidine in 36 patients with painful bladder disease demonstrated improvements in symptoms, including suprapubic pain and nocturia [28]. However, histological examination of bladder biopsies showed no qualitative change in the GAG layer, the basement membrane or in muscle collagen deposition. There was a minor decrease in the T cell infiltrate in the cimetidine-treated patients.

AMITRIPTYLINE

A small uncontrolled study of IC patients, treated with amitriptyline for 3 weeks, reported significant improvement in pain and daytime frequency and even total remission of symptoms in a few patients [29].

L-ARGININE

A randomized, double-blind, placebo-controlled trial compared L-arginine (500 mg tds) for 3 months, with placebo, in the treatment of IC [30]. In the intention-to-treat analysis no significant differences were highlighted between the two groups. In a more recent randomized, double-blind, placebo-controlled, crossover trial of L-arginine, at a total dose of 2.4 g per day, a statistically significant improvement in the IC symptom index was reported [31]. This effect was small and the authors felt it unlikely to be of clinical significance.

BACILLUS CALMETTE–GUÉRIN

A randomized, double-blind, placebo-controlled trial reported a 60% response rate in the intravesical bacillus Calmette–Guérin (BCG) group compared with a 27% response rate in the placebo group [32]. Follow-up of these patients at 27 months indicated that > 90% of initial responders experienced sustained improvement in symptoms [33].

CYCLOSPORIN

In a small study of the use of cyclosporin in the treatment of IC 11 patients were given 2.5–5.0 mg/kg/day for 3 months [34]. Results showed decreased frequency, increased voided volume and a reduction or cessation of pain in ten patients. However, following the end of treatment improvements were not sustained and symptoms returned in the majority of patients.

HEPARIN

A study of 48 patients with IC, receiving self-administered intravesical heparin, 3 times a week for 3 months, reported that 56% of patients had a significant improvement in their symptoms [35].

MISOPROSTOL

A small study of 25 patients, given oral misoprostol (600 µg/day) reported a 56% improvement rate at 3 months and 48% sustained improvement at 9 months [36].

MONTELUKAST

A small study of ten patients with IC, on a once-daily regimen for 3 months, found a statistically significant reduction in pain, urinary frequency and nocturia [37]. No significant side-effects were reported.

Future developments

SUPLATAST TOSILATE

This experimental agent is an immune regulator that suppresses cytokine production in helper T cells, IgE synthesis, inflammatory mediator release from mast cells and eosinophilic recruitment [38]. A preliminary study of 14 patients with non-ulcerative IC, receiving 300 mg/day for 1 year, has shown significant increases in bladder capacity and decreased urgency, frequency and pain as assessed by the IC symptom index [39]. No placebo-controlled trials have yet been reported.

VANILLOID RECEPTOR ANTAGONISTS

C-fibres in the bladder mediate pain. One area of current research is focusing on the rationale that if these fibres, and therefore pain sensation, can be blocked, then treatment will be effective regardless of the aetiology underlying the condition. The vanilloid receptor-1 (VR-1) is activated by agents such as capsaicin (applied intravesically). Vanilloids act by decreasing the temperature threshold for activation of the receptor to levels that permit channel-gating at normal body temperature. Desensitization, via continuous application of VR-1 agonists, occurs via the depletion of substance P at nerve terminals and leads to the cessation of pain. A randomized, placebo-controlled trial of 36 IC patients compared $10\,\mu mol/L$ capsaicin twice weekly for 1 month with placebo [40]. Results indicated significant improvement in frequency and nocturia in patients receiving capsaicin. However, both groups experienced a significant reduction in pain and there was no statistical difference between the two groups. The main side-effect reported was a burning or warm sensation at the time of instillation that caused significant discomfort in some patients.

RESINIFERATOXIN

The capsaicin analogue resiniferatoxin (RTX) has been studied in a randomized, placebo-controlled trial in 18 patients with hypersensitive disorder of the lower urinary tract [41]. RTX was administered intravesically at a dose of 10 nmol/L. Patients were assessed at 30 days and 3 months. Results showed a significant improvement in frequency and nocturia at 30 days that was sustained at 3 months (although to a lesser degree). Pain score improvements were only significant at 30 days and were not sustained.

BOTULINUM TOXIN (BTX®, BOTOX®)

Botulinum toxin (BTX) probably works by inducing detrusor paralysis via the inhibition of acetylcholine release [42]. The effects are temporary but treatment can be repeated. Its possible use in the treatment of urethral and bladder conditions, such as detrusor overactivity, has been summarized elsewhere [43]. Very little has been published on its use in the management of IC [44].

GENE THERAPY

The use of gene therapy to deliver opioid precursors, such as preproencephalin (PPE), to the peripheral nerves of the bladder is currently under investigation [45].

References

1 Gillenwater J, Wein AJ. Summary of the National Institute of Arthritis, Diabetes, Digestive and Kidney Diseases workshop on interstitial cystitis. *J Urol* 1988; **140**: 203.

2 Hanno PM, Landis JR, Mathews-Cook Y *et al*. Diagnosis of interstitial cystitis revisited: lessons learnt from the National Institutes of Health Interstitial Cystitis Database study. *J Urol* 1999; **161**: 553–7.

3 MillerJL, Rothman I, Bavendam TG *et al*. Prostatodynia and interstitial cystitis: one and the same? *Urology* 1995; **45**(4): 587–90.

4 Nickel J. Interstitial cystitis: characterisation and management of an enigmatic urological syndrome. *Rev Urol* 2002; **4**(3): 112–21.

5 Lukban JC, Parkin MD, Holzberg AS *et al*. Interstitial cystitis and pelvic floor dysfunction: a comprehensive review. *Pain Med* 2001; **2**(1): 60–71.

6 Held PJ, Hanno PM, Wein AJ *et al*. Epidemiology of interstitial cystitis. In: Hanno PM, Staskin DR, Krane RJ *et al*. eds. *Interstitial Cystitis*. New York: Springer-Verlag, 1990: 29–48.

7 Wesselman U. Interstitial cystitis: a chronic visceral pain syndrome. *Urology* 2001; 57(Suppl. 6a): 32–9.

8 Hanno PM, Levin RM, Monson FC. Diagnosis of interstitial cystitis. *J Urol* 1990; **143**: 278–81.

9 Ratner V. Current controversies that adversely affect interstitial cystitis patients. *Urology* 2001; 57(Suppl. 6a): 89–94.

10 Agarwal M, O'Reilly PH, Dixon RA. Intersitial cystitis – a time for revision of name and diagnostic criteria in the new millennium? *BJU Int* 2001; **87**: 348–50.

11 Kusek JW, Nyberg LM. The epidemiology of interstitial cystitis: is it time to expand our definition? *Urology* 2001; 57(Suppl. 6a): 95–9.

12 Sant GR, Theoharides TC. Interstitial cystitis. *Curr Opin Urol* 1999; **9**: 297–302.

13 Ehren I, Lundberg JO, Adolfsson J *et al*. Effects of L-arginine treatment on symptoms and bladder nitric oxide levels in patients with interstitial cystitis. *Urology* 1998; **52**(6): 1026–9.

14 Kanwar S, Wallace JL, Befus D, Kubes P. Nitric oxide synthesis inhibition increases epithelial permeability via mast cells. *Am. J Physiol* 1994; **266**: G222.

15 Palmer RMJ, Ferrige AG, Moncada S. Nitric oxide release accounts for the biological activity of endothelium-derived relaxing factor. *Nature* 1987; **327**: 524–6.

16 Davies NM, Longstreth J, Jamali F. Misoprostol therapeutics revisited. *Pharmacotherapy* 2001; **21**: 60–73.

17 Theoharides TC, Sant GR. New agents for the medical treatment of interstitial cystitis. *Expert Opin Invest Drugs* 2001; **10**: 521–46.

18 Hanno PM. Amitriptyline in the treatment of interstitial cystitis. *Urol Clin North Am* 1994; **21**: 89–91.

19 Parsons CL, Benson G, Childs SJ *et al.* A quantitatively controlled method to study prospectively interstitial cystitis and demonstrate the efficacy of pentosan polysulphate. *J Urol* 1993; **150**: 845–8.

20 Hanno PM. Analysis of long-term Elmiron therapy for interstitial cystitis. *Urology* 1997; **49**(Suppl. 5a): 93–9.

21 Nickel J, Barkin J, Forrest J *et al.* Randomised, double-blind, dose-ranging study of pentosan polysulfate sodium (PPS) for interstitial cystitis (IC). *J Urol* 2001; **165**(Suppl. 5): 67 (Abstract).

22 Sant GR, Propert KR, Hanno PM *et al.* A pilot clinical trial of oral pentosan polysulphate and oral hydroxyzine in patients with interstitial cystitis. *J Urol* 2003; **170**(3): 810–15.

23 Porru D, Campus G, Tudino D *et al.* Results of treatment of refractory interstitial cystitis with intravesical hyaluronic acid. *Urol Int* 1997; **59**: 26–9.

24 Nordling J, Jorgensen S, Kallestrup E. Cystistat for the treatment of interstitial cystitis: a 3-year follow-up study. *Urology* 2001; **57**(Suppl. 6): 123 (Abstract).

25 Perez-Marrero R, Emerson LE, Feltis JT. A controlled study of dimethyl sulfoxide in interstitial cystitis. *J Urol* 1988; **140**: 36–9.

26 Peeker R, Haghsheno MA, Holmang S *et al.* Intravesical bacillus Calmette–Guerin and dimethyl sulfoxide for the treatment of classic and non-ulcer interstitial cystitis: a prospective randomised double-blind study. *J Urol* 2000; **164**: 1912–16.

27 Theoharides TC, Sant GR. Hydroxyzine therapy for interstitial cystitis. *Urology* 1997; **49**: 108–110.

28 Thilagarajah R, Witherow RO, Walker MM. Oral cimetidine gives effective symptom relief in painful bladder disease: a prospective, randomised, double-blind, placebo controlled trial. *BJU Int* 2001; **87**: 207–12.

29 Hanno PM, Beuhler J, Wein AJ. Use of amitriptyline in the treatment of interstitial cystitis. *J Urol* 1989; **141**: 846–8.

30 Korting GE, Smith SD, Wheeler MA *et al.* A randomized double-blind trial of oral L-arginine for treatment of interstitial cystitis. *J Urol* 1999; **61**: 558–65.

31 Cartledge JJ, Davies AM, Eardley I. A randomised double-blind placebo-controlled cross-over trial of the efficacy of L-arginine in the treatment of interstitial cystitis. *BJU Int* 2000; **85**: 421–6.

32 Peters KM, Diokno AC, Steinert BW *et al.* The efficacy of intravesical Tice strain bacillus Calmette–Guérin in the treatment of interstitial cystitis: a double-blind, prospective, placebo-controlled trial. *J Urol* 1997; **157**: 2090–94.

33 Peters KM, Diokno AC, Steinert BW, Gonzalez JA. The efficacy of intravesical bacillus Calmette–Guérin in the treatment of interstitial cystitis: long term follow-up. *J Urol* 1998; **159**: 483–7.

34 Forsell T, Ruutu M, Isoniemi H *et al.* Cyclosporine in severe interstitial cystitis. *J Urol* 1996; **155**: 1591–3.

35 Parsons CL, Housley T, Schmidt JD *et al.* Treatment of interstitial cystitis with intravesical heparin. *Br J Urol* 1994; **73**: 504–507.

36 Kelly JD, Young MR, Johnston SR *et al.* Clinical response to an oral prostaglandin analogue in patients with interstitial cystitis. *Eur Urol* 1998; **34**: 53–6.

37 Bouchelouche K, Nordling J, Hald T *et al.* The cysteinyl leukotriene D4 receptor antagonist montelukast for the treatment interstitial cystitis. *J Urol* 2001; **166**: 1734–7.

38 Ueda T, Tamaki M, Ogawa O *et al.* Improvement of interstitial cystitis symptoms and problems that developed during treatment with oral IPD-1151T. *J Urol* 2000; **164**: 1917–20.

39 O'Leary MP, Sand GR, Fowler FJ Jr *et al.* The interstitial cystitis symptom index and problem index. *Urology* 1997; **49**: 58–63.

40 Lazzeri M, Beneforti P, Benaim G *et al.* Intravesical capsaicin for treatment of severe bladder pain: a randomised, placebo-controlled study. *J Urol* 1996; **156**: 947–52.

41 Lazzeri M, Beneforti M, Spinelli A *et al.* Intravesical resiniferatoxin for the treatment of hypersensitive disorder: A randomised placebo controlled study. *J Urol* 2000; 676–9.

42 Smith CP, Franks ME, McNeil BK *et al.* Effect of botulinum toxin A on the autonomic nervous system of the rat lower urinary tract. *J Urol* 2003; **169**: 1896–900.

43 Reitz A, von Tobel J, Stohrer M *et al.* European experience of 184 cases treated with botulinum-A toxin injections into detrusor muscle for neurogenic incontinence. *Neurourol Urodyn* 2002; **21**: 427–428 (Abstract).

44 Chancellor MB, Yishimura N. Treatment of interstitial cystitis. *Urology* 2004; **63**(Suppl. 3A): 85–92.

45 Yoshimura N, Franks ME, Sasaki K *et al.* Gene therapy of bladder pain with herpes simplex virus (HSV) vectors expressing preproenkephalin (PPE). *Urology* 2001; **57**(Suppl. 1): 116 (Abstract).

Part 2
Urinary Tract Infection

5: Treatment of Simple Urinary Tract Infection

Dana Stieber & Kalpana Gupta

Introduction

Urinary tract infections (UTIs) are the most common bacterial infections in women. The majority of these are simple UTIs, also known as acute uncomplicated cystitis. Acute uncomplicated cystitis is defined as infection of the bladder in an otherwise healthy adult woman without known anatomical or functional abnormalities of the urinary tract and no predisposition to infection. Acute uncomplicated cystitis most commonly affects young sexually active women and accounts for more than 8 million physician visits per year in the USA [1]. Twenty-five to thirty-five per cent of women between the ages of 20 and 40 have experienced symptoms described as a UTI [2] and the majority of women will experience at least one UTI during their lifetime. With an estimated cost of $92–120 per treated infection, acute uncomplicated cystitis confers an economic burden of nearly $1 billion to the health care system annually [3]. In addition, UTIs are associated with significant morbidity, with each episode estimated to result in 6 symptom days, and approximately 1 day lost from work [4]. Thus, appropriate management of this common infection is essential.

Acute cystitis is an infection localized to the bladder mucosa and caused by bacterial attachment to the mucosa or urethra resulting in a local inflammatory response. The vast majority of acute cystitis cases are caused by bacterial ascension following perineal colonization. Symptoms are quite classic and include an abrupt onset of dysuria, frequency, urgency and/or suprapubic pain [1]. Diagnosis is commonly based on the presence of these clinical symptoms. Ideally, a clean midstream urine sample is collected for urinalysis. The presence of pyuria on microscopy or leucocyte esterase testing confirms the diagnosis. In most settings, urine culture is not routinely performed in acute uncomplicated cystitis unless the patient is non-responsive to empiric antimicrobial therapy or symptoms return within 2 weeks. If a urine culture is performed, bacteriuria in a quantity of $\geqslant 10^2$ colony-forming units of bacteria per millilitre in symptomatic patients is considered significant [1].

General principles of therapy

The selection of an appropriate antimicrobial agent in the treatment of acute UTI depends on several of the following factors [5–7]. Principally, agents with activity against the most common uropathogens and with specific pharmacokinetic parameters that support high urine concentrations and infrequent dosing intervals are preferred. Ideally, the agents should also be well tolerated, with few adverse effects, dosed once to twice daily to maximize patient compliance, and be cost-effective. Due to the fact that uropathogen susceptibility profiles vary by geographical location, the susceptibility profile of local community-acquired uropathogens should help guide initial empiric antimicrobial selection. Other factors such as the antimicrobial effect on the faecal and vaginal flora, which can influence recurrence rates, and patient-specific factors should also be considered [6]. Acquisition cost of the drug is also an important variable to account for. A comparison of retail prescription prices in US dollars for the most commonly used antimicrobials is provided in Fig. 5.1.

In vitro activity

Traditionally, management of acute uncomplicated cystitis has been simplified by the predictability of the spectrum of causative organisms and of the susceptibility patterns of these organisms. The uropathogens most commonly causing community-acquired UTI in order of decreasing prevalence include *Escherichia coli* (75–90%), *Staphylococcus saprophyticus* (5–15%) and enterococci and non–*E. coli* aerobic Gram-negative rods such as *Klebsiella* species and *Proteus mirabilis* (5–10%) [6,8]. This spectrum has been quite consistent across studies as well as over time. Thus empiric therapy,

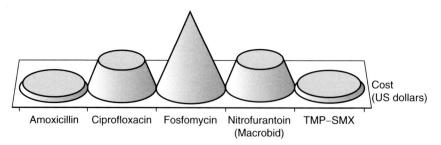

Figure 5.1 Comparative cost of antimicrobials used in acute urinary tract infection (UTI). Costs (in US dollars) were determined using average US retail pricing at the time of writing (2002). The costs were calculated for the optimal dose and duration of each drug for treatment of acute uncomplicated cystitis: amoxicillin 250 mg PO BID × 7 days, ciprofloxacin 250 mg PO BID × 3 days, fosfomycin 3 g PO × 1 dose, nitrofurantoin (Macrobid®) 100 mg PO BID × 7 days, trimethoprim/sulphamethoxazole 800/160 mg PO BID × 3 days.

i.e. without urine culture or susceptibility testing, with a 3-day regimen of trimethoprim–sulphamethoxazole (TMP–SMX), has been the standard management approach employed by many clinicians. However, with increasing rates of antimicrobial resistance among the common pathogens in community-acquired infections, including uncomplicated cystitis, management with narrow-spectrum, inexpensive agents has become a less viable option [9]. Recent Infectious Diseases Society of America (IDSA) guidelines recommend the use of a 3-day course of TMP–SMX to empirically treat acute uncomplicated UTI except in situations where the rate of resistance to TMP–SMX is greater than 10–20% [1]. This is supported by economic analyses, suggesting that it becomes more cost-effective to use fluoroquinolone rather than TMP–SMX for treatment of UTI when the TMP–SMX resistance prevalence is greater than 22% [3].

Defining *in vitro* resistance as it pertains to the urinary tract is not easy since the US National Committee for Clinical Laboratory Standards bases susceptibility and breakpoint information on serum concentrations, except for nitrofurantoin and fosfomycin, which are agents used solely in the treatment of cystitis. Breakpoint minimum inhibitory concentrations are established to efficiently separate biologically susceptible strains of organisms from intermediate or non-susceptible strains, and to predict if a particular antimicrobial will be effective in the treatment of the associated organism [10]. As noted in the Table 5.1, antimicrobial agents often achieve urinary concentrations that far exceed serum concentrations. The correlation of mean inhibitory concentration (MIC) with clinical outcomes that are associated with different sites of infection, such as the urine, may result in different breakpoint concentrations. If an organism is labelled as 'resistant' by laboratory susceptibility information that is based upon serum concentrations, it may not necessarily translate into therapeutic failure. It is recognized that serum concentrations do not correlate well with urinary bacterial eradication rates, especially in acute cystitis. Therefore, susceptibility information should be interpreted with caution and closer evaluation of 'resistant' organisms should focus on the MIC value compared with achievable urine, rather than serum, concentrations. A recent treatment trial specifically designed to address this issue demonstrated that 50–60% of women who were treated with TMP–SMX in the setting of a TMP–SMX–resistant uropathogen had clinical and bacteriological failures [11], providing solid evidence that *in vitro* susceptibility does correlate with treatment outcomes.

Many studies have reported on *in vitro* susceptibility rates among UTI isolates, but few have focused specifically on acute uncomplicated cystitis. A population-based study of outpatient women with an ICD9 code diagnosis of cystitis demonstrated increasing rates of resistance among *E. coli* isolates

Table 5.1 Concentrations of antimicrobial agents

Antimicrobial agent	Oral dose (mg)*	Oral bioavailability (%)	Peak serum concentration (μg/ml)	Serum half-life (h)	Urine concentration (μg/ml)	Renal excretion (%)	Reference
Amoxicillin	250	89	3.5–5	0.7–1.4	305–865	50–70	[17,18]
	500		5.5–11		772		
Cephalexin	250	~ 100	9	0.5–1.2	830	69–100	[19]
	500		15–18		1100		
Ciprofloxacin	250	60–80	0.94–1.53	3–5	105 ± 30.1	40.8	[20,21]
	500		1.6–2.9		350		
Fosfomycin	3000	10–30 (calcium salt); 34–58 (tromethamine salt)	26	5.7	1053–4415	18–60	[22]
Gatifloxacin	400	96	3.4	5.5–7.3	239.4 ± 51.8	76.9	[20]
Gemifloxacin	320	75–95	N/A	2.6–5	20–144	29.7	[23]
Levofloxacin	500	99	5.7	6–8	434.7 ± 93.8	75.9	[20]
Moxifloxacin	200	90	N/A	7.5–10.8	303.8 ± 112.7	9.27	[20]
Nitrofurantoin	100	87 (fasting) 90 (food)	< 2	0.3	50–250	34–40	[24]
Ofloxacin	400	90–98	1.96	5–7.5	93–427	84.3	[23]
TMP–SMX	160/80	90–100	1–2/40–60	8–15/7–12	75/190	50–60/50–75	[25]
Trimethoprim	100	90–100	—	8–15	13–136	50–60	[25,26]
Trovafloxacin	400	88–90	1.1–3.3 (for 100 and 300 mg)	7–13.7	146.3 ± 40.6	19.9	[20]

*All oral doses represent single doses, except trimethoprim (100 mg PO BID × 4 days).

to ampicillin, cephalothin and TMP–SMX from 1992 to 1996 [12]. Resistance to ciprofloxacin and nitrofurantoin was 1–2% and did not increase during the study period. In a nationwide analysis of data collected from the Surveillance Network Database (USA), a surveillance system that collects antimicrobial susceptibility results from nine geographic regions of the USA, similar trends were found [12]. The analyses were restricted to urine cultures obtained from outpatient women aged 15–50 and over 50 years old in order to focus on community-acquired UTIs. Ampicillin resistance among *E. coli* and non–*E. coli* isolates was as high as 40% nationwide. TMP–SMX resistance patterns varied across the USA, with rates as low as 10% in northeastern states and as high as 22% in western USA. Resistance to fluoroquinolones and nitrofurantoin was found to be minimal, and did not vary across geographical regions.

The general susceptibility pattern of uropathogens in Europe differs slightly from the USA. Fluit *et al.* recently reported results from the SENTRY Antimicrobial Surveillance Program, consisting of 20 hospitals across Europe, analysing data collected during a 3-month period in 1997. The distribution of uropathogens was found to be similar to the USA, with

E. coli representing the majority of cases, followed by *Enterococcus* (12%), *Klebsiella* (7%), *Proteus* (7%), *Pseudomonas* (7%) and *Enterobacter* (5%) [13]. *E. coli* isolates were resistant to penicillins in 40% of cases, although almost uniformly susceptible to cephalosporins, carbapenems, and piperacillin/tazobactam. In contrast to the USA, observed resistance to fluoroquinolones was between 11% and 12%, with highest observed resistance rates in England, Portugal, Italy and the Netherlands. These results, although not specific to acute cystitis, point to increasing fluoroquinolone resistance among UTI isolates in Europe. Low levels of resistance to nitrofurantoin have renewed interest in this agent for empiric therapy in certain patient populations. Analysis of Canadian uropathogens demonstrates patterns of susceptibility similar to those in the USA. The most common organisms found in 2000 outpatient UTI samples during 1998 were *E. coli*, *K. pneumoniae*, *P. mirabilis*, *Enterococcus* and *S. saprophyticus*, with *E. coli* representing 80% of uropathogens [14]. Susceptibility to ampicillin, TMP–SMX, nitrofurantoin and ciprofloxacin was performed using National Committee for Clinical Laboratory Standards (NCCLS) standards. High levels of resistance were demonstrated to ampicillin (41%) and TMP–SMX (19.2%). TMP–SMX resistance was high when tested against ciprofloxacin-and ampicillin-resistant *E. coli*, whereas nitrofurantoin and ciprofloxacin activity was preserved *in vitro* against ampicillin-and TMP–SMX-resistant *E. coli* [14].

General pharmacological considerations

Several pharmacokinetic and pharmacodynamic properties are important in determining the efficacy of antimicrobial agents used in the treatment of acute uncomplicated cystitis [15]. Pharmacokinetics refers to the disposition of the drug in the body, with respect to absorption, distribution, metabolism and elimination. Pharmacodynamics describes the action of a drug based on physiological, chemical or molecular observations. The antimicrobial concentration at the affected site is crucial to the treatment of infection, and drugs that reliably concentrate in the urine for extended periods of time are necessary to adequately treat acute UTI. Oral absorption and urinary elimination are two pharmacokinetic measures that predict the efficacy of agents used in UTI. Adequate oral bioavailability is necessary to achieve therapeutic serum concentrations, and a high percentage of renal elimination with reliable concentration in the renal tubule ensures the presence of drug at the site of infection. Factors that affect drug concentration and thus the rate of excretion are the glomerular filtration rate (GFR) and active tubular secretion. Drugs such as sulphonamides are filtered and not secreted, so urinary concentrations decrease as the GFR decreases. Active secretion into the renal tubular transport system facilitates urine drug concentrations up to 150 times that of serum concentrations [16]. Agents with a low pKa (i.e. strong acids) are reliably secreted in the renal tubule and achieve high urine concentrations. Drugs such as fluoroquinolones and β-lactams are filtered and actively secreted; consequently, urinary concentrations are unaffected by changes in the GFR or protein binding. The length of time that the urinary concentration remains above the organism's MIC predicts adequate killing of the organism and may explain why rapidly excreted drugs like β-lactam antibiotics are less efficacious when used in short-course therapy [6]. The elimination half-life aids in determining the dosing interval necessary to maintain therapeutic serum concentrations, and thus therapeutic urine concentrations of the antimicrobial (Table 5.1). It is reasonable to prolong dosing intervals to once or twice daily for agents with longer half-lives that are able to sustain therapeutic urine concentrations [6]. With respect to length of therapy, in general, the average duration of therapy employed for acute uncomplicated cystitis has shortened over the last 2 decades. Success rates with shortened courses of agents used in acute UTI, combined with the reduced cost and improved patient compliance, have prompted 3-day regimens to replace traditional 5-to 14-day courses of treatment [27].

Drugs in use

Trimethoprim–sulphamethoxazole

TMP–SMX has historically been an effective and inexpensive 'gold standard' in the treatment of acute cystitis and chronic suppressive therapy. The agents have activity against the majority of uropathogens implicated in acute UTI, such as *E. coli*, *S. saprophyticus* and *K. pneumoniae*. Thus, TMP–SMX has been used in the treatment of cystitis since the early 1980s and continues to be used today, although changing microbial resistance patterns are redefining its place in therapy.

TMP–SMX is a synthetic antimicrobial containing a 1:5 ratio of TMP to SMZ. The individual components of TMP–SMX are proposed to act synergistically *in vitro*, but there is no clear evidence that *in vivo* synergy exists [28]. The sulphonamide component inhibits bacterial synthesis of dihydrofolic acid by inhibition of dihydropteroate synthase (*dhps*), whereas trimethoprim blocks the production of tetrahydrofolic acid from dihydrofolic acid by reversible, competitive inhibition of dihydrofolate reductase (*dhfr*). Humans do not possess *dhps*, and human *dhfr* is inherently resistant to TMP, lending selectivity in treating bacterial infection. Theoretically, using these agents together takes advantage of the sequential inhibition of reactions necessary for the bacterial production of nucleic acids and proteins, leading to cell death (Septra Product Info 2000). TMP–SMX has been shown to have synergistic activity against a host of uropathogens, including aerobic Gram-negative rods such as *E. coli* [12].

Resistance has become a more prevalent problem as these agents have been used with increasing frequency over the past 20 years. Chromosomal patterns of change in the structure and regulation of the *dhps* and *dhfr* genes demonstrate the evolutionary adaptation to the presence of TMP–SMX [28]. Plasmid-encoded, drug-resistant *dhfr*s in bacteria are constantly increasing. For example, a highly resistant isolate of *E. coli* exhibited more than 100-fold increased production of chromosomal *dhfr* resulting in an MIC of $> 1\,\mu g/ml$ [28]. In some communities in the USA, resistance now exceeds 20%, and, globally, resistance is also on the rise, with resistance reported to be as high as 60% in Central America and Asia [28].

The pharmacokinetics of TMP–SMX are ideal for treating acute cystitis. The components follow first-order kinetics; they are readily absorbed, attaining high serum concentrations, and are reliably concentrated and excreted to sufficient levels in the urine. Colonization of the vaginal introitus by *E. coli* is a precursor of acute cystitis and may lead to higher rates of recurrence. Thus, effective treatment of the infection may depend partially on successful eradication of uropathogens from the vaginal flora [29]. TMP–SMX was found to remarkably reduce vaginal colonization by *E. coli* during and up to 30 days after therapy [29].

Adverse effects with TMP–SMX are generally mild and include sun sensitivity, nausea and diarrhoea. Since a significant proportion of the TMP component is excreted in the urine, caution should be exercised in patients with renal impairment, and the dose of TMP–SMX should be adjusted to avoid crystalluria. Serious, yet infrequent, haematological adverse effect may occur in patients with glucose-6-phosphate dehydrogenase (G6PD) deficiency. The sulphamethoxazole component of TMP–SMX has been shown to induce haemolytic anaemia in patients with G6PD deficiency, and should be avoided in the subset of patients who are known to be deficient or have a high likelihood of deficiency (persons of Mediterranean descent) [30]. In general, short-course therapy for cystitis tends to be well tolerated.

Trimethoprim

Trimethoprim alone has been a successful agent used in the treatment of acute cystitis, and is an option in patients with allergies to sulphamethoxazole. In some European countries, it is the drug of choice for acute uncomplicated cystitis. Trimethoprim is 50–60% excreted in the urine, with concentrations dependent on renal blood flow and pH since trimethoprim is a weak base. However, the agent reliably concentrates in the urine with levels significantly higher than in the serum. Patients with renal impairment require dose adjustments when the creatinine clearance is below 30 ml/min to avoid crystalluria. Trimethoprim also achieves higher concentrations in vaginal fluids than does SMZ alone [29], although the significance of this finding for suppressive therapy has not been determined.

Beta-lactam antibiotics

Beta-lactam-derived antibiotics are not routinely used as empiric treatment for acute cystitis. The pharmacokinetics of these agents is not favourable for treating cystitis; however, these agents do remain an option for specific patients and in the treatment of enterococcal UTI.

Beta-lactam agents share a common mechanism of action. They disrupt the transpeptidation reaction responsible for cross-linkage of the peptido-glycan structure and interrupt cell wall synthesis. Binding to penicillin-binding proteins (PBPs), which are associated with the cell wall membrane, disrupts the cell wall integrity and leads to bacteriostatic or bactericidal effects, depending on the concentration of the agent and the pathogen. The spectrum of different β-lactams is affected by their relative affinity to PBPs, and resistance is a function of β-lactamase hydrolysis. Several parameters are unfavourable to therapeutic success with these agents. They are rapidly absorbed and attain high serum and urine concentrations. However, the relatively short elimination half-lives of these agents (0.5–2 h) does not allow therapeutic urine concentrations to persist for an adequate amount of time above the uropathogen MIC. This may be a reason why short-course treatment with a β-lactam is less successful than treatment of the same duration with TMP–SMX [31]. Adverse effects with these agents tend to be mild, including diarrhoea, nausea and abdominal cramping. Beta-lactams are disruptive to the vaginal microbial flora and therapy can result in genital itching, vaginitis and occasionally yeast infection [32].

Nitrofurantoin

Nitrofurantoin is an agent that is well established in the treatment of uncomplicated UTIs. It is an agent that has been used for over 20 years in practice, and has recently gained attention again due to low-resistance patterns. Nitrofurantoin is dependent on enzymatic reduction to be active and is unique among antimicrobials due to multiple mechanisms of actions. The agent works by interfering with several bacterial enzyme systems including DNA and RNA synthesis, carbohydrate metabolism and other metabolic enzyme proteins [33]. Multiple mechanisms of action may explain why over time relatively no resistance has developed to this agent. For example, nitrofurantoin is very active against *E. coli* strains, with resistant rates < 2%, as well as other aerobic Gram-negative rods, and Gram-positive organisms [33].

Nitrofurantoin is a weak acid, and is excreted in the kidney via glomerular filtration and tubular secretion, attaining high urinary concentrations that are somewhat dependent upon pH. Since it is a weak acid, the presence of acidic urine increases the amount of drug reabsorbed from the renal tubule; conversely, alkaline urine results in decreased drug reabsorption, and the vast amount is then excreted, leading to higher urine concentrations [33]. It is rapidly metabolized in all bodily tissues, resulting in very low serum concentrations relative to urine, and the inactive metabolite may tint the urine brown. Ingesting the medication with food has been shown to increase the bioavailability by approximately 40%. The elimination half-life in patients with normal renal function is 20 min to 1 h, and approximately half is excreted in the active unchanged form. Patients with renal insufficiency, defined as a creatinine clearance less than 50 ml/min, should avoid nitrofurantoin to prevent crystalluria and the potential adverse effects of drug accumulation.

There are two different formulations of nitrofurantoin, the macrocrystalline form that must be dosed four times daily and a modified monohydrate-macrocrystal form that allows for twice-daily dosing [12]. The macrocrystalline form provides delayed release and slightly decreased bioavailability from the gastrointestinal tract, while the modified monohydrate form delays gastric uptake via a unique gel matrix and allows prolongation of the dosing interval [33]. Side-effects with this agent are most notably nausea and vomiting, which are usually dose-related. The delayed release forms are associated with a lower incidence of nausea compared with the microcrystal form, and taking the medication with food has dual benefits of reducing nausea and improving bioavailability. More serious adverse effects, such as peripheral neuropathy, have been reported infrequently and precipitating factors are unclear. Proposed risk factors include older age, higher dose, extended duration of therapy and renal insufficiency. Major, yet infrequent, adverse events including chronic pulmonary reactions, hepatic injury and hypersensitivity reaction have been reported over the last 30 years [34]. These are most likely to occur in patients on low-dose, chronic suppression therapy (longer than 6 months) [33]. Patients on chronic suppression therapy should have liver function tests performed periodically, although chances of hepatic injury are low. Nitrofurantoin has been shown to cause clinically significant haemolytic anaemia in G6PD-deficient patients, and should be avoided in patients with known or highly suspected G6PD deficiency [30].

Fosfomycin

Fosfomycin is the only single-dose treatment that is Food and Drug Administration (FDA)–approved for treatment UTI of acute uncomplicated cystitis. Fosfomycin is a phosphonic acid bactericidal agent, with a mechanism of action and chemical structure that are unique among the other antimicrobials used to treat acute UTI. Fosfomycin is a bactericidal agent that inhibits peptidoglycan synthesis in the bacterial cell wall [22]. The agent has Gram-positive and Gram-negative microbial coverage, including the most common pathogens of acute cystitis (*E. coli*, *Serratia*, *Klebsiella* and *Enterococcus*). Resistance to fosfomycin is relatively rare in practice, occurring by chromosomal or rarely by plasmid-mediated mechanisms. Cross-resistance between fosfomycin and the antimicrobials commonly used in acute UTI has seldom been reported. Fosfomycin was reformulated recently as an oral tromethamine salt, to improve bioavailability to approximately 34–41% compared with 10% for the calcium salt [22].

The tromethamine form achieves significantly higher serum and urine concentrations as a result of improved solubility and acid stability in the gastrointestinal tract [35]. It is not metabolized *in vivo* and is eliminated 35–40% on average (range 10–60%) by the kidney and up to 20% in the faeces. The elimination half-life is approximately 6 h, with oral administration aiding in increasing the serum elimination half-life. Fosfomycin is filtered and secreted by the kidney, achieving reliable therapeutic concentrations in the urine.

The normal dose given for acute cystitis is a one-time dose of 3 g orally as a sachet. The sachet is an orange-flavoured product that must be mixed with 4 oz of water and ingested immediately. Therapeutic urinary concentrations occur within 4 h, achieving levels $> 128\,\mu g/ml$, which are above the MIC of most organisms, and generally persist for 24–48 h [22]. Adverse effects of the single-dose treatment include nausea, diarrhoea, headache and changes in the vaginal flora.

Fluoroquinolones

Fluoroquinolones have emerged as efficacious, alternative first-line agents for the empiric treatment of acute UTI, especially in the setting of high TMP–SMX resistance levels. In the USA, uropathogen resistance to these agents has remained low. However, in Europe, as previously mentioned, resistance to fluoroquinolones has been rising, and their place in empiric treatment under these circumstances is less clear.

There are numerous fluoroquinolones that have been studied in the treatment of acute UTI, dating back over 40 years to the first quinolone, nalidixic acid [36]. Agents in this class differ not only in their antimicrobial spectrum, but also in their specific pharmacokinetic and pharmacodynamic properties. Renal excretion varies among the available agents. Agents with high renal excretion ($\geqslant 75\%$) include gatifloxacin, levofloxacin, lomefloxacin and ofloxacin. Ciprofloxacin and fleroxacin have intermediate rates of renal excretion (40–74%) and agents with a low rate of renal excretion (<40%) include trovafloxacin, gemifloxacin, moxifloxacin and norfloxacin. [37]. Levofloxacin, moxifloxacin, gatifloxacin and ofloxacin all possess excellent oral bioavailability, penetrate well into tissues and body fluids and have extended elimination half-lives that allows for once-daily dosing in patients without renal impairment [38]. Levofloxacin and gatifloxacin are mainly excreted unchanged in the urine, whereas moxifloxacin undergoes hepatic metabolism but still achieves acceptable urinary concentrations [38].

Since the fluoroquinolones exhibit concentration-dependent killing, the concentration achieved at the site of infection will predict the efficacy of these agents. Agents that are not excreted to an intermediate or high degree in the urine do not reliably achieve concentrations high enough to be effective in the treatment of acute UTI. The antimicrobial spectrum must also be taken into account. In general, fluoroquinolones have excellent Gram-negative activity. The Gram-positive spectrum improves with each subsequent generation, with second-generation agents such as ciprofloxacin having the least activity, third-generation agents such as gatifloxacin and moxifloxacin having good Gram-positive activity and fourth-generation agents such as trovafloxacin having good Gram-positive as well as anaerobic activity. Recent *in vitro* studies comparing MIC values among uropathogens have found that a bimodal distribution exists for all fluoroquinolones, with a significant number of staphylococcal and enterococcal strains 'resistant' to ciprofloxacin and ofloxacin. In these studies, the MICs of gatifloxacin and moxifloxacin against Gram-positive cocci were found to be 2–3 dilutions lower than ciprofloxacin and ofloxacin [10]. It is not clear how these data will translate into clinical outcomes, especially in acute uncomplicated cystitis, which is predominantly a Gram-negative infection. The ideal fluoroquinolones for treatment of acute uncomplicated cystitis have intermediate or high renal excretion and are highly active against Enterobacteriaceae.

Clinical trials

There are numerous clinical studies aimed at identifying either the optimal drug, duration or dosing for treatment of acute uncomplicated cystitis. However, in a recent attempt to identify randomized treatment trials that appropriately defined acute uncomplicated cystitis and prospectively evaluated bacteriological response rates, thousands of abstracts were reviewed and only 337 studies met criteria for closer evaluation. Of these, only 76 met criteria for contribution to the IDSA guideline development. Thus, one must be careful about basing therapeutic choices on the results of any single study. The aggregate results of select studies evaluating optimal treatment durations and antimicrobial agents are summarized below.

Duration of treatment

Treatment duration of acute uncomplicated cystitis has evolved from single- to multiple-dose therapy based on several clinical studies evaluating efficacy and side-effects of varying durations of treatment. In general, studies have found that single-dose therapy is not as efficacious as longer-course regimens. The one exception to this rule is when fosfomycin is used for treatment of acute uncomplicated cystitis, since it is only approved for single-dose therapy. In a subanalysis of a study involving both men and women, treatment of UTI in women with 2 or 3 days of fosfomycin 3 g daily did not result in higher efficacy as compared with a single 3-g dose [39]. Diarrhoea was more frequent in patients treated with multiple doses. Thus, a single-dose of fosfomycin is preferred when it is used for treatment of acute uncomplicated cystitis.

Trials comparing single-dose TMP–SMX therapy to ⩾7 day day courses of therapy demonstrated that longer therapy was significantly more effective in eradicating initial bacteriuria, with average rates of 87% with single-dose therapy and 94% with longer therapy. In addition, rates of recurrence were not significantly different. However, the benefit of longer therapy was maximized at 3 days; after this time, the rate of side-effects increases without an appreciable increase in cure rates. Meta-analysis of two trials comparing 3-day treatment with TMP–SMX to longer duration found that eradication rates were equivalent (93–94%) with shorter therapy and the incidence of adverse effects was significantly lower (18% vs 30% with longer course) [1]. Thus, when TMP–SMX is used for treatment of acute uncomplicated cystitis, a 3-day dosing regimen is considered optimal. Similarly, meta-analyses of studies of trimethoprim alone have found that single-dose therapy is less effective than multiple-day therapy (83% vs 93% eradication rates). Adverse events also increase with longer than 3 days of therapy [1].

The optimal duration of treatment with nitrofurantoin is somewhat uncertain due to a lack of well-designed clinical trials. A trial comparing single-dose treatment with 10 days of treatment was of insufficient power to detect a difference in eradication rate; however, short-term therapy had significantly lower rates of adverse effects [40]. Similarly, most other studies comparing short-course regimens with 7-day therapy have not been adequately powered to demonstrate a difference in therapeutic outcomes, and larger, controlled trials with this drug are needed. Therefore, based on limited evidence, most experts agree that a 3-day treatment regimen of nitrofurantoin is likely of insufficient duration, and 7-day therapy is necessary to achieve eradication rates comparable with TMP–SMX.

Trials of single-dose versus longer-duration therapy with β-lactams demonstrate that single-dose treatment is significantly less effective in eradicating uropathogens, although the incidence of side-effects is reduced [1]. Clinical trials have shown 3-day treatment with β-lactam to be less efficacious than 5 days or more of treatment [31]. Thus, when these agents are used as treatment options in acute cystitis, duration of treatment should be at least 5–7 days.

Several clinical trials have been done to determine the ideal treatment duration for fluoroquinolones. The IDSA reports four studies of norfloxacin, ciprofloxacin and fleroxacin comparing single-dose with longer-duration durations [1]. Individually, it was shown that all three agents had significantly lower eradication rates with single-dose therapy than with longer durations. Two smaller studies demonstrated high rates of bacterial eradication with single-dose therapy of ofloxacin and pefloxacin [41,42]. Studies comparing 3-day treatment with longer durations (5 or 7 days) of various quinolones have not shown a therapeutic benefit in terms of bacterial eradication [43–45]. Thus, a 3-day treatment regimen is optimal when using a fluoroquinolone for the treatment of acute uncomplicated cystitis.

Antimicrobial efficacy

Since TMP–SMX is the drug of choice and the most well studied antimicrobial for acute uncomplicated cystitis, studies comparing other antimicrobials with TMP–SMX are of greatest interest and use. Studies comparing antimicrobial agents within the same class but of different spectrum or pharmacokinetics are also instructive. The main outcome of interest evaluated in most of these studies is bacterial eradication, although rates of adverse effects and recurrence are also important.

Trimethoprim alone is considered to be equivalent in efficacy to TMP–SMX by most practitioners. Meta-analysis of two trials comparing 7-day regimens of trimethoprim alone to TMP–SMX demonstrated that eradication of initial bacteriuria and adverse effect rates were equivalent [46,47]. Interestingly, the eradication rates in these studies were 88% for each drug, somewhat lower than the 93% demonstrated in 3-day studies of TMP–SMX and 5-day studies of trimethoprim.

In general, most β-lactams are less effective than TMP–SMX, TMP alone or fluoroquinolones in eradicating initial bacteriuria, with rates typically approximately 10% lower with amoxicillin compared with TMP–SMX [1]. Beta-lactams may also predispose patients to higher rates of recurrence. When compared with TMP–SMX in a 3-day treatment regimen, cefadroxil and amoxicillin had the least effect on *E. coli* eradication in vaginal fluids, possible explaining the poorer outcomes with these latter drugs [31]. These agents have a place in therapy when pregnancy is suspected in a patient, and should be used as first-line therapy in this situation. Beta-lactams remain a good agent to use for enterococcal UTI, and most strains causing acute uncomplicated cystitis have been reported to be highly susceptible.

A 3-day regimen of nitrofurantoin macrocrystal (given four times daily) has been directly compared with a 3-day regimen of TMP–SMX in one study. Despite a small sample size, it demonstrated a statistically significant lower rate of initial bacterial eradication in the nitrofurantoin arm (84%) versus the TMP–SMX arm (98%) [31]. In another study comparing 7-day regimens of nitrofurantoin monohydrate crystal with TMP–SMX and TMP, similar initial bacterial eradication rates were achieved (77–83%), although the power to show a statistical difference between the regimens was limited by the sample size [46]. In addition, the overall rates of eradication in this study were lower than expected from other studies. Thus, the rate of bacterial cure to be expected with a 7-day course of nitrofurantoin is not very well defined, but probably lies between 85% and 95%.

There are several trials evaluating fosfomycin single-dose treatment for acute uncomplicated cystitis, and many of these show equal eradication rates between fosfomycin and agents such as trimethoprim, TMP–SMX, nitrofurantoin and some fluoroquinolones. However, many of these studies are not powered to actually show a statistically significant difference in eradication, even in meta-analyses [1]. A meta-analysis of two trials comparing fosfomycin single-dose treatment and norfloxacin 5- or 7-day treatment did demonstrate a significantly higher incidence of adverse effects with the former agent [1,48,49]. In general, rates of eradication with this drug should be expected to fall in the range of 77–82%, much lower than those expected with TMP–SMX, fluoroquinolones and even nitrofurantoin. Cost may also be a significant factor in treatment determination, as this agent is generally 10-fold more expensive than TMP–SMX.

The fluoroquinolones are, in general, considered to be the only class of drug equal in efficacy to TMP–SMX in a 3-day regimen for treatment of acute uncomplicated cystitis. Ofloxacin is the fluoroquinolone that is best studied in comparison with TMP–SMX. In three trials, ofloxacin and TMP–SMX given for 3 or more days of therapy were equivalent in initial bacterial eradication rates (95–96%), recurrence rates (8–9%) and adverse effects

(23–25%) [1]. A randomized trial of ciprofloxacin, ofloxacin and TMP–SMX also demonstrated similar cure rates (93–97%) [8], as did a trial of nitrofurantoin and TMP–SMX (7-day regimens) compared with 3 days of low-dose ciprofloxacin [50]. There have been many studies comparing various fluoroquinolones, especially some of the newer broader-spectrum agents with more traditional fluoroquinolones such as ciprofloxacin and levofloxacin. Variation in dosing, duration and outcome ascertainment makes it difficult to directly compare these studies. However, most show equivalence in eradication between older and newer fluoroquinolones. Clinical trials of agents with longer half-lives, pefloxacin and rufloxacin, have also demonstrated equivalence in bacterial eradication with TMP–SMX [42,51], although adverse events may be higher with the newer agents. A recently published trial compared single-dose gatifloxacin with 3-day courses of either gatifloxacin or ciprofloxacin [52]. Using a 97.5% confidence interval, no differences were found between single-dose gatifloxacin and 3-day treatment with gatifloxacin or ciprofloxacin. Thus, the current standard of practice is to use a 3-day regimen of a fluoroquinolone when TMP–SMX cannot be used. Traditional quinolones such as ciprofloxacin and levofloxacin are the most widely used. Emerging clinical trials with newer fluoroquinolones testing single-dose therapy may change standard practice in the future, but results need to be validated in large, controlled trials.

Future developments

Since antimicrobial resistance will continue to evolve and complicate the treatment of acute uncomplicated cystitis, much research is aimed at identifying novel non-antimicrobial-based methods of prevention. Use of cranberry juice or solids for prevention of UTI is the strategy with the strongest body of evidence published to date [53,54]. As *in vitro* studies have demonstrated, cranberry products contain proanthocyanadins, compounds that competitively inhibit the attachment of *E. coli* to uroepithelial cells. In terms of clinical trials, Avorn *et al.* demonstrated that the ingestion of cranberry juice decreased the incidence of asymptomatic bacteriuria and pyuria in a group of elderly institutionalized women. Importantly, the incidence of symptomatic urinary infections was not significantly reduced. More recent randomized controlled studies of younger women have demonstrated a reduction in the rate of recurrent UTIs with ingestion of cranberry–lingonberry juice and with use of a solid cranberry product [55,56]. Thus, there is a fair amount of evidence supporting the use of cranberry products for prevention of acute cystitis; however, there is no published literature supporting the use of cranberry products for the treatment of acute cystitis. In addition, the optimal dosing, route and formulation of cranberry and the expected duration and durability of efficacy in the prevention of acute uncomplicated cystitis have not been elucidated.

Another strategy being studied for prevention of UTI involves development of a lactobacillus probiotic to replenish the normal vaginal flora and reduce colonization with uropathogens, thus reducing subsequent rates of UTI. This has been effective in small non-randomized trials but requires validation in a placebo-controlled randomized study. Finally, anti-adhesin-based vaccines and topically applied carbohydrates that inhibit bacterial attachment are other strategies for preventing UTI that may be feasible in the near future.

Conclusion

The therapy of acute cystitis has become more complex due to changing antimicrobial susceptibility patterns. However, there are several drugs with favourable pharmacokinetic properties that are still active against the predominant uropathogens causing acute uncomplicated cystitis. The choice of antimicrobial should involve knowledge of these pharmacokinetic properties and of local susceptibility patterns and consideration of patient variables such as the likelihood of having a resistant organism, history of drug allergy and severity of symptoms. With these issues in mind, empiric antimicrobial therapy for acute uncomplicated cystitis can continue to be a safe and effective management approach, even in the setting of evolving antimicrobial resistance.

References

1   Warren JW, Abrutyn E, Hebel JR, Johnson JR, Schaeffer AJ, Stamm WE. Guidelines for antimicrobial treatment of uncomplicated acute bacterial cystitis and acute pyelonephritis in women. Infectious Diseases Society of America (IDSA). *Clin Infect Dis* 1999; **29**(4): 745–58.

2   Kunin CM. Urinary tract infections in females. *Clin Infect Dis* 1994; **18**(1): 1–10, quiz 11–12.

3   Le TP, Miller LG. Empirical therapy for uncomplicated urinary tract infections in an era of increasing antimicrobial resistance: a decision and cost analysis. *Clin Infect Dis* 2001; **33**(5): 615–21.

4   Foxman B. Epidemiology of urinary tract infections: incidence, morbidity, and economic costs. *Am J Med* 2002; **113**(Suppl. 1A): 5S–13S.

5   Echols RM, Tosiello RL, Haverstock DC, Tice AD. Demographic, clinical, and treatment parameters influencing the outcome of acute cystitis. *Clin Infect Dis* 1999; **29**(1): 113–19.

6   Hooton TM, Stamm WE. Diagnosis and treatment of uncomplicated urinary tract infection. *Infect Dis Clin North Am* 1997; **11**(3): 551–81.

7   Brown PD. Antibiotic selection for urinary tract infection: new microbiologic considerations. *Curr Infect Dis Rep* 1999; **1**(4): 384–8.

8   McCarty JM, Richard G, Huck W, Tucker RM, Tosiello RL, Shan M *et al.* A randomized trial of short-course ciprofloxacin, ofloxacin, or trimethoprim/sulfamethoxazole for the treatment of acute urinary tract infection in women. Ciprofloxacin Urinary Tract Infection Group. *Am J Med* 1999; **106**(3): 292–9.

9   Gupta K, Hooton TM, Stamm WE. Increasing antimicrobial resistance and the management of uncomplicated community-acquired urinary tract infections. *Ann Intern Med* 2001; **135**(1): 41–50.

10   Naber KG, Hollauer K, Kirchbauer D, Witte W. In vitro activity of gatifloxacin compared with gemifloxacin, moxifloxacin, trovafloxacin, ciprofloxacin and ofloxacin against uropathogens cultured from patients with complicated urinary tract infections. *Int J Antimicrob Agents* 2000; **16**(3): 239–43.

11   Raz R, Chazan B, Kennes Y, Colodner R, Rottensterich E, Dan M *et al.* Empiric use of trimethoprim-sulfamethoxazole (TMP-SMX) in the treatment of women with uncomplicated urinary tract infections, in a geographical area with a high prevalence of TMP-SMX-resistant uropathogens. *Clin Infect Dis* 2002; **34**(9): 1165–9.

12   Gupta K, Sahm DF, Mayfield D, Stamm WE. Antimicrobial resistance among uropathogens that cause community-acquired urinary tract infections in women: a nationwide analysis. *Clin Infect Dis* 2001; **33**(1): 89–94.

13   Fluit AC, Jones ME, Schmitz FJ, Acar J, Gupta R, Verhoef J. Antimicrobial resistance among urinary tract infection (UTI) isolates in Europe: results from the SENTRY Antimicrobial Surveillance Program 1997. *Antonie Van Leeuwenhoek* 2000; **77**(2): 147–52.

14   Zhanel GG, Karlowsky JA, Harding GK, Carrie A, Mazzulli T, Low DE *et al.* A Canadian national surveillance study of urinary tract isolates from outpatients: comparison of the activities of trimethoprim-sulfamethoxazole, ampicillin, mecillinam, nitrofurantoin, and ciprofloxacin. The Canadian Urinary Isolate Study Group. *Antimicrob Agents Chemother* 2000; **44**(4): 1089–92.

15   Amsden GW, Duran JM. Interpretation of antibacterial susceptibility reports: in vitro versus clinical break-points. *Drugs* 2001; **61**(2): 163–6.

16   Sommers DK. Pharmacological principles in the treatment of urinary tract infections. *S Afr Med J* 1983; **64**(4): 123–6.

17   Arancibia A, Guttmann J, Gonzalez G, Gonzalez C. Absorption and disposition kinetics of amoxicillin in normal human subjects. *Antimicrob Agents Chemother* 1980; **17**(2): 199–202.

18   Cole M, Ridley B. Absence of bioactive metabolites of ampicillin and amoxycillin in man. *J Antimicrob Chemother* 1978; **4**(6): 580–2.

19   Nightingale CH, Greene DS, Quintiliani R. Pharmacokinetics and clinical use of cephalosporin antibiotics. *J Pharm Sci* 1975; **64**(12): 1899–926.

20   Lubasch A, Keller I, Borner K, Koeppe P, Lode H. Comparative pharmacokinetics of ciprofloxacin, gatifloxacin, grepafloxacin, levofloxacin, trovafloxacin, and moxifloxacin after single oral administration in healthy volunteers. *Antimicrob Agents Chemother* 2000; **44**(10): 2600–603.

21   Vance-Bryan K, Guay DR, Rotschafer JC. Clinical pharmacokinetics of ciprofloxacin. *Clin Pharmacokinet* 1990; **19**(6): 434–61.

22   Patel SS, Balfour JA, Bryson HM. Fosfomycin tromethamine. A review of its antibacterial activity, pharmacokinetic properties and therapeutic efficacy as a single-dose oral treatment for acute uncomplicated lower urinary tract infections. *Drugs* 1997; **53**(4): 637–56.

23   Naber CK, Hammer M, Kinzig-Schippers M, Sauber C, Sorgel F, Bygate EA *et al.* Urinary excretion and bactericidal activities of gemifloxacin and ofloxacin after a single oral dose in healthy volunteers. *Antimicrob Agents Chemother* 2001; **45**(12): 3524–30.

24 Mannisto P. The effect of crystal size, gastric content and emptying rate on the absorption of nitrofurantoin in healthy human volunteers. *Int J Clin Pharmacol Biopharm* 1978; **16**(5): 223–8.

25 Patel RB, Welling PG. Clinical pharmacokinetics of co-trimoxazole (trimethoprim-sulphamethoxazole). *Clin Pharmacokinet* 1980; **5**(5): 405–23.

26 Kasanen A, Anttila M, Elfving R, Kahela P, Saarimaa H, Sundquist H *et al.* Trimethoprim. Pharmacology, antimicrobial activity and clinical use in urinary tract infections. *Ann Clin Res* 1978; **10**(Suppl. 22): 1–39.

27 Tice AD. Short-course therapy of acute cystitis: a brief review of therapeutic strategies. *J Antimicrob Chemother* 1999; **43**(Suppl. A): 85–93.

28 Huovinen P, Sundstrom L, Swedberg G, Skold O. Trimethoprim and sulfonamide resistance. *Antimicrob Agents Chemother* 1995; **39**(2): 279–89.

29 Tartaglione TA, Johnson CR, Brust P, Opheim K, Hooton TM, Stamm WE. Pharmacodynamic evaluation of ofloxacin and trimethoprim-sulfamethoxazole in vaginal fluid of women treated for acute cystitis. *Antimicrob Agents Chemother* 1988; **32**(11): 1640–43.

30 Beutler E. G6PD deficiency. *Blood* 1994; **84**(11): 3613–36.

31 Hooton TM, Winter C, Tiu F, Stamm WE. Randomized comparative trial and cost analysis of 3-day antimicrobial regimens for treatment of acute cystitis in women. *JAMA* 1995; **273**(1): 41–5.

32 Reeves DS. A perspective on the safety of antibacterials used to treat urinary tract infections. *J Antimicrob Chemother* 1994; **33**(Suppl. A): 111–20.

33 Guay DR. An update on the role of nitrofurans in the management of urinary tract infections. *Drugs* 2001; **61**(3): 353–64.

34 D'Arcy PF. Nitrofurantoin. *Drug Intell Clin Pharm* 1985; **19**(7–8): 540–47.

35 Reeves DS. Fosfomycin trometamol. *J Antimicrob Chemother* 1994; **34**(6): 853–8.

36 Tolkoff-Rubin NE, Rubin RH. Ciprofloxacin in management of urinary tract infection. *Urology* 1988; **31**(4): 359–67.

37 Naber KG. Which fluoroquinolones are suitable for the treatment of urinary tract infections? *Int J Antimicrob Agents* 2001; **17**(4): 331–41.

38 Rodvold KA, Neuhauser M. Pharmacokinetics and pharmacodynamics of fluoroquinolones. *Pharmacotherapy* 2001; **21** (10 Pt 2): 233S–52S.

39 Moroni M. Monuril in lower uncomplicated urinary tract infections in adults. *Eur Urol* 1987; **13**(Suppl. 1): 101–104.

40 Gossius G, Vorland L. A randomised comparison of single-dose vs. three-day and ten-day therapy with trimethoprim-sulfamethoxazole for acute cystitis in women. *Scand J Infect Dis* 1984; **16**(4): 373–9.

41 Hooton TM, Johnson C, Winter C, Kuwamura L, Rogers ME, Roberts PL *et al.* Single-dose and three-day regimens of ofloxacin versus trimethoprim-sulfamethoxazole for acute cystitis in women. *Antimicrob Agents Chemother* 1991; **35**(7): 1479–83.

42 Leelarasamee A, Leelarasamee I. Comparative efficacies of oral pefloxacin in uncomplicated cystitis. Single dose or 3-day therapy. *Drugs* 1995; **49**(Suppl. 2): 365–7.

43 Double-blind comparison of 3-day versus 7-day treatment with norfloxacin in symptomatic urinary tract infections. The Inter-Nordic Urinary Tract Infection Study Group. *Scand J Infect Dis* 1988; **20**(6): 619–24.

44 Iravani A, Tice AD, McCarty J, Sikes DH, Nolen T, Gallis HA *et al.* Short-course ciprofloxacin treatment of acute uncomplicated urinary tract infection in women. The minimum effective dose. The Urinary Tract Infection Study Group [corrected]. *Arch Intern Med* 1995; **155**(5): 485–94.

45 Neringer R, Forsgren A, Hansson C, Ode B. Lomefloxacin versus norfloxacin in the treatment of uncomplicated urinary tract infections: three-day versus seven-day treatment. The South Swedish Lolex Study Group. *Scand J Infect Dis* 1992; **24**(6): 773–80.

46 Spencer RC, Moseley DJ, Greensmith MJ. Nitrofurantoin modified release versus trimethoprim or co-trimoxazole in the treatment of uncomplicated urinary tract infection in general practice. *J Antimicrob Chemother* 1994; **33**(Suppl. A): 121–9.

47 Comparison of trimethoprim at three dosage levels with co-trimoxazole in the treatment of acute symptomatic urinary tract infection in general practice. *J Antimicrob Chemother* 1981; **7**(2): 179–83.

48 Boerema JB, Willems FT. Fosfomycin trometamol in a single dose versus norfloxacin for seven days in the treatment of uncomplicated urinary infections in general practice. *Infection* 1990; **18**(Suppl. 2): S80–88.

49 de Jong Z, Pontonnier F, Plante P. Single-dose fosfomycin trometamol (Monuril) versus multiple-dose norfloxacin: results of a multicenter study in females with uncomplicated lower urinary tract infections. *Urol Int* 1991; **46**(4): 344–8.

50 Iravani A, Klimberg I, Briefer C, Munera C, Kowalsky SF, Echols RM. A trial comparing low-dose, short-course ciprofloxacin and standard 7 day therapy with co-trimoxazole or nitrofurantoin in the treatment of uncomplicated urinary tract infection. *J Antimicrob Chemother* 1999; **43**(Suppl. A): 67–75.

51 Jardin A, Cesana M. Randomized, double-blind comparison of single-dose regimens of rufloxacin and pefloxacin for acute uncomplicated cystitis in women. French Multicenter Urinary Tract Infection-Rufloxacin Group. *Antimicrob Agents Chemother* 1995; **39**(1): 215–20.

52 Richard GA, Mathew CP, Kirstein JM, Orchard D, Yang JY. Single-dose fluoroquinolone therapy of acute uncomplicated urinary tract infection in women: results from a randomized, double-blind, multicenter trial comparing single-dose to 3-day fluoroquinolone regimens. *Urology* 2002; **59**(3): 334–9.

53 Howell AB, Foxman B. Cranberry juice and adhesion of antibiotic-resistant uropathogens. *JAMA* 2002; **287**(23): 3082–3.

54 Howell AB, Vorsa N, Der Marderosian A, Foo LY. Inhibition of the adherence of P-fimbriated Escherichia coli to uroepithelial-cell surfaces by proanthocyanidin extracts from cranberries. *N Engl J Med* 1998; **339**(15): 1085–6.

55 Stothers L. A randomized trial to evaluate effectiveness and cost effectiveness of naturopathic cranberry products as prophylaxis against urinary tract infection in women. *Can J Urol* 2002; **9**(3): 1558–62.

56 Kontiokari T, Sundqvist K, Nuutinen M, Pokka T, Koskela M, Uhari M. Randomised trial of cranberry-lingonberry juice and Lactobacillus GG drink for the prevention of urinary tract infections in women. *BMJ* 2001; **322**(7302): 1571.

6: New Concepts in Antimicrobial Treatment for Complicated Urinary Tract Infections: Single Daily Aminoglycoside Dosing and 'Switch' Therapy

Richard A. Santucci & John N. Krieger

Introduction

This chapter presents two 'new' approaches to treatment of patients with complicated urinary tract infections (UTIs): once-daily therapy with aminoglycosides (AGs) and oral 'switch' therapy. The information is important because it may help us improve treatment of patients most commonly seen in urology. We begin by defining complicated UTI, then we briefly outline the theoretical basis of the two treatment strategies that have proven worthy of adding to your armamentarium. We emphasize the clinically relevant aspects of the therapies and make clear, specific recommendations.

Complicated urinary tract infection

Complicated UTIs are a heterogeneous group of diseases defined as infection with compromising factors that may be anatomical, structural, functional or in patients with underlying disease [1]. Anatomical abnormalities include aberrations that cause retention of urine, such as ureteropelvic junction obstruction, pelvic kidney, ureteral stricture, ureterocele, cystocele, bladder diverticuli, prostatic obstruction and urethral stricture. Nonobstructing anatomical abnormalities may also compromise host defense against UTI, for example polycystic kidneys, stones, transplant kidneys, vesicoureteral reflux, fistulae and pregnancy. Other anatomical abnormalities that complicate UTI include ureteral stents, bladder catheters, percutaneous nephrostomy tubes, kidney stones and tumours. Functional alterations that compromise normal host defenses against UTI include neurological disorders that interfere with voiding and renal insufficiency that impairs urinary excretion of antimicrobials. Compromising medical conditions that place the patient in the complicated UTI group include extreme age, sickle cell disease, diabetes, cancer, liver disease, immunosuppression, neutropenia and HIV infection [2]. The importance of such factors is illustrated by studies suggesting that elderly patients with UTI may have up to a 26% incidence of septic shock, and are clearly at higher risk for prolonged illness and even death [3]. Finally, infections occurring after genitourinary surgery are often complicated. Relative resistance to treatment, a tendency to make the patient more ill than simple UTI and relapse of infection by the same strain are hallmarks of 'complicated' UTI.

Patients with complicated UTI also have a tendency towards resistant organisms and multiple organisms [4]. These characteristics make complicated UTIs difficult to treat. Often, complicating factors must also be addressed, and this treatment often determines the outcome for the patient. Patients with complicated UTI are more likely to suffer sequelae and renal damage than those without compromising factors [5].

This chapter emphasizes the issues surrounding antimicrobial treatment of complicated UTI. We acknowledge that there is much more to effective treatment of these patients, most of it a part of basic, competent urologic care. Discussion of imaging to determine anatomical abnormalities, drainage of abscesses, need to ensure adequate drainage of the urinary tract and the changing of catheters or stents that may be coated with microbial 'biofilm' are beyond the scope of this chapter. We have chosen to emphasize some new concepts in antimicrobial treatment.

Once-daily AG therapy for complicated UTIs

Since their development in the 1940s the AGs have been mainstays of antimicrobial therapy, especially in complicated UTIs. Gentamicin, the most frequently used AG, was discovered in 1963 and remains the most widely used AG in most hospitals in the USA and Britain [6,7], despite the availability of other drugs including amikacin, netilmicin, kanamycin, tobramicin and other AGs available outside the USA (e.g. dibekacin, paromomycin and isepamicin).

Gentamicin remains popular because it is effective. Antimicrobial resistance is uncommon, and when it occurs, resistance can often be overcome by the addition of β-lactam antibiotics, such as penicillins or cephalosporins [8]. Gentamicin is also inexpensive and familiar, both in its dosing and side-effects. Despite concerns about toxicity and the inconvenience of having to monitor serum levels, gentamicin often represents the antimicrobial of choice for 'serious' Gram-negative infections [9,10], or as an important component of wide-spectrum empiric coverage for extremely ill patients [11].

Standards for gentamicin have been revolutionized with two relatively simple dosing modifications. These changes result in better efficacy, improved safety, more convenience and lower costs (sometimes dramatically). The first modification is single daily dosing (SDD), where gentamicin (or another AG) is given in infrequent large doses, such as 5 mg/kg of gentamicin once a day. The second modification is 'switch' therapy, where an initial dose of AG is followed immediately by oral antimicrobials. The plan is to manage the infection on an outpatient basis, often after as few as one intravenous (IV) AG dose.

Single daily dosing of AGs

Definition

The concept of SDD is not new. However, it is gaining wide clinical acceptance only now. SDD was first proposed in 1974 [12] as a way to decrease toxicity and costs of gentamicin while increasing convenience. Despite numerous studies, clinical acceptance of SDD has been slow, perhaps owing to its somewhat contrary approach of decreasing toxicity by amassing the toxic substance (the AG) into a larger dose than is customary.

SDD is also known as 'extended interval', 'once-daily', and 'skip' dosing. The theory is that a single large dose results in a higher peak and lower trough levels that achieve more effective microbial killing while reducing toxicity. SDD is given as a single IV gentamicin dose of 5–7 mg/kg every 24 h. More than 60 clinical studies [12–40] and a large number of animal studies [20,41–48] document that SDD provides equal or superior efficacy to standard dosing. Further, the data suggest that SDD is safer and less expensive than traditional multiple daily dosing regimens [8,10,11,13,27, 49–64]. The rationale for SDD hinges on the potential to achieve a lower rate of antimicrobial resistance, better bacterial killing, less toxicity, more convenience and lower costs than classical dosing regimens (Table 6.1). SDD has become standard in many medical centres [65], including at least 40% of teaching hospitals worldwide [13]. Some early critics cited concerns that studies of adequate statistical power have not been conducted, and that there are inadequate data to assess toxicity [66,67]. These criticisms become less concerning as studies of SDD continue to appear in the literature.

Rationale for SDD in complicated UTIs

In 1974 the first SDD report reasoned that infrequent AG dosing would be ideal for patients with UTI because AGs are eliminated almost entirely by the kidneys with prolonged high urinary levels [12]. Subsequent studies confirmed the efficacy of SDD for treating complicated UTIs and pyelonephritis [17,18,24,27,31,37,68,69]. As with other strategies, patients with concomitant urinary tract obstruction have lower clinical and bacteriological responses to SDD. Thus, careful monitoring of urine cultures during

Table 6.1 Potential benefits of gentamicin single daily dosing (SDD)

Properties of SDD	Resulting benefits
Simplified dosing calculations	Fewer dosing errors, increased ease of use
Guaranteed high peak serum concentrations	Improved antimicrobial and clinical efficacy
Improved post-antibiotic effect	Improved antimicrobial killing
High concentrations overwhelm 'killer enzymes' that cause resistance	Improved antimicrobial killing, less resistance
Less 'adaptive resistance'	Improved antimicrobial killing, less resistance
Improved drug delivery to abscesses, bronchi	Improved antimicrobial killing
Less (or equal) nephrotoxicity	Less renal damage
Less (or equal) ototoxicity	Less ear damage
Simple monitoring	Less expense, more accurate serum levels
Less frequent need to administer drug	Less expense, more convenience, simpler home-based therapy

treatment is mandatory [68]. Because poorly functioning kidneys excrete significantly less AG [27], special attention is also required in patients with diseased kidneys, including those with unilateral obstructive or reflux nephropathy. However, there is no published evidence that such patients have lower cure rates. The rationale for SDD may be summarized as providing three clinical advantages: decreased antimicrobial resistance, improved bacterial killing and decreased patient toxicity. In addition, SDD reduces costs and increases convenience for patient and caregiver.

DECREASED ANTIMICROBIAL RESISTANCE AND IMPROVED KILLING

First, SDD is theoretically more potent because higher serum drug concentrations are obtained than with standard dosing. SDD improves bacterial elimination because these high serum levels directly counter antimicrobial resistance strategies. This is because the long time interval between doses ensures that so-called 'adaptive resistance' reverts back to a non-resistant state [60,70]. (Adaptive resistance is a rapidly developing but reversible temporary resistance that happens after the first exposure to AG, but rapidly reverts in a few hours [71].) Also, the high serum levels can be expected to overwhelm bacterial AG-inactivating enzymes (review [11]).

SDD also ensures a potent 'first pass effect', efficiently killing a large percentage of bacteria upon first contact (review [11]). Additionally, SDD achieves a longer 'post-antibiotic effect' than 8-h doses (review [54,60,62]).

(This post-antibiotic effect is a special consequence of AGs that results in several extra hours of antimicrobial activity even at serum levels far below the minimum inhibitory concentration [52,72].) Lastly, SDD improves tissue penetration, especially in those areas that take up drugs poorly [73]. In combination, these benefits of SDD translate into improved clinical outcomes [73,74].

LESS TOXICITY

Many clinicians find it difficult to conceive that gentamicin could be less toxic when given in larger boluses. The reason that SDD is less toxic is that AG uptake into the kidney [21] and ear [75] are both saturable processes (review [54]). When low gentamicin doses are administered, these organs become fully saturated; but, when high doses are administered these organs are no more saturated than with lower doses. The result is that with SDD, critical target organs are saturated only once every 24 h. With standard multiple daily doses, target organs are saturated three times every 24 h. Paradoxically, infrequent large doses prove less toxic than frequent small doses. In animal studies this principle holds true: the most toxic AG dosing regimens involve continuous drug infusion [20].

Nephrotoxicity

Although acute renal damage is difficult to assess, animal [20,41,62,76,77] and clinical [10,16,21,53,56,78–81] studies suggest that SDD has the same or a better nephrotoxicity safety profile than more frequent dosing. In adults [17,25,30,31,82–85], non-neutropenic children [36,78,86] and neutropenic children [18], studies report no differences in serum creatinine between SDD and standard multiple daily dosing regimens. Some studies even showed that the incidence [56,81] and severity [87] of nephrotoxicity decrease with SDD. When clinical nephrotoxicity is detected with SDD, its onset is 3 days later than nephrotoxicity observed with multiple daily dosing [81]. This advantage is so significant that patients with early nephrotoxicity on standard dosing regimens improved after switching to SDD [16]. After treatment of over 2000 patients with SDD at one centre, the nephrotoxicity rate was only 1% [33].

Toxicity is most associated with prolonged gentamicin therapy, even when SDD is used (Table 6.2). In one large series, the rate of nephrotoxicity was 2% after 6 days and 3.3% after 11 days of treatment [33]. Age > 61 years also slightly increases the risk of nephrotoxicity with SDD, from 1% to 1.6%. Although nephrotoxicity with SDD is rare, special care must be taken in older patients and in those who require prolonged therapy.

Table 6.2 Toxicities associated with AG therapy

Toxicity	Reported rate (%)	Risk factors
Nephrotoxicity	1–55	Other nephrotoxic drugs [58]
		Hydrocortisone/ACE inhibitors/ hypercalcemia
		Dosing frequency (MDD > SDD) [54]
		Prolonged duration of therapy > 9 days [8]
		Pre-existing renal disease [58]
		Recent prior AG use [58]
		Severity of concomitant disease
		AG used (gentamicin > amikacin) [58]
		Volume depletion [58]
Ototoxicity, hearing loss	2–45	Other ototoxic drugs [155]
		Older age [155]
		Dosing frequency (standard dosing > SDD) [54]
		Prolonged duration of therapy [54]
		AG used (gentamicin > tobramycin > amikacin > netilmicin) [64]
		Recent prior AG use [58]
		Exposure to loud noises
		Genetic susceptibility to AG toxicity [156]
Vestibular damage	1–4	Older age [155]
		Other ototoxic drugs
Other toxicities		
Neuromuscular blockade	Rare	Other skeletal muscle relaxants
B6 depletion	Rare	
Anaphylaxis	Rare	
Convulsions	Rare	
Neuritis	Rare	
Tremor	Rare	
Nausea	Rare	
Vomiting	Rare	
Stomatitis	Rare	
Elevated liver enzymes	Rare	
Headache	Rare	
Lethargy	Rare	
Skin necrosis after intramuscular use	Rare	Repeated injections at same site

Ototoxicity

Human data show no difference in serial audiograms or electronystagmograms (a sensitive test for ototoxicity) between SDD and standard multiple daily dosing regimens [16,83]. The rate of clinically apparent ototoxicity is also felt to be generally comparable [10,80]. In eight meta-analyses covering a large proportion of the available literature, SDD showed lower ototoxicity than traditional regimens in one analysis and equal ototoxicity in the seven other analyses [88]. Animal studies also found lower ototoxicity rates with SDD than with multiple daily AG dosing [89] (review [10]).

Some clinicians might be concerned about the safety of SDD because they were (wrongly) taught an adage that 'high peaks hurt ears.' Available data do not support this conclusion [75,83,90]. Rather, long duration of therapy, repeated courses of treatment or high cumulative doses appear critical (Table 6.2).

Truly, the field of AG-induced ototoxicity is complex. Good data are hard to obtain. How one measures ototoxicity also greatly influences results, because toxicity usually occurs in the high-frequency range, beyond the range of normal speech [60,91]. While the incidence of AG-associated hearing loss ranges widely in studies from 2% to 45% [29,60,91–93], it largely depends on how toxicity is measured. Guidelines for monitoring ototoxicity are also not well established [94]. Audiometric tests are used most commonly [58] but other newer tests such as otoacoustic emissions [95] or high-frequency audiograms also are reported in the literature [96]. Finally, it is difficult to control studies for concurrent illnesses and medications that may also be associated with hearing loss [97]. For example, studies of ill patients not treated with AGs showed a 13% [92] to 24% [98] incidence of hearing loss.

COST AND CONVENIENCE

Gentamicin itself is extremely inexpensive (< $1.00 per 80-mg vial). Most expenses are incurred in nursing, pharmacy and monitoring fees. SDD gentamicin dosing greatly reduces these costs of administration [28]. Our survey of two Seattle hospitals showed that traditional multiple daily dosing was 250% more expensive than SDD. Over 1 week, SDD could save up to $700 per patient ($500 compared with $1200) in 1996 [99]. Others confirmed significant dollar savings with SDD [32,81,82]. Additional savings occur by limiting adverse events [81], simplifying monitoring and increasing the potential for early hospital discharge followed by home IV therapy.

EFFICACY

In vitro [60,62], animal [11,20,41,42,61,62,76,100] and clinical [12–40] studies support the efficacy of extended interval gentamicin dosing. By 1997, more than 50 studies found SDD more effective than traditional multiple daily dosing regimens [13]. Among 29 early reports, seven (24%) showed superior results with SDD, and the rest (76%) showed equal efficacy [62]. Meta-analysis of 18 randomized clinical trials involving 2317 patients concluded that SDD is more effective (odds ratio = 1.47) and less nephrotoxic (odds ratio = 0.60) than multiple daily dosing [64]. More recent meta-analyses of 22 [80] and 26 [10] of the best-designed studies concluded that SDD is as effective as multiple daily dosing, with similar toxicity. An ambitious 'meta-analysis of meta-analyses' concluded that SDD decreased mortality, clinical failure, and microbiological failure in six of eight of the reviewed meta-analyses [88]. These studies include patients with many conditions treated by urologists, including abdominal infection [84,101], pelvic inflammatory disease [16], 'severe' infections [26,30], Gram-negative infections [24,25] and UTIs [12,14,24,37,38,68,80,85,102].

In immunocompromised patients, β-lactam antimicrobials are combined with SDD AG because of the concern for bacterial regrowth during the long dosing interval. Meta-analysis of studies evaluating AG plus β-lactam combinations in immunocompromised adults found no difference in efficacy of SDD versus traditional dosing regimens [56]. There are few studies examining the efficacy of 24-h dosing of AGs for surgical prophylaxis. However, one found similar infection rates with SDD and twice-daily gentamicin plus metronidazole in patients who were undergoing colorectal surgery [103].

Studies involving children also demonstrate the efficacy of SDD. SDD avoids underdosing, which occurs in 14% of children receiving standard multiple daily AG dosing [104]. In children, SDD AG proved effective for pyelonephritis [37,38,105] and for serious Gram-negative infections [36,106] (review [11]). Neutropenic children receiving SDD or multiple daily AG plus β-lactam combinations had similar clinical outcomes [18] (review [60]).

SDD is not recommended for everyone

Some authorities suggest that SDD should not be used in conditions resulting in unpredictable drug clearance, including pregnancy [80,88], dialysis, neonates [80,107], and in patients with severe ascites [80] (review [13]). Others feel that more clinical trials are also needed to evaluate SDD in patients with *Pseudomonas* infections [80] and endocarditis [54,80,88, 107], because these diseases have the potential for bacterial regrowth during the long dosing interval. However, animal studies suggest that SDD gentamicin plus ampicillin is effective against endocarditis [47,108,109]. Future studies are likely to elucidate the role of SDD in these populations. It is axiomatic that SDD AG should not be chosen for patients with bacteria that are unlikely to be sensitive to gentamicin (such as most Gram-positive organisms). Some authorities expand this prohibition of SDD therapy to patients with Gram-positive infections, even when the AG is combined with penicillin and is intended to provide synergy against the Gram-positive pathogens [13].

Basics of dosing

In adults, the simplest gentamicin SDD schedule is 5–7 mg/kg IV once every 24 h. The US Food and Drug Administration–approved maximum is 5 mg/kg [56,88], while 7 mg/kg is suggested by some authorities [33,107]. This 7 mg/kg dose achieves a peak of roughly 20 µg/ml in most patients, ten-fold greater than the minimum inhibitory concentration of *Pseudomonas aeruginosa*, the most serious life-threatening pathogen.

SDD offers a marked advantage over divided daily dosing for patients who are massively infected, not improving as expected, or who have partially resistant organisms. In such cases, the SDD dose can be increased further to achieve a peak 10–20 times the mean inhibitory concentration (MIC) of the target organism to ensure excellent coverage.

SDD must be modified for patients that are very thin (< 25% below ideal body weight) or obese (> 25% above ideal body weight) [110] (Table 6.3). Because gentamicin is provided in a concentration of 40 mg/ml, doses can be rounded to increments of 20 mg (0.5 ml) to ensure ease of preparation [90]. In fact, whenever possible, we round the dose of gentamicin to the nearest 80 mg, so that entire vials are used.

Table 6.3 Recommendations for calculating single daily dosing (SDD) of gentamicin

Calculate initial dose	Usual 5–7 mg/kg (round to nearest 40 mg) or Increase dose until peak is 10–20 times MIC of target organism (rarely required against resistant organisms)
Decrease initial dose for very thin or obese patients < 25% or > 25% lean body weight	> 75% lean body weight (thin): increase dose by 12% > 125% lean body weight (obese): decrease dose by 20% times the excess body weight > 175% lean body weight (obese): decrease dose by 40% times the excess body weight
Increase dosing interval for renal failure [157]	Every 24 h if creatinine clearance ≥ 60 ml/min 40–60 ml/min dose every 36 h 20–40 ml/min dose every 48 hours < 20 ml/min redose when trough = 0, consider not using AGs, or use standard dosing
Monitor	Obtain trough before next dose and arbitrarily increase dosing interval if > 0.5 g/ml or Use nomogram (Fig. 6.1)

The usual gentamicin SDD dosing interval is 24 h. This interval must be extended in patients with renal insufficiency [57] (Table 6.3). We agree with the recommendation that gentamicin should be avoided in anephric patients or in patients with severe renal insufficiency (< 20 ml/min) [107], although some advocate its use even in these patients [80].

Monitoring

Monitoring of SDD is controversial [111]. All authorities agree that peak serum AG determinations are unnecessary because SDD produces very high peaks [107], which in all but the most extreme cases are therapeutic. Whether to obtain serum AG trough levels, and how often, is highly controversial. We recommend obtaining a gentamicin serum trough level immediately before the second AG dose. If the trough is less than 0.5 μg/ml then we institute no dosage changes—if it is higher we increase the dosage interval. (We have chosen a trough level of 0.5 μg/ml because in studies of amikacin (which generally runs levels double that of gentamicin), levels below 1.1 μg/ml were associated with no nephrotoxicity. Halving this 1.1 figure to achieve roughly 0.5 μg/ml, we come up with an experimentally safe trough level [26].) We check the trough level daily for 2–3 days, then every third day thereafter. Baseline serum creatinine is obtained at the start of therapy, then rechecked every 3–7 days during treatment [13].

Alternatives to this monitoring approach have been suggested. Some authors suggest a trough cut-off of 1.0 μg/ml [8,15] and still others suggest a trough not exceeding 0.05 μg/ml [107], which is below the limit of detection of the most commonly used assays, and therefore not clinically useful. Another approach is to obtain a gentamicin level 6–14 h after SDD, then use nomograms to calculate the dosing interval [33,57,80,112] (Fig. 6.1). This technique allows the second AG dose to be individualized, while a trough obtained 24 h after the first dose does not allow individualization until the third dose. Some authorities recommend checking the trough daily [113], others advocate a check once every 3 days, and still others obtain serum AG levels only in select patients (e.g. creatinine clearance < 60 ml/min, receiving nephrotoxic agents including contrast media, quadriplegics, amputees, intensive care unit (ICU) patients, those older than 60 years or receiving more than 5 days of AG [33,82]).

Some authors have advocated using a therapeutic monitoring service comprising pharmacists to dictate gentamicin dosing. They cite lower complication rates, shorter duration of therapy and more appropriate gentamicin levels when such a service is used instead of clinicians monitoring all their own patients [114]. Although the incidence of nephrotoxicity after SDD is low, monitoring serum creatinine levels before therapy and

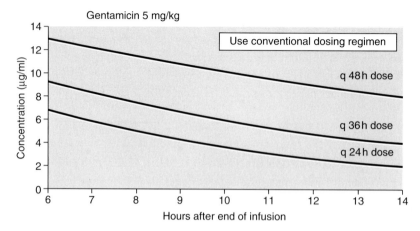

Figure 6.1 Single daily dosing (SDD) gentamicin trough nomogram. (Reprinted with permission from the author [80]. (Appears online at http://www.cop.ufl.edu/safezone/pat/pha5128/nomogram.htm.)

every 2–3 days is still suggested while the patient is taking AGs [13,58]. More frequent serum creatinine determinations are recommended only for patients with multiple risk factors for nephrotoxicity (pre-existing renal insufficiency, dehydration, nephrotoxins, etc.) [57].

Switch therapy

Definition

Switch therapy is a strategy for initiating treatment of patients with serious infections with IV antimicrobials, then changing to an appropriate oral agent once the patient improves. On many occasions, this means after only one parenteral dose, especially in cases of acute uncomplicated pyelonephritis. Switch therapy is one of many 'antibiotic streamlining' approaches. This approach was also termed 'sequential therapy' and 'transitional therapy' before the term 'switch' therapy was accepted [115]. As many as 50% of patients hospitalized for serious infections may be switch therapy candidates [116], yet in some hospitals records show that no more than one out of ten (and probably less) are being offered switch therapy [117].

Switch therapy, often after a single daily dose of AG, is commonly used to treat pyelonephritis [118,119], capitalizing on the 100-h half-life of AGs in the urine [27]. However, switch therapy has also been used to treat pneumonia [120–122] and other serious infections [123–125], including complicated UTI [126–129]. Generally, it has a low failure rate [116,122] and can result in great cost saving [125,130,131].

Rationale

Despite undeniable advantages, such as less expense, greater convenience, the potential for earlier hospital discharge and fewer IV catheter-related complications, switch therapy remains dramatically underutilized. The most important reason may be the mistaken impression that oral antimicrobials are somehow less effective than IV antimicrobials. This is not true. In fact, many antimicrobials have near-identical serum levels when given orally or intravenously, and the 'area under the curve', which is a measure of potency that reflects both serum drug levels and drug half-lives, are identical for a wide range of oral and IV antimicrobials: metronidazole, clindamycin, ciprofloxacin and amoxicillin/clavuluronic acid [130]. Fluroquinolones, which are the most frequently used antimicrobials in urology have proven equal efficacy between oral and IV routes [132]. Oral antimicrobial therapy is effective even when the doses are not taken on time. In one study, patients taking twice-daily oral ciprofloxacin at home seldom took the doses at the exact time prescribed, yet efficacy was still quite high [125].

A second reason for underuse of switch therapy is the perverse incentive provided by insurance plans that require IV therapy as continued justification for hospitalization. Some physicians are reluctant to use switch therapy in patients they want to continue to observe in the hospital. This trend may be countered by reimbursement plans that pay fixed reimbursement based on diagnosis favouring an early switch to oral antimicrobials. Some authorities propose a system of vigorous intervention to promote switch therapy, including the use of automatic stop orders for IV medications, education programmes and reminder stickers placed onto charts to break old prescribing habits [133]. One study showed that only one-on-one meetings with physicians by knowledgeable pharmacists changed prescribing habits (cited in [130]).

EFFICACY

A large number of studies have shown that an early switch from parenteral to oral antimicrobials is as effective as staying on IV medications for a variety of infections, including many serious infections with associated septicemia [27,117–125,134,135]. Generally, switch therapy has a low failure rate, in the 2–5% range [116,122]. In urology, most of the reported evidence for the efficacy of switch therapy is in patients with uncomplicated pyelonephritis [118,119]. There is limited but compelling evidence for efficacy in complicated UTI [126,127]. For example, studies show that switch therapy using oral instead of IV quinolones was effective against pyelonephritis and other complicated UTIs, with efficacy rates in the

85–100% range [136]. Davis [137] reported success with switching to oral ciprofloxacin therapy after 3 days of IV ciprofloxacin in 148 patients, at least 23 of whom had complicated UTIs. Freifeld treated at least eight patients and Kern another ten patients with urinary tract complicated by neutropenia during cancer chemotherapy with good results [128,129]. Our experience with switch therapy has been so positive, that we favour switch therapy in complicated UTIs despite the relatively low numbers of published studies confirming the efficacy of this approach.

COST SAVINGS

Switch therapy can result in great cost savings. For example, ciprofloxacin costs $74/day when administered intravenously and $6/day when administered orally, a 13-fold difference [138]. Drug costs may be decreased by almost $300 a day using switch therapy [125]. More extensive cost savings result from earlier hospital discharge, which may occur in 50% of treated patients [130] and can average 1 day less in the hospital per admission [135]. Further savings are realized by the lack of need for IV access, which in one study is 4 days less per patient [139]. Total cost savings have been estimated to be as high as $1000 [130] to $1200 per day [125,131].

DECREASED HOSPITAL STAY

Switch therapy has been shown to decrease the number of IV medications used in a hospital by a dramatic 43% [140] and generally results in decreased hospital stays. Up to 50% of patients treated with switch therapy may be discharged home earlier, resulting in hospital stays that are between 1 [135] and 1.5 [117] days shorter. When used against pneumonia in one study, hospital stay decreased by a remarkable 3 days [139].

OTHER BENEFITS

Switch therapy may also be safer than conventional parenteral therapy. In one study, switching from parenteral AG/β-lactam therapy to oral therapy decreased ototoxicity from 30% to 17% [118]. Switch therapy holds the potential to decrease the number of days patients receive AGs, and therefore to decrease toxicity significantly [8,90]. In general, the oral ciprofloxacin should result in a low complication rate: only 8% of patients will have side-effects and these will largely be mild gastrointestinal complaints [141]. Hazards of oral quinolones are rare, for example, they can increase theophylline levels dangerously and levels should be monitored in patients who are taking both drugs.

Patient selection

Obviously, patients who cannot take oral medications are not candidates for switch therapy. These may include those who are at risk for aspiration, who need total bowel rest or who have bowel obstruction. Some patients will have unreliable absorption of medications, including those with severe vomiting, nasogastric suction, malabsorption syndromes and who recently have had chemotherapy [142,143]. Patients with nasogastric suction, for example, had only minimal absorption of a 750-mg oral test dose of ciprofloxacin, with malabsorption persisting for 2 days in up to 30% of the patients [144]. Quinolone absorption is impaired in those receiving oral calcium, magnesium or sucralphate supplementation [145,146].

Switch therapy can be used safely in neutropenic patients [128,129], but it is not recommended in cases of meningitis and endocarditis [133]. Switch therapy appears to be efficacious in children [131], although a large number of studies have yet to be completed.

Basics of dosing

Switch therapy can be instituted immediately in those patients who can tolerate oral ingestion, even before clinical improvement is documented, by starting an oral quinolone following a single high-dose bolus of gentamicin [118]. There is no need to observe the patient on IV antibiotics before starting oral agents [119], and it is not necessary that the patient be afebrile before starting oral therapy [147]. This approach is often successful, with the exception of infections from enterococcus, which can have a high failure rate (44%) when oral ciprofloxacin is used. Confirming the success of therapy is mandatory when enterococcus is involved [141].

Generally, the ideal oral antimicrobial is the same agent that was given intravenously, although this is not always possible [147]. Most oral antimicrobials, ultimately, will be acceptable candidates for switch therapy if they have greater than 50% oral bioavailability (this includes most available oral agents [148]). Several antimicrobials are considered ideal candidates for switch therapy because of excellent absorption and bioavailability: fluoroquinolones, cefaclor, cefpodoxime, cefixime, azithromycin, doxycycline [133], metronidazole, clindamycin, co-trimoxazole, amoxycillin/clavuluronate [130], doxycycline, metronidazole, trimethoprim–sulphamethoxazole and clindamycin [138]. Quinolones tend to be most used by urologists. These agents have the added advantage that they are excreted in the urine in such high concentrations that they may overwhelm antimicrobial resistance to urinary tract pathogens. Levofloxacin, for instance, has a peak urinary concentration of $1000\,\mu g/ml$ and ciprofloxacin has a concentration of

400 µg/ml [149]. Compared with the MIC of 4 µg/ml that usually defines 'resistance' in standard laboratory testing, the quinolones have urinary concentrations several-hundred fold more than the MIC of the target organism, and in theory may be more efficacious despite being used against a 'resistant' organism. (Antibiotic concentrations of five times the MIC are generally associated with clinical and bacteriological response rates [133].) Although this tendency towards high concentrations of antimicrobial in the urine may allow for successful early treatment even in 'resistant' organisms, it must be remembered that resistance is associated with higher clinical failure rates [150] and therapy should likely still be changed to an antimicrobial to which the pathogens are susceptible, once cultures are available.

For most Gram-negative UTIs, switch therapy using quinolones is suggested. In cases of polymicrobial infection, the quinolone can be added to second agents such as oral clindamycin, amoxicillin or metronidazole. (Amoxycillin should be used cautiously because of the potential for resistance, which approaches 43% [136]) When Gram-positive organisms are present, the addition of a β-lactam agent is appropriate [130]. Some complicated UTIs should be treated for longer than is standard. Acute uncomplicated pyelonephritis, for example, is treated for 7 days, while in patients with spinal cord injuries and UTIs some authors advocate treatment of relapsing infections for 14 days [151]. Others advocate treating all complicated UTIs for 10 [152] to 14 [2] days, although limited data are available on treatment duration.

Pregnancy

UTIs in pregnancy can theoretically be treated with switch therapy [153]. However, some authors advocate inpatient treatment of pyelonephritis in pregnancy because of a reported 2% incidence of acute respiratory distress that occurs after the initiation of antimicrobial therapy in these patients [5,154]. In addition, quinolones, one of the major drug classes for switch therapy, are not recommended in pregnancy because of the potentially harmful effect on fetaltendon development. Alternative agents to quinolones that can be used for switch therapy in pregnant women include clavulanic acid plus ampicillin, cephalexin, aztreonam and trimethoprim/sulphamethoxazole (except in the last trimester).

Conclusions

Gentamicin and other AGs remain crucial parts of the urologist's armamentarium. New strategies, such as SDD, offer the potential to decrease costs and toxicity while improving efficiency. Primary renal excretion and a urinary half-life of > 4 days ensure persistent high urinary levels, allowing early conversion to oral antimicrobials with switch therapy. Switch therapy facilitates outpatient management of complicated UTIs with equal efficacy to standard IV therapy. SDD AG dosing and switch therapy are underused strategies that should be added to our everyday tools.

References

1 Wagenlehner FME, Naber KG. Hospital-acquired urinary tract infection. *J Hosp Infect* 2000; **46**: 171–1.
2 Nicolle LE. Urinary tract pathogens in complicated infection and in elderly individuals. *J Infect Dis* 2001; **183**(Suppl. 1): S5–8.
3 Gleckman RA, Bradley PJ, Roth RM, Hibert DM. Bacteremic urosepsis: a phenomenon unique to elderly women. *J Urol* 1985; **133**(2): 174–5.
4 Nicolle LE. A practical guide to antimicrobial management of complicated urinary tract infection. *Drugs Aging* 2001; **18**(4): 243–54.
5 Roberts JA. Management of pyelonephritis and upper urinary tract infections. *Urol Clin North Am* 1999; **26**(4): 753–63.
6 Phillips I, King A, Shannon K. Prevalence and mechanisms of aminoglycoside resistance. A ten-year study. *Am J Med* 1986; **80**(Suppl. 6B): 48–55.
7 KEP, PAK, LAF, SBS, SAK. Epidemiological studies of aminoglycoside resistance in the U.S.A. *J Antimicrob Chemother* 1981; **8**(Suppl. A): 89–105.
8 Beaucaire G. The role of aminoglycosides in modern therapy. *J Chemother* 1995; **7**(Suppl. 2): 111–23.
9 Marik PE, Havlik I, Monteagudo FS, Lipman J. The pharmacokinetic of amikacin in critically ill adult and paediatric patients: comparison of once-versus twice-daily dosing regimens. *J Antimicrob Chemother* 1991; **27**(Suppl. C): 81–9.
10 Ali MZ, Goetz MB. A meta-analysis of the relative efficacy and toxicity of single daily dosing versus multiple daily dosing of aminoglycosides. *Clin Infect Dis* 1997; **24**(5): 796–809.
11 Lortholary O, Tod M, Cohen Y, Petitjean O. Aminoglycosides. *Med Clin North Am* 1995; **79**(4): 761–87.
12 Labovitz E, Levison ME, Kaye D. Single-dose daily gentamicin therapy in urinary tract infection. *Antimicrob Agents Chemother* 1974; **6**(4): 465–70.
13 Anaizi N. Once-daily dosing of aminoglycosides. A consensus document. *Int J Clin Pharmacol Ther* 1997; **35**(6): 223–6.
14 Lee SS, Liu YC, Wann SR, Lin WR, Tsai TH, Lin HH *et al.* Once daily isepamicin treatment in complicated urinary tract infections. *J Microbiol Immunol Infect* 1999; **32**(2): 105–10.
15 Cooke RP, Grace RJ, Gover PA. Audit of once-daily dosing gentamicin therapy in neutropenic fever. *Int J Clin Pract* 1997; **51**(4): 229–31.
16 Tulkens PM. Pharmacokinetic and toxicological evaluation of a once-daily regimen versus conventional schedules of netilmicin and amikacin. *J Antimicrob Chemother* 1991; **27**(Suppl. C): 49–61.
17 Vanhaeverbeek M, Siska G, Herchuelz A. Pharmacokinetics of once-daily amikacin in elderly patients. *J Antimicrob Chemother* 1993; **31**(1): 185–7.
18 Zeitany RG, el Saghir NS, Santhosh-Kumar CR, Sigmon MA. Increased aminoglycoside dosage requirements in hematologic malignancy. *Antimicrob Agents Chemother* 1990; **34**(5): 702–708.

19 Hoepelman IM, Rozenberg-Arska M, Verhoef J. Comparison of once daily ceftriaxone with gentamicin plus cefuroxime for treatment of serious bacterial infections. *Lancet* 1988; **1**(8598): 1305–309.

20 Powell SH, Thompson WL, Luthe MA, Stern RC, Grossniklaus DA, Bloxham DD *et al.* Once-daily vs. continuous aminoglycoside dosing: efficacy and toxicity in animal and clinical studies of gentamicin, netilmicin, and tobramycin. *J Infect Dis* 1983; **147**(5): 918–32.

21 Gilbert DN, Lee BL, Dworkin RJ, Leggett JL, Chambers HF, Modin G *et al.* A randomized comparison of the safety and efficacy of once-daily gentamicin or thrice-daily gentamicin in combination with ticarcillin-clavulanate. *Am J Med* 1998; **105**(3): 182–91.

22 Lai MN, Kao MT, Chen CC, Cheung SY, Chung WK. Intraperitoneal once-daily dose of cefazolin and gentamicin for treating CAPD peritonitis. *Perit Dial Int* 1997; **17**(1): 87–9.

23 Maller R, Emanuelsson BM, Isaksson B, Nilsson L. Amikacin once daily: a new dosing regimen based on drug pharmacokinetics. *Scand J Infect Dis* 1990; **22**(5): 575–9.

24 Maller R, Ahrne H, Eilard T, Eriksson I, Lausen I. Efficacy and safety of amikacin in systemic infections when given as a single daily dose or in two divided doses. Scandinavian Amikacin Once Daily Study Group. *J Antimicrob Chemother* 1991; **27**(Suppl. C): 121–8.

25 Maller R, Ahrne H, Holmen C, Lausen I, Nilsson LE, Smedjegard J. Once-versus twice-daily amikacin regimen: efficacy and safety in systemic Gram-negative infections. Scandinavian Amikacin Once Daily Study Group. *J Antimicrob Chemother* 1993; **31**(6): 939–48.

26 ter Braak EW, de Vries PJ, Bouter KP, van der Vegt SG, Dorrestein GC, Nortier JW *et al.* Once-daily dosing regimen for aminoglycoside plus beta-lactam combination therapy of serious bacterial infections: comparative trial with netilmicin plus ceftriaxone. *Am J Med* 1990; **89**(1): 58–66.

27 Bailey RR, Peddie B. Tobramycin in the treatment of severe and complicated urinary tract infections. *Med J Aust* 1977; **2**(Pt 3, Suppl. 2): 34–7.

28 Mitra AG, Whitten MK, Laurent SL, Anderson WE. A randomized, prospective study comparing once-daily gentamicin versus thrice-daily gentamicin in the treatment of puerperal infection. *Am J Obstet Gynecol* 1997; **177**(4): 786–92.

29 Meunier F, Van der Auwera P, Aoun M, Ibrahim S, Tulkens PM. Empirical antimicrobial therapy with a single daily dose of ceftriaxone plus amikacin in febrile granulocytopenic patients: a pilot study. *J Antimicrob Chemother* 1991; **27**(Suppl. C): 129–39.

30 Sturm AW. Netilmicin in the treatment of Gram-negative bacteremia: single daily versus multiple daily dosage. *J Infect Dis* 1989; **159**(5): 931–7.

31 Koo J, Tight R, Rajkumar V, Hawa Z. Comparison of once-daily versus pharmacokinetic dosing of aminoglycosides in elderly patients. *Am J Med* 1996; **101**(2): 177–83.

32 Del Priore G, Jackson-Stone M, Shim EK, Garfinkel J, Eichmann MA, Frederiksen MC. A comparison of once-daily and 8-hour gentamicin dosing in the treatment of postpartum endometritis. *Obstet Gynecol* 1996; **87**(6): 994–1000.

33 Nicolau DP, Freeman CD, Belliveau PP, Nightingale CH, Ross JW, Quintiliani R. Experience with a once-daily aminoglycoside program administered to 2,184 adult patients. *Antimicrob Agents Chemother* 1995; **39**(3): 650–55.

34 Lye WC, Wong PL, van der Straaten JC, Leong SO, Lee EJ. A prospective randomized comparison of single versus multidose gentamicin in the treatment of CAPD peritonitis. *Adv Perit Dial* 1995; **11**: 179–81.

35 de Vries PJ, Verkooyen RP, Leguit P, Verbrugh HA. Prospective randomized study of once-daily versus thrice-daily netilmicin regimens in patients with intraabdominal infections. *Eur J Clin Microbiol Infect Dis* 1990; **9**(3): 161–8.

36 Kafetzis DA, Sianidou L, Vlachos E, Davros J, Bairamis T, Papandreou Y *et al.* Clinical and pharmacokinetic study of a single daily dose of amikacin in paediatric patients with severe Gram-negative infections. *J Antimicrob Chemother* 1991; **27**(Suppl. C): 105–12.

37 Vigano A, Principi N. A randomised comparison of isepamicin and amikacin in the treatment of bacterial infections in paediatric patients. *J Chemother* 1995; **7**(Suppl. 2): 95–101.

38 Carapetis JR, Jaquiery AL, Buttery JP, Starr M, Cranswick NE, Kohn S *et al.* Randomized, controlled trial comparing once daily and three times daily gentamicin in children with urinary tract infections. *Pediatr Infect Dis J* 2001; **20**(3): 240–46.

39 Bates RD, Nahata MC, Jones JW, McCoy K, Young G, Cox S *et al.* Pharmacokinetics and safety of tobramycin after once-daily administration in patients with cystic fibrosis. *Chest* 1997; **112**(5): 1208–13.

40 Beaucaire G, Leroy O, Beuscart C, Karp P, Chidiac C, Caillaux M. Clinical and bacteriological efficacy, and practical aspects of amikacin given once daily for severe infections. *J Antimicrob Chemother* 1991; **27**(Suppl. C): 91–103.

41 Herscovici L, Grise G, Thauvin C, Lemeland JF, Fillastre JP. Efficacy and safety of once daily versus intermittent dosing of tobramycin in rabbits with acute pyelonephritis. *Scand J Infect Dis* 1988; **20**(2): 205–12.

42 Kapusnik JE, Hackbarth CJ, Chambers HF, Carpenter T, Sande MA. Single, large, daily dosing versus intermittent dosing of tobramycin for treating experimental pseudomonas pneumonia. *J Infect Dis* 1988; **158**(1): 7–12.

43 Gerber AU, Kozak S, Segessenmann C, Fluckiger U, Bangerter T, Greter U. Once-daily versus thrice-daily administration of netilmicin in combination therapy of *Pseudomonas aeruginosa* infection in a man-adapted neutropenic animal model. *Eur J Clin Microbiol Infect Dis* 1989; **8**(3): 233–7.

44 Ahmed A, Paris MM, Trujillo M, Hickey SM, Wubbel L, Shelton SL *et al.* Once-daily gentamicin therapy for experimental *Escherichia coli* meningitis. *Antimicrob Agents Chemother* 1997; **41**(1): 49–53.

45 Campbell BG, Bartholow S, Rosin E. Bacterial killing by use of once daily gentamicin dosage in guinea pigs with *Escherichia coli* infection. *Am J Vet Res* 1996; **57**(11): 1627–30.

46 Bugnon D, Potel G, Xiong YQ, Caillon J, Kergueris MF, Le Conte P *et al.* In vivo antibacterial effects of simulated human serum profiles of once-daily versus thrice-daily dosing of amikacin in a *Serratia marcescens* endocarditis experimental model. *Antimicrob Agents Chemother* 1996; **40**(5): 1164–9.

47 Gavalda J, Cardona PJ, Almirante B, Capdevila JA, Laguarda M, Pou L *et al.* Treatment of experimental endocarditis due to *Enterococcus faecalis* using once-daily dosing regimen of gentamicin plus simulated profiles of ampicillin in human serum. *Antimicrob Agents Chemother* 1996; **40**(1): 173–8.

48 Schwank S, Blaser J. Once-versus thrice-daily netilmicin combined with amoxicillin, penicillin, or vancomycin against *Enterococcus faecalis* in a pharmacodynamic in vitro model. *Antimicrob Agents Chemother* 1996; **40**(10): 2258–61.

49 Grassi C, Ginesu F, Pozzi E, Rimoldi R, Crimi N, Periti P. Once-daily tobramycin therapy in lower respiratory tract infections. *J Chemother* 1995; **7**(4): 371–9.

50 Freeman CD, Strayer AH. Mega-analysis of meta-analysis: an examination of meta-analysis with an emphasis on once-daily aminoglycoside comparative trials. *Pharmacotherapy* 1996; **16**(6): 1093–102.

51 Freeman CD, Nicolau DP, Belliveau PP, Nightingale CH. Once-daily dosing of aminoglycosides: review and recommendations for clinical practice. *J Antimicrob Chemother* 1997; **39**(6): 677–86.

52 Craig WA. Once-daily versus multiple-daily dosing of aminoglycosides. *J Chemother* 1995; **7**(Suppl. 2): 47–52.

53 Zhanel GG, Ariano RE. Once daily aminoglycoside dosing: maintained efficacy with reduced nephrotoxicity? *Ren Fail* 1992; **14**(1): 1–9.

54   Bates RD, Nahata MC. Once-daily administration of aminoglycosides. *Ann Pharmacother* 1994; **28**(6): 757–66.

55   Gilbert DN. Once-daily aminoglycoside therapy. *Antimicrob Agents Chemother* 1991; **35**(3): 399–405.

56   Hatala R, Dinh T, Cook DJ. Once-daily aminoglycoside dosing in immunocompetent adults: a meta-analysis. *Ann Intern Med* 1996; **124**(8): 717–25.

57   Deamer RL, Dial LK. The evolution of aminoglycoside therapy: a single daily dose. *Am Fam Physician* 1996; **53**(5): 1782–6.

58   Periti P. Preclinical and clinical evaluation of once-daily aminoglycoside chemotherapy. *J Chemother* 1995; **7**(4): 311–37.

59   Periti P. Pharmacoeconomic evaluation of once-daily aminoglycoside treatment. *J Chemother* 1995; **7**(4): 380–94.

60   Preston SL, Briceland LL. Single daily dosing of aminoglycosides. *Pharmacotherapy* 1995; **15**(3): 297–316.

61   Pechere JC, Craig WA, Meunier F. Once daily dosing of aminoglycoside: one step forward. *J Antimicrob Chemother* 1991; **27**(Suppl. C): 149–52.

62   Barclay ML, Begg EJ, Hickling KG. What is the evidence for once-daily aminoglycoside therapy? *Clin Pharmacokinet* 1994; **27**(1): 32–48.

63   Barza M, Ioannidis JP, Cappelleri JC, Lau J. Single or multiple daily doses of aminoglycosides: a meta-analysis. *BMJ* 1996; **312**(7027): 338–45.

64   Ferriols-Lisart R, Alos-Alminana M. Effectiveness and safety of once-daily aminoglycosides: a meta-analysis. *Am J Health Syst Pharm* 1996; **53**(10): 1141–50.

65   Schumock GT, Raber SR, Crawford SY, Naderer OJ, Rodvold KA. National survey of once-daily dosing of aminoglycoside antibiotics. *Pharmacotherapy* 1995; **15**(2): 201–209.

66   Bertino JS, Jr., Rotschafer JC. Single daily dose of aminoglycosides – a concept whose time has not yet come. *Clin Infect Dis* 1997; **24**(5): 820–23.

67   Rotschafer JC, Rybak MJ. Single daily dosing of aminoglycosides: a commentary. *Ann Pharmacother* 1994; **28**(6): 797–801.

68   Landes RR. Single daily doses of tobramycin in therapy of urinary tract infections. *J Infect Dis* 1976; **134** (Suppl.): S142–5.

69   Van der Auwera P, Meunier F, Ibrahim S, Kaufman L, Derde MP, Tulkens PM. Pharmacodynamic parameters and toxicity of netilmicin (6 milligrams/kilogram/day) given once daily or in three divided doses to cancer patients with urinary tract infection. *Antimicrob Agents Chemother* 1991; **35**(4): 640–47.

70   Barclay ML, Begg EJ. Aminoglycoside adaptive resistance: importance for effective dosage regimens. *Drugs* 2001; **61**(6): 713–21.

71   Daikos GL, Lolans VT, Jackson GG. First-exposure adaptive resistance to aminoglycoside antibiotics *in vivo* with meaning for optimal clinical use. *Antimicrob Agents Chemother* 1991; **35**(1): 117–23.

72   Zhanel GG, Craig WA. Pharmacokinetic contributions to postantibiotic effects. Focus on aminoglycosides. *Clin Pharmacokinet* 1994; **27**(5): 377–92.

73   Moore RD, Smith CR, Lietman PS. The association of aminoglycoside plasma levels with mortality in patients with Gram-negative bacteremia. *J Infect Dis* 1984; **149**(3): 443–8.

74   Moore RD, Smith CR, Lietman PS. Association of aminoglycoside plasma levels with therapeutic outcome in Gram-negative pneumonia. *Am J Med* 1984; **77**(4): 657–62.

75   Tran Ba Huy P, Bernard P, Schacht J. Kinetics of gentamicin uptake and release in the rat. Comparison of inner ear tissues and fluids with other organs. *J Clin Invest* 1986; **77**(5): 1492–500.

76   Wood CA, Norton DR, Kohlhepp SJ, Kohnen PW, Porter GA, Houghton DC *et al.* The influence of tobramycin dosage regimens on nephrotoxicity, ototoxicity, and antibacterial efficacy in a rat model of subcutaneous abscess. *J Infect Dis* 1988; **158**(1): 13–22.

77 Olier B, Viotte G, Morin JP, Fillastre JP. Influence of dosage regimen on experimental tobramycin nephrotoxicity. A biochemical approach. *Chemotherapy* 1983; **29**(6): 385–94.

78 Hayani KC, Hatzopoulos FK, Frank AL, Thummala MR, Hantsch MJ, Schatz BM *et al.* Pharmacokinetics of once-daily dosing of gentamicin in neonates. *J Pediatr* 1997; **131** (1 Pt 1): 76–80.

79 Christensen S, Ladefoged K, Frimodt-Moller N. Experience with once daily dosing of gentamicin: considerations regarding dosing and monitoring. *Chemotherapy* 1997; **43**(6): 442–50.

80 Bailey TC, Little JR, Littenberg B, Reichley RM, Dunagan WC. A meta-analysis of extended-interval dosing versus multiple daily dosing of aminoglycosides. *Clin Infect Dis* 1997; **24**(5): 786–95.

81 Hitt CM, Klepser ME, Nightingale CH, Quintiliani R, Nicolau DP. Pharmacoeconomic impact of once-daily aminoglycoside administration. *Pharmacotherapy* 1997; **17**(4): 810–14.

82 Nicolau DP, Wu AH, Finocchiaro S, Udeh E, Chow MS, Quintiliani R *et al.* Once-daily aminoglycoside dosing: impact on requests and costs for therapeutic drug monitoring. *Ther Drug Monit* 1996; **18**(3): 263–6.

83 Nordstrom L, Ringberg H, Cronberg S, Tjernstrom O, Walder M. Does administration of an aminoglycoside in a single daily dose affect its efficacy and toxicity? *J Antimicrob Chemother* 1990; **25**(1): 159–73.

84 Hollender LF, Bahnini J, De Manzini N, Lau WY, Fan ST, Hermansyur K *et al.* A multi-centric study of netilmicin once daily versus thrice daily in patients with appendicitis and other intra-abdominal infections. *J Antimicrob Chemother* 1989; **23**(5): 773–83.

85 Van der Auwera P. Pharmacokinetic evaluation of single daily dose amikacin. *J Antimicrob Chemother* 1991; **27**(Suppl. C): 63–71.

86 Miron D. Once daily dosing of gentamicin in infants and children. *Pediatr Infect Dis J* 2001; **20**(12): 1169–73.

87 Prins JM, Buller HR, Kuijper EJ, Tange RA, Speelman P. Once versus thrice daily genta-micin in patients with serious infections. *Lancet* 1993; **341**(8841): 335–9.

88 Gilbert DN. Meta-analyses are no longer required for determining the efficacy of single daily dosing of aminoglycosides. *Clin Infect Dis* 1997; **24**(5): 816–19.

89 Pettorossi VE, Ferraresi A, Errico P, Draicchio F, Dionisotti S. The impact of different dosing regimens of the aminoglycosides netilmicin and amikacin on vestibulotoxicity in the guinea pig. *Eur Arch Otorhinolaryngol* 1990; **247**(5): 277–82.

90 McCormack JP, Jewesson PJ. A critical reevaluation of the "therapeutic range" of amino-glycosides. *Clin Infect Dis* 1992; **14**(1): 320–39.

91 Brummett RE, Fox KE. Aminoglycoside-induced hearing loss in humans. *Antimicrob Agents Chemother* 1989; **33**(6): 797–800.

92 Smith CR, Lipsky JJ, Laskin OL, Hellmann DB, Mellits ED, Longstreth J *et al.* Double-blind comparison of the nephrotoxicity and auditory toxicity of gentamicin and tobramy-cin. *N Engl J Med* 1980; **302**(20): 1106–109.

93 Kahlmeter G, Dahlager JI. Aminoglycoside toxicity – a review of clinical studies published between 1975 and 1982. *J Antimicrob Chemother* 1984; **13**(Suppl. A): 9–22.

94 Janknegt R. Aminoglycoside therapy. Current use and future prospects. *Pharm Week Sci* 1990; **12**(3): 81–90.

95 Stavroulaki P, Apostolopoulos N, Dinopoulou D, Vossinakis I, Tsakanikos M, Douniada-kis D. Otoacoustic emissions – an approach for monitoring aminoglycoside induced ototoxicity in children. *Int J Pediatr Otorhinolaryngol* 1999; **50**(3): 177–84.

96 Fausti SA, Henry JA, Helt WJ, Phillips DS, Frey RH, Noffsinger D *et al.* An individualized, sensitive frequency range for early detection of ototoxicity. *Ear Hear* 1999; **20**(6): 497–505.

97   Govaerts PJ, Claes J, Van de Heyning PH, Derde MP, Kaufman L, Marquet JF *et al.* Effect of isepamicin dosing scheme on concentration in cochlear tissue. *Antimicrob Agents Chemother* 1991; **35**(11): 2401–406.

98   Davey PG, Jabeen FJ, Harpur ES, Shenoi PM, Geddes AM. A controlled study of the reliability of pure tone audiometry for the detection of gentamicin auditory toxicity. *J Laryngol Otol* 1983; **97**(1): 27–36.

99   Santucci RA, Krieger JN. Once-daily dosing of aminoglycosides: you can teach an old dog new tricks. In: Northwest Urological Society Annual Meeting; 1996.

100   Gerber AU, Craig WA, Brugger HP, Feller C, Vastola AP, Brandel J. Impact of dosing intervals on activity of gentamicin and ticarcillin against Pseudomonas aeruginosa in granulocytopenic mice. *J Infect Dis* 1983; **147**(5): 910–17.

101   Fan ST, Lau WY, Teoh-Chan CH, Lau KF, Mauracher EH. Once daily administration of netilmicin compared with thrice daily, both in combination with metronidazole, in gangrenous and perforated appendicitis. *J Antimicrob Chemother* 1988; **22**(1): 69–74.

102   Limson BM, Mendoza MT. Single daily injection of tobramycin in the therapy of urinary tract infections. *Phil J Intern Med* 1979; **17**: 179–183.

103   Mendes da Costa P, Kaufman L. Amikacin once daily plus metronidazole versus amikacin twice daily plus metronidazole in colorectal surgery. *Hepatogastroenterology* 1992; **39**(4): 350–54.

104   Skopnik H, Heimann G. Once daily aminoglycoside dosing in full term neonates. *Pediatr Infect Dis J* 1995; **14**(1): 71–2.

105   Tod MM, Padoin C, Petitjean O. Individualising aminoglycoside dosage regimens after therapeutic drug monitoring: simple or complex pharmacokinetic methods? *Clin Pharmacokinet* 2001; **40**(11): 803–14.

106   Trujillo H, Robledo J, Robledo C, Espinal D, Garces G, Mejia J *et al.* Single daily dose amikacin in paediatric patients with severe Gram-negative infections. *J Antimicrob Chemother* 1991; **27**(Suppl. C): 141–7.

107   Begg EJ, Barclay ML, Duffull SB. A suggested approach to once-daily aminoglycoside dosing. *Br J Clin Pharmacol* 1995; **39**(6): 605–609.

108   Blatter M, Fluckiger U, Entenza J, Glauser MP, Francioli P. Simulated human serum profiles of one daily dose of ceftriaxone plus netilmicin in treatment of experimental streptococcal endocarditis. *Antimicrob Agents Chemother* 1993; **37**(9): 1971–6.

109   Saleh-Mghir A, Cremieux AC, Vallois JM, Muffat-Joly M, Devine C, Carbon C. Optimal aminoglycoside dosing regimen for penicillin-tobramycin synergism in experimental *Streptococcus adjacens* endocarditis. *Antimicrob Agents Chemother* 1992; **36**(11): 2403–407.

110   Traynor AM, Nafziger AN, Bertino JS, Jr. Aminoglycoside dosing weight correction factors for patients of various body sizes. *Antimicrob Agents Chemother* 1995; **39**(2): 545–8.

111   Begg EJ, Barclay ML, Kirkpatrick CM. The therapeutic monitoring of antimicrobial agents. *Br J Clin Pharmacol* 2001; **52**(Suppl. 1): 35S–43S.

112   Finnell DL, Davis GA, Cropp CD, Ensom MH. Validation of the Hartford nomogram in trauma surgery patients. *Ann Pharmacother* 1998; **32**(4): 417–21.

113   Kirkpatrick CM, Duffull SB, Begg EJ. Once-daily aminoglycoside therapy: potential ototoxicity. *Antimicrob Agents Chemother* 1997; **41**(4): 879–80.

114   Hansen M, Christrup LL, Jarlov JO, Kampmann JP, Bonde J. Gentamicin dosing in critically ill patients. *Acta Anaesthesiol Scand* 2001; **45**(6): 734–40.

115   Quintiliani R, Nightingale C. Transitional antibiotic therapy. *Infect Dis Clin Pract* 1994; **3**(Suppl. 3): S161–7.

116   Ahkee S, Smith S, Newman D, Ritter W, Burke J, Ramirez JA. Early switch from intravenous to oral antibiotics in hospitalized patients with infections: a 6-month prospective study. *Pharmacotherapy* 1997; **17**(3): 569–75.

117 Przybylski KG, Rybak MJ, Martin PR, Weingarten CM, Zaran FK, Stevenson JG *et al*. A pharmacist-initiated program of intravenous to oral antibiotic conversion. *Pharmacotherapy* 1997; **17**(2): 271–6.

118 Bailey RR, Begg EJ, Smith AH, Robson RA, Lynn KL, Chambers ST *et al*. Prospective, randomized, controlled study comparing two dosing regimens of gentamicin/oral ciprofloxacin switch therapy for acute pyelonephritis. *Clin Nephrol* 1996; **46**(3): 183–6.

119 Caceres VM, Stange KC, Kikano GE, Zyzanski SJ. The clinical utility of a day of hospital observation after switching from intravenous to oral antibiotic therapy in the treatment of pyelonephritis. *J Fam Pract* 1994; **39**(4): 337–9.

120 Ramirez JA, Bordon J. Early switch from intravenous to oral antibiotics in hospitalized patients with bacteremic community-acquired *Streptococcus pneumoniae* pneumonia. *Arch Intern Med* 2001; **161**(6): 848–50.

121 Ramirez JA. Managing antiinfective therapy of community-acquired pneumonia in the hospital setting: focus on switch therapy. *Pharmacotherapy* 2001; **21** (7 Pt 2): 79S–82S.

122 Rhew DC, Hackner D, Henderson L, Ellrodt AG, Weingarten SR. The clinical benefit of in-hospital observation in 'low-risk' pneumonia patients after conversion from parenteral to oral antimicrobial therapy. *Chest* 1998; **113**(1): 142–6.

123 Gentry LO, Rodriguez GG. Oral ciprofloxacin compared with parenteral antibiotics in the treatment of osteomyelitis. *Antimicrob Agents Chemother* 1990; **34**(1): 40–43.

124 Cohn SM, Lipsett PA, Buchman TG, Cheadle WG, Milsom JW, O'Marro S *et al*. Comparison of intravenous/oral ciprofloxacin plus metronidazole versus piperacillin/tazobactam in the treatment of complicated intraabdominal infections. *Ann Surg* 2000; **232**(2): 254–62.

125 Paladino JA, Sperry HE, Backes JM, Gelber JA, Serrianne DJ, Cumbo TJ *et al*. Clinical and economic evaluation of oral ciprofloxacin after an abbreviated course of intravenous antibiotics. *Am J Med* 1991; **91**(5): 462–70.

126 Gelfand MS, Simmons BP, Craft RB, Grogan J, Amarshi N. A sequential study of intravenous and oral fleroxacin in the treatment of complicated urinary tract infection. *Am J Med* 1993; **94**(3A): 126S-130.

127 DeGier R, Karperien A, Bouter JK. A sequential study of intravenous and oral fleroxacin for 7 or 14 days in the treatment of complicated urinary tract infections. *Int J Antimicrob Agents* 1995; **6**: 27–30.

128 Freifeld A, Marchigiani D, Walsh T, Chanock S, Lewis L, Hiemenz J *et al*. A double-blind comparison of empirical oral and intravenous antibiotic therapy for low-risk febrile patients with neutropenia during cancer chemotherapy. *N Engl J Med* 1999; **341**(5): 305–11.

129 Kern WV, Cometta A, De Bock R, Langenaeken J, Paesmans M, Gaya H. Oral versus intravenous empirical antimicrobial therapy for fever in patients with granulocytopenia who are receiving cancer chemotherapy. International Antimicrobial Therapy Cooperative Group of the European Organization for Research and Treatment of Cancer. *N Engl J Med* 1999; **341**(5): 312–18.

130 Nathwani D, Tillotson G, Davey P. Sequential antimicrobial therapy – the role of quinolones. *J Antimicrob Chemother* 1997; **39**(4): 441–6.

131 Rice HE, Brown RL, Gollin G, Caty MG, Gilbert j, Skinner MA *et al*. Results of a pilot trial comparing prolonged intravenous antibiotics with sequential intravenous/oral antibiotics for children with perforated appendicitis. *Arch Surg* 2001; **136**: 1391–5.

132 Mombelli G, Pezzoli R, Pinoja-Lutz G, Monotti R, Marone C, Franciolli M. Oral vs intravenous ciprofloxacin in the initial empirical management of severe pyelonephritis or complicated urinary tract infections: a prospective randomized clinical trial. *Arch Intern Med* 1999; **159**(1): 53–8.

133   Lelekis M, Gould IM. Sequential antibiotic therapy for cost containment in the hospital setting: why not? *J Hosp Infect* 2001; **48**(4): 249–57.

134   Gangji D, Jacobs F, de Jonckheer J, Coppens L, Serruys E, Hanotte F *et al.* Randomized study of intravenous versus sequential intravenous/oral regimen of ciprofloxacin in the treatment of Gram-negative septicemia. *Am J Med* 1989; **87**(5A): 206S–208S.

135   Partsch DJ, Paladino JA. Cost-effectiveness comparison of sequential ofloxacin versus standard switch therapy. *Ann Pharmacother* 1997; **31**(10): 1137–45.

136   Blondeau JM. Clinical utility of the new fluoroquinolones for treating respiratory and urinary tract infections. *Expert Opin Investig Drugs* 2001; **10**(2): 213–37.

137   Davis C. Sequential intravenous/oral ciprofloxacin as an empiric antimicrobial therapy: results of a Canadian multicenter study. The Canadian Collaborative Investigational Group. *Clin Ther* 1994; **16**(3): 505–21.

138   Cunha BA. Intravenous-to-oral antibiotic switch therapy. A cost-effective approach. *Postgrad Med* 1997; **101**(4): 111–12, 115–18, 122–3 passim.

139   Laing RB, Mackenzie AR, Shaw H, Gould IM, Douglas JG. The effect of intravenous-to-oral switch guidelines on the use of parenteral antimicrobials in medical wards. *J Antimicrob Chemother* 1998; **42**(1): 107–11.

140   Sevinc F, Prins JM, Koopmans RP, Langendijk PN, Bossuyt PM, Dankert J *et al.* Early switch from intravenous to oral antibiotics: guidelines and implementation in a large teaching hospital. *J Antimicrob Chemother* 1999; **43**(4): 601–606.

141   Krcmery S, Naber KG. Ciprofloxacin once versus twice daily in the treatment of complicated urinary tract infections. German Ciprofloxacin UTI Study Group. *Int J Antimicrob Agents* 1999; **11**(2): 133–8.

142   Johnson EJ, MacGowan AP, Potter MN, Stockley RJ, White LO, Slade RR *et al.* Reduced absorption of oral ciprofloxacin after chemotherapy for haematological malignancy. *J Antimicrob Chemother* 1990; **25**(5): 837–42.

143   Brown NM, White LO, Blundell EL, Chown SR, Slade RR, MacGowan AP *et al.* Absorption of oral ofloxacin after cytotoxic chemotherapy for haematological malignancy. *J Antimicrob Chemother* 1993; **32**(1): 117–22.

144   Cohn SM, Cohn KA, Rafferty MJ, Smith AH, Degutis LC, Kowalsky SF *et al.* Enteric absorption of ciprofloxacin during the immediate postoperative period. *J Antimicrob Chemother* 1995; **36**(4): 717–21.

145   Polk RE. Drug–drug interactions with ciprofloxacin and other fluoroquinolones. *Am J Med* 1989; **87**(5A): 76S–81S.

146   Stein GE. Drug interactions with fluoroquinolones. *Am J Med* 1991; **91**(6A): 81S–6S.

147   Barlow GD, Nathwani D. Sequential antibiotic therapy. *Curr Opin Infect Dis* 2000; **13**(6): 599–607.

148   Quintiliani R, Cooper BW, Briceland LL, Nightingale CH. Economic impact of streamlining antibiotic administration. *Am J Med* 1987; **82**(4A): 391–4.

149   Baden LR, Horowitz G, Jacoby H, Eliopoulos GM. Quinolones and false-positive urine screening for opiates by immunoassay technology. *JAMA* 2001; **286**(24): 3115–19.

150   Talan DA, Stamm WE, Hooton TM, Moran GJ, Burke T, Iravani A *et al.* Comparison of ciprofloxacin (7 days) and trimethoprim-sulfamethoxazole (14 days) for acute uncomplicated pyelonephritis pyelonephritis in women: a randomized trial. *JAMA* 2000; **283**(12): 1583–90.

151   Biering-Sorensen F, Bagi P, Hoiby N. Urinary tract infections in patients with spinal cord lesions: treatment and prevention. *Drugs* 2001; **61**(9): 1275–87.

152   MacMillan RD. Complicated urinary tract infections in patients with voiding dysfunction. *Can J Urol* 2001; **8**(Suppl. 1): 13–17.

153 Angel JL, O'Brien WF, Finan MA, Morales WJ, Lake M, Knuppel RA. Acute pyelonephritis in pregnancy: a prospective study of oral versus intravenous antibiotic therapy. *Obstet Gynecol* 1990; **76**(1): 28–32.

154 Cunningham FG. Urinary tract infections complicating pregnancy. *Baillieres Clin Obstet Gynaecol* 1987; **1**(4): 891–908.

155 Govaerts PJ, Claes J, van de Heyning PH, Jorens PG, Marquet J, De Broe ME. Aminoglycoside-induced ototoxicity. *Toxicol Lett* 1990; **52**(3): 227–51.

156 Fischel-Ghodsian N. Genetic factors in aminoglycoside toxicity. *Ann N Y Acad Sci* 1999; **884**: 99–109.

157 Gonzalez P, Aguado JM, Martin MA, Fernandez-Chacon T, Ortuno B. Once-daily aminoglycoside dosing. *Lancet* 1993; **341**(8849): 895.

7: Prostatitis

Martin Ludwig & Wolfgang Weidner

Principles of therapy

The term prostatitis or 'prostatitis syndrome' covers numerous pathological conditions that recently have been classified with new definitions by the consensus conference of the National Institute of Diabetes and Digestive and Kidney Diseases (NIDDK) [1] (Table 7.1). As different types of prostatitis syndrome require different therapeutic strategies in drug treatment each category is covered separately in this chapter.

Acute bacterial prostatitis (cat. I)

Acute bacterial prostatitis *always* causes an acute urinary tract infection (UTI) and is caused by common uropathogens. Antimicrobial substances represent the hallmarks of therapy. The most common etiologic cause of acute bacterial prostatitis is Gram-negative bacteria, predominantly strains of *Escherichia coli* that have been identified in 65–80% of infections [2,3]. *Pseudomonas aeruginosa*, *Serratia*, *Klebsiella*, and *Enterobacter aerogenes* have been isolated in 10–15% of cases [2]. *Enterococcus faecalis* also may cause acute bacterial prostatitis [4]. Sporadic incidence of *Staphylococcus saprophyticus*, hemolytic streptococci [2], *Staphylococcus aureus* and *coagulase-negative* staphylococci [5], as well as *Neisseria gonorrhoeae*, *Mycobacterium tuberculosis*, *Salmonella*, *Clostridia* and parasitic organisms and fungi, has been reported. However, immunocompromised states, particularly HIV infection and clinical stages of AIDS, may well lead to an increase of bacterial forms of acute prostatitis and also to an increasing significance of uncommon pathogens.

Although most antimicrobials achieve adequate urinary levels after administration, sufficient drug tissue penetration into the prostate gland is relevant for eradicating the pathogens and minimizing the risk of development of chronic bacterial prostatitis. In acute prostatitis even antimicrobials that normally diffuse poorly into prostatic secretions lead to symptomatic relief and result in the eradication of the pathogen. The intense inflammatory reaction that occurs in this disease apparently permits therapeutic levels of drugs that are normally unable to accumulate in prostatic secretions and prostatic stroma [6]. Therefore, a broader spectrum of antimicro-

Table 7.1 The new NIH classification of the prostatitis syndrome [1]

Category	Name	Description
I	Acute bacterial prostatitis	Acute infection of the prostate gland
II	Chronic bacterial prostatitis	Recurrent infection of the prostate
III	Chronic abacterial prostatitis/ chronic pelvic pain syndrome	No demonstrable infection
IIIA	Inflammatory chronic pelvic pain syndrome	White cells in semen, expressed prostatic secretions or post-prostatic massage urine
IIIB	Non-inflammatory chronic pelvic pain syndrome	No white cells in semen, expressed prostatic secretions or post-prostatic massage urine
IV	Asymptomatic inflammatory prostatitis	No subjective symptoms, detected either by prostate biopsy or by the presence of white cells in expressed prostatic secretions or semen during evaluation for other disorders

bials is available in this disease as compared with chronic bacterial prostatitis, depending on the susceptibility of the pathogen. Initially, intravenous application followed by oral medication of the antimicrobial for 4–6 weeks has been recommended; however, comparative data from prospective studies are not available to date [7]. With the administration of adequate antimicrobial substances associated with symptomatic relief from the acute infection, the percentage of development of chronic bacterial prostatitis is low.

Chronic bacterial prostatitis (cat. II)

Etiologically, the same pathogens responsible for cat. I prostatitis may cause chronic bacterial prostatitis. Antimicrobial treatment is the most powerful part of the treatment concept for this disease. In contrast to cat. I prostatitis, antimicrobials must fulfil the following prerequisites to be effective in the treatment of bacterial prostatitis: lipid solubility, low protein binding, dissociation constant close to plasma pH and a pH gradient between 7.4 and 6.4 for plasma and prostatic secretions [8]. The duration of therapy depends on the antimicrobial drug used and is detailed in Table 7.2 [9]. The use of α-receptor blockers has been described mainly in men with chronic pelvic pain syndrome (CPPS) (see 'Chronic pelvic pain syndrome (cat. IIIA and IIIB)'). However, their administration in combination with antimicrobials seems to improve symptomatic relief and decrease recurrence rates of the responsible pathogen even in chronic bacterial prostatitis [10].

Three major problems appear to be responsible for treatment failures:

Table 7.2 Suggestions for antimicrobial therapy in cat. II prostatitis [6,9]

	Substance	Duration	Remarks
First-line therapy	Fluoroquinolones, i.e. ciprofloxacin, ofloxacin, levofloxacin	2–4 weeks	Cure rate about 70%
Second-line therapy	Trimethoprim or trimethoprim– sulphamethoxazole	3 months	Cure rate 50%, hampered diffusion into alkaline inflammatory prostate secretions
Long-term therapy	Trimethoprim, nitrofurantoin	3–6 months	Suppression of recurrent urinary tract infections

- In the infected human (alkaline) prostatic secretions not every antimicrobial substance is available in sufficient concentrations. This is clearly different in the dog model system [8].
- Hampered antimicrobial diffusion into infected calcified prostatic calculi may lead to recurrent UTIs. However, men with prostatic calculi did not demonstrate decreased eradication rates of the pathogen as compared with patients without calculi in our own series [11].
- Bacterial microcolonies in the prostate gland may be protected by a glycocalix slime and thereby reduce diffusion of antimicrobials [12].

Recurrent UTIs typically occur in chronic bacterial prostatitis when antimicrobial therapy fails to eradicate the pathogen. In these men a long-term antibiotic suppression over 3–6 months is recommended to prevent recurrent UTI [6].

Two alternative treatment modalities have been discussed (overview in [13]):
- The transperineal injection of antimicrobials, usually with amikacin. Long-term results with regard to bacteriological cure are disappointing.
- In an immunological approach a cell vaccine made from several inactivated uropathogenic bacteria has been used without convincing results.

The role of *Chlamydia* (C.) *trachomatis* and mycoplasms, particularly *Ureaplasma* (U.) *urealyticum*, in some cases of chronic bacterial prostatitis remains highly equivocal. Some authors were able to associate the finding of *C. trachomatis* and high numbers of *U. urealyticum* in prostatic secretions with symptomatic disease whereas others did not confirm these results (overviews in [2,14]). However, when these pathogens are suspected as etiologically involved in the patient's symptoms, a specific antimicrobial therapy is justified.

Chronic pelvic pain syndrome (cat. IIIA and IIIB)

In contrast to bacterial prostatitis, the etiopathology of most cases of CPPS remains unclear. Although some pathogenic mechanisms have been identified, therapeutic strategies often remain empirical. Particularly, in this type of prostatitis syndrome, drug treatment is only one of several options that can be supplemented by physical, invasive, behavioural and surgical treatment strategies.

Most authors agree that in cat. III, especially in cat. IIIA CPPS, one empirical trial with antimicrobial treatment is justified even though evidence for bacterial infection is lacking. The idea behind this strategy is that bacteria might not have been demonstrated either because their number was too low or because fastidious or, etiologically, cryptic bacteria that escape the routine diagnostic process may be involved [15]. This theory has been supported by a non-blinded study resulting in symptomatic improvement in about 50% of the patients regardless of demonstration of an inflammation or infection [16]. New molecular biology amplification methods of bacterial DNA expressed in prostatic secretions and prostatic tissue might help to resolve this problem in the future [17]. It has been emphasized that conventional antimicrobial treatment should be discontinued when a symptomatic improvement cannot be achieved after 2 weeks of administration [9]. A combination of antimicrobial treatment with repetitive prostatic massage has been suggested in order to assist in the drainage of infected material and in antimicrobial penetration within potentially obstructed cavities [18].

Bladder voiding disturbances have been suspected in a various percentage of men with CPPS. Whereas a significant bladder outlet obstruction as assessed by a complete urodynamic evaluation has been found in only a few patients [19], functional bladder voiding disturbances causing high-pressure turbulent voiding seem to be prevalent in 30–40% of men with CPPS [20]. Bladder neck dysfunction has been claimed to represent a major pathogenic factor. Additionally, video urodynamic studies have indicated an increased maximum urethral closure pressure recorded at the distal prostatic and membranous urethral segments [10], possibly due to an adrenergic increase of the pelvic floor muscle tension. Chronic pain may be caused by increased muscle tension and by consecutive influx of urine and particularly urinary urate and creatinine into the prostatic ducts [21]. This hypothesis has been fuelled further by evidence of a significantly increased intraprostatic pressure in men with cat. IIIA than in those with cat. IIIB prostatitis and controls [22]. Consecutively, three basic therapeutic strategies have evolved:

1 Alpha-1-receptor antagonism of the bladder neck will cause smooth muscle relaxation in the base of the bladder, the proximal urethra and the prostate and possibly will reduce hypertrophied smooth muscle. This therapeutic option is supposed to particularly relieve voiding complaints of an irritative nature in men with CPPS [20].

2 The second option is to reduce the influx of purine and pyrimidine base–containing metabolites into the prostatic ducts that have been hypothesized to cause pelvic pain by facilitating the initiation of an inflammatory reaction in the prostatic duct [21]. Thus, allopurinol as the most widespread drug to decrease urate in serum (and therefore in urine) has been suggested to relief symptoms [23]. However, further evaluation of this trial does not confirm the beneficial effects of this substance [24].

3 Reduction of the urethral pressure profile by decreasing the tone of the striated pelvic floor muscles [25].

5-alpha-reductase-inhibitors have been found beneficial in the treatment of symptomatic benign prostatic hyperplasia (BPH). As lower urinary tract symptoms associated with BPH may resemble symptoms of CPPSs in men, a Finnish study group has evaluated finasteride in men with cat. IIIA CPPS and subsequently has stated a significant decrease in symptom severity in these men [26]. The authors hypothesized reduction of prostatic oedema, reduction of prostatic volume in the area where the prostatic inflammation is localized, anti-inflammatory effects and the shrinking of the prostate gland to be the pathomechanisms relevant for improvement in symptoms.

Some years ago, a similarity of symptoms was stated between women diagnosed with interstitial cystitis and men with CPPS [27]: both entities are characterized by pain and voiding symptoms associated with non-specific inflammation of the lower urinary tract. Subsequently, some of the diagnostic criteria for interstitial cystitis have been applied for men with non-inflammatory CPPS. The authors found a symptomatic relief after hydrodistension in those men in whom cystoscopically petechial haemorrhage was present analogous to interstitial cystitis; however, only 20 patients have been included in this protocol. The authors have hypothesized that CPPS in men and interstitial cystitis in women may have a similar pathogenesis. These results have led to the idea of evaluating therapeutic strategies in men with CPPS, which has turned out to be effective in patients with interstitial cystitis. Until today, only pentosan polysulphate (PPS), an exogenous glycosaminoglycane, has been investigated in men with inflammatory CPPS [28]. The rationale for the use of this substance is to enforce the protective layer covering the epithelium of the urinary tract.

It has been theorized that in a subset of men with CPPS an inflammatory dysregulation of the injury response may be present, leading to persistent upregulation of proinflammatory cytokines, immune cell infiltration, oxidant stress and cellular injury [29,30]. The finding that the prostate gland is capable of both a humeral and a cellular immune response is not new and was first proved in the 1960s [31]. Since then, various authors have worked on antigen-specific antibodies, antibody-coated bacteria, cellular immune mechanisms and resulting immune therapies (overview in [32]). However, particularly in the last years, some important breakthroughs have been achieved:

● In a number of studies, various cytokines in prostatic secretions and seminal fluid have increased in cat. IIIA vs cat. IIIB vs controls [33–40], indicating the relevance of a persisting upregulated immune reaction in the absence of pathogenic pathogens and even of leucocytes in prostatic secretions.

● In some men with CPPS, an evidence of a proliferative CD4 T cell response to prostate-specific antigen (PSA) has been identified as a potential antigen in this disease [41].

The complex immune mechanisms involved in the pathogenesis of chronic prostatitis/CPPS have evolved into therapeutic strategies for reducing pain by interfering with the specific and non-specific immune system:

● Theoretically, phytotherapy may provide symptomatic relief by anti-inflammatory effects. However, additional effects independent of the immune system have been ascribed to these substances, particularly 5-α-reductase activity, and positive effects on bladder voiding. Best investigated are bioflavonoids. Documented properties include activity as an antioxidant and as an anti-inflammatory by blocking both chemokines and cytokines. Additionally, they interfere with tyrosine kinase enzyme activation, inhibiting the division and growth of T cells (overview in [30]). Pollen extract has been found to inhibit the biosynthesis of prostaglandins and leucotriens *in vitro*, and inhibitory effects on the contraction of the urethra and prostate growth have been described in animal models (overview in [42]). Until today, double-blind randomized prospective trials only exist for bioflavonoids [30], providing evidence for a symptomatic improvement in some cases.

● Traditionally, non-steroidal anti-inflammatory drugs (NSAIDs) have been tried with some symptomatic success (overview in [43]). However, the majority of studies are based on non-controlled data. Thus, prospective blinded randomized clinical trials for judging the efficiency of these drugs in CPPS are lacking.

● The use of immune modulators such as cytokine inhibitors or COX-2 inhibitors is promising. Although prospective blinded randomized trials are under way. Use of these drugs cannot be recommended until results from

definitive research trials are present due to their potential of causing deleterious side-effects.

Further therapeutic strategies, such as analgesics, antidepressants, and the
combination of the different therapeutic options detailed above, are based
on unpublished data or represent reports from personal experience of
investigators involved in this disease [15]. Their 'evidence-based value' is
low. In 1998, the International Prostatitis Collaborative Network (ICPN)
suggested a priorization of treatments for chronic prostatitis (Table 7.3),
but, on the other hand, emphasized that this list of proposed treatments
should evolve over time according to research results [44].

Asymptomatic prostatitis (cat. IV)

Generally, asymptomatic prostatitis does not require therapy. However, in
about 30% [45] to 100% [46] of men with increased PSA, prostatic biopsy
may reveal the histological finding of prostatic inflammation. Several hypoth-
eses have been controversially discussed to explain elevated blood PSA levels
in men with histological inflammation of the prostate (overview in [47]):

• Leakage of PSA from acini and ductal lumina to the circulation, caused
by disruption of anatomical barriers, particularly the glandular epithelium,
due to inflammation.

• Release of PSA stored in epithelial cells into stromal tissue following
epithelial cellular injury and cell death, consecutively followed by leakage
into the general circulation as a result of increased vascularization and
vascular permeability of the prostate during inflammation.

Table 7.3 Prioritization of treatments for chronic prostatitis [44]

Rank	Treatment category
1	Antimicrobials
2	Alpha-blockers
3	(Repetitive) prostatic massage
4	Anti-inflammatories (NSAIDs, hydroxyzine)
5	Pain control measures
6	Biofeedback
7	Alpha-reductase inhibitors
8	Muscle relaxants
9	Devices (e.g. TUMT, TUNA)
10	Physical therapy
11	Psychotherapy
12	Alternate therapy (e.g. meditation, coping skills, acupuncture)
13	Allopurinol, surgery (TURBN, TURP, radical prostatectomy)

About 42% of asymptomatic men with elevated PSA have been found to have elevated leucocyte counts in their prostatic secretions [48]. Therapeutic strategies in these men are aimed at reducing the PSA value in order to better differentiate between men with prostatic carcinoma and men with prostatic inflammation and consecutive increase of PSA.

Drugs available

Acute bacterial prostatitis (cat. I)

Acute bacterial prostatitis always represents a complicated infection and an acute severe systemic illness. Keeping these facts in mind, the following treatment options have been suggested:
- For patients requiring parenteral therapy: antimicrobial treatment covering the organisms likely involved, such as a high-dose broad-spectrum cephalosporin (e.g. cefuroxime, cefotaxime (2 g/day), ceftriaxone (1 g/day)) plus gentamicin (dosage according to renal function) until apyrexia, followed by a switch to oral quinolone therapy for a further 4–6 weeks or according to sensitivities of isolated bacteria [7,49].
- Ofloxacin or ciprofloxacin intravenously until apyrexia, followed by a switch to oral therapy for a further 4–6 weeks [7] or orally for 4 weeks [49]. Dosage: ciprofloxacin 500 mg twice daily; ofloxacin 200 mg twice daily.
- Trimethoprim–sulphamethoxazole (orally) for 4–6 weeks [7]. Dosage: 960 mg twice daily.

Chronic bacterial prostatitis (cat. II)

Drugs available for curative antimicrobial treatment in case of infection with common UTI pathogens and symptomatic suppression of concomitant UTI are summarized in Table 7.2 [6,9]. Therapeutical guidelines for the rare cases of chronic bacterial prostatitis caused by Gram-positive pathogens (*enterococci*) have not been standardized. Trials with quinolones, cotrimoxazole, tetracyclines and makrolides should strongly be linked to sensitivities. New third-generation quinolones like gatifloxacin may provide better sensitivity profiles in these cases.

In patients with a medical history of urethritis or with associated infection with *C. trachomatis* or *U. urealyticum*, oral treatment with tetracycline or erythromycin should be initiated. The suggested duration of therapy is 2 weeks. Azithromycin, a novel azalide antimicrobial, represents an interesting alternative because of its effectiveness against *C. trachomatis*, its excellent bioavailability and its sustained high tissue levels. However, experience only exists in the treatment of chlamydial [50] and non-gonococcal urethritis

[51] whereas comparable data in the treatment of prostatitis syndrome is lacking. Recurrent infections with these pathogens require the evaluation and, if necessary, the treatment of the patient's sexual partner. However, the symptomatic effect of all these treatment options has never been sufficiently assessed and therefore remains unclear.

Chronic pelvic pain syndrome (cat. IIIA and IIIB)

Detailed information about drugs available in the treatment of CPPS is provided in Table 7.4 [10,16,20,23,25,28,30,42,52–54].

Asymptomatic prostatitis (cat. IV)

Asymptomatic prostatitis does not necessarily require treatment, as indicated in the previous sections; however, in men with increased PSA values and evidence of prostatitis [48,55,56], a reduction of PSA due to treatment may reduce the probability that prostate cancer is present. As elevation of PSA may be a consequence of inflammation and/or silent infection, antimicrobials and anti-inflammatory drugs can be administered. However, most studies use different types of antimicrobials in combination with different types of anti-inflammatory drugs, thus making an evaluation of these drugs more difficult (Table 7.5). The basic problem remains that prostate cancer has been found in 10% of men with asymptomatic prostatitis and PSA decline following antimicrobial therapy, [55], thus complicating a therapeutic algorithm on the basis of PSA reduction in men with asymptomatic prostatitis.

Relevant trials

Acute bacterial prostatitis (cat. I)

Relevant trials in the treatment of acute prostatitis should give an answer to the following most critical questions:
• *The antimicrobial problem:* the decision regarding which antimicrobial substance is best suited for initial therapy is followed by the question of which mode of application (orally or intravenously) should be favoured. Finally, if intravenous treatment has been started, the optimal point has to be chosen to switch to oral administration.
• *The urinary drainage problem:* it is undisputed that patients with high residual volume require urinary diversion. However, it has to be decided at which amount of residual volume a suprapubic or urethral catheter is recommended.

Table 7.4 Drugs available in cat. IIIA and B chronic pelvic pain syndrome

Drug classification	Substance/dosage/duration	Evaluated in category	Kind of trial	Effect	Remarks	Authors
Antimicrobials	Ofloxacin (2 × 300 mg; 3 months)	II, IIIA, IIIB	p, nc	Symptomatic improvement in all categories		Nickel et al. 2001 [16]
	Ciprofloxacin (dosage not described; 1 month)	II, IIIA	p, r, c	Symptomatic improvement	Combination with α-blockers enhances performance, individualized study design	Barbalias et al. 1993 [10]
Alpha-blockers	Terazosin (5 mg/day; 2 months), tamsulosin 0.4 mg/day; 2 months)	IIIA	p, r, pc, db	Symptomatic improvement of both α-blockers vs placebo		Lacquaniti et al. 1999 [52]
	Alfuzosin (2,5 mg/day; 6 weeks)	IIIA, IIIB	p, r, pc, db	Symptomatic improvement in α-blocker treatment vs placebo	All patients with urodynamic abnormalities, only 20 patients	de la Rosette et al. 1992 [20]
	Terazosin (2–10 mg/day; 4 weeks)	IIIA, IIIB	p, nc	Symptomatic improvement of CPPS patients vs controls		Neal et al. 1994 [53]
Muscle relaxants	Baclofen (3 × 5 mg; 3 days then 3 × 10 mg; 1 month)	NIH IIIB	p, r, pc, db	Effective but inferior to α-blocker (phenoxybenzamine)	Crossed treatment design	Osborn et al. 1981 [25]
Uricostatics	Allopurinol (1–2 × 300 mg; 8 months)	IIIA	p, r, pc, db	Significant symptom relief vs placebo	Study design doubtful [Nickel et al. 1996]	Persson et al. 1996 [23]

(Continued)

Table 7.4 *Continued*

Drug classification	Substance/dosage/duration	Evaluated in category	Kind of trial	Effect	Remarks	Authors
5-α-reductase-inhibitors	Finasteride (5 mg/day; 12 months)	IIIA	p, r, pc, db	Significant symptom relief vs placebo		Leskinen *et al.* 1999 [26]
Treatment strategies against interstitial cystitis	Pentosan polysulphate (3 × 100 mg; 6 months)	IIIA	p, nc	Significant symptom relief vs baseline		Nickel *et al.* 2000 [28]
Phytotherapy	Quercetin (2 × 500 mg; 1 month)	IIIA, IIIB	p, r, pc, db	Significant symptom relief vs placebo		Shoskes *et al.* 1999 [30]
	Pollen extract (Cernilton® N; 1 tablet *tid*; 6 months)	IIIA, IIIB	p, nc	Symptom relief		Rugendorff *et al.* 1993 [42]
NSAID	Nimesulide (2 × 100 mg; 1 month)	NIH IIIA	p, nc	Symptom relief	Substance not available in Germany; other NSAIDs not investigated	Canale *et al.* 1993 [54]

p, prospective; r, randomized; nc, non-controlled; c, controlled; pc, placebo-controlled; db, double-blind; sb, single-blind.

Table 7.5 Drug administration in cat. IV prostatitis in order to reduce PSA value

Authors	Antimicrobials	Non-antimicrobials	Evaluated in category	Remarks	Biopsies in case of PSA reduction
Potts 2000 [48]	Trimethoprim–sulphamethoxazole, quinolones (4 weeks)	None	IV	Exact drug administration not described	No
Karazanashvili and Managadze 2001 [55]	Ofloxacin (400 mg, 2 times daily, 15 days)	Phytotherapy (*Hypericum perforatum, Helichrysum arenarium, Matricaria chamomilla*)	IV		Yes
Bozeman et al. 2002 [56]	Quinolones, trimethoprim–sulphamethoxazole, doxycycline (4 weeks)	Ibuprofen, celecoxib	IIIA, IV	Patients' distribution cat. IIIA vs IV not described, exact drug administration not described	No

• *The hospitalization problem:* although it is clear that men with absolute indications for close nursing interventions like sepsis, potential need for fluid replacement, cardiopulmonary monitoring and similar conditions require hospitalization, the medical outcome of inpatient treatment is unclear and the decision may depend on economic grounds as well.

Unfortunately, clinical data to definitely answer these questions on the basis of prospective randomized trials do not exist. Data available are mostly based on non-comparative trials or expert opinion (overview in [57]). Despite these unsolved problems recommendations for treatment strategies do exist [7].

Chronic bacterial prostatitis (cat. II)

In cat. II prostatitis, similar problems as in cat. I prostatitis have to be faced: due to the extremely low prevalence of these diseases, comparative data are lacking. Keeping in mind that due to their pharmacodynamic properties quinolones represent the therapy of choice, several non-controlled studies detail the application of quinolones [11,58–61], the follow-up and bacterial cure rates (Table 7.6). Current proposals for the treatment of cat. II prostatitis have therefore emphasized the need for further standardized evaluation [9].

Chronic pelvic pain syndrome (cat. IIIA and IIIB)

Relevant trials have been summarized in Table 7.4. It is, however, obvious that only a few trials meet the guidelines demanded in the recent consensus statement of the IPCN [44]. Particularly, antimicrobials representing the group of drugs prescribed most frequently in the treatment of this disease

Table 7.6   Relevant trials in chronic bacterial prostatitis

Author	Substance	Daily dosage (mg)	Duration of therapy (days)	*n*	Follow-up	Cure rate (%)
Pust *et al.* 1989 [58]	Ofloxacin	400	14	21	6–2 months	67
Schaeffer *et al.* 1990 [59]	Norfloxacin	800	28	14	6 months to 2 years	64
Weidner *et al.* 1991 [60]	Ciprofloxacin	1000	28	28	Median 30 months; maximum 36 months	63
Weidner *et al.* 1999 [11]	Ciprofloxacin	1000	28	40	Maximum 24 months	70–80
Naber *et al.* 2000 [61]	Ciprofloxacin	1000	28	65	9 months	60

[62] are inadequately investigated. Currently, a first prospective multicentre, randomized, blinded placebo-controlled trial has started comparing the most frequent therapeutic strategies in cat. III prostatitis: administration of antimicrobials and α-blockers. The initiators of this investigation have recently detailed the setting of the study in order to provide an example for a design according to IPCN and Chronic Prostatitis Collaborative Research Network (CPCRN) guidelines [63]. On the other hand, therapeutic strategies like repetitive prostatic massage and psychotherapy may be extremely useful, but are nearly impossible to be reasonably conducted as blinded studies.

Asymptomatic prostatitis (cat. IV)

Relevant trials to reduce PSA in asymptomatic prostatitis in order to differentiate between men with inflammation and those with prostatic carcinoma are summarized in Table 7.5.

Future developments

Acute and chronic bacterial prostatitis (cat. I and II)

Although numerous investigations are performed in order to develop new antimicrobial substances with high penetration rates into the prostatic tissue and with broad-spectrum efficacy against all etiologically involved pathogens, it is questionable that major breakthroughs will be made possible by this therapeutic strategy. Existing fluoroquinolones to date do possess these characteristics. The problem is not so much bacterial resistance but recurrence rates of about 30% in cases of chronic bacterial infection (Table 7.6). Therefore, further work-up has to integrate:
- alternative modes of application in order to achieve prolonged high tissue penetration of efficacious antimicrobials [64];
- the combination of antimicrobial treatment with methods to enhance the bactericidal performance of the antimicrobial substance [65];
- investigations evaluating supportive therapeutic strategies like enhancement of the specific and non-specific immune system.

Current literature analysing these items has reached either the level of *in vitro* studies or of animal models. Studies in humans are insufficiently designed to date.

Chronic pelvic pain syndrome (cat. IIIA and IIIB)

The most exciting advances are expected in the treatment of the CPPS. Under the auspices of the National Institute of Health (NIH) and following the constitution of the IPCN and CPCRN scientific research in this field has not only been accelerated but has standardized. Studies investigating this subject have to use the same classification system, acknowledged inclusion/exclusion criteria and symptomatic outcome measures [44,63]. Basic research studies will hopefully give new insights into the mostly unknown etiopathology of this disease and lead to new therapeutic strategies. Although now a number of prospective randomized double-blind studies exist to facilitate a reasonable therapy in this disease, symptomatic results often remain disappointing for both physicians and patients. Thus, advances in scientific research are urgently needed and should be made possible considering high standards of quality. As has been emphasized in this chapter, drug treatment can only represent one branch in the therapeutic strategy to be complemented by physical, invasive, manual, behavioural and surgical treatment options (Table 7.3) that even may require unconventional approaches to this disease.

Asymptomatic prostatitis (cat. IV)

The basic problem is to differentiate asymptomatic men with elevated PSA due to inflammation from those with prostatic cancer. Therefore, in the future, the critical question will be to provide a treatment algorithm both feasible to handle and sensitive enough to safely exclude prostatic carcinoma.

References

1 Nickel JC. Prostatitis: myths and realities. *Urology* 1998; **51**: 362–6.
2 Weidner W, Schiefer HG, Krauss H, Jantos C, Friedrich HJ, Altmannsberger M. Chronic prostatitis: a thorough search for etiologically involved microorganisms in 1461 patients. *Infection* 1991; **19**(Suppl. 3): 119–25.
3 Lopez-Plaza I, Bostwick DG. Prostatitis. In: Bostwick DG, ed. *Pathology of the prostate.* New York: Churchill Livingstone, 1990: 15–30.
4 Bergman B. On the relevance of gram-positive bacteria in prostatitis. *Infection* 1994; **22**(Suppl. 1): S22.
5 Nickel JC, Costerton JW. Coagulase-negative staphylococcus in chronic prostatitis. *J Urol* 1992; **147**: 398–401.
6 Meares EM. Acute and chronic prostatitis and prostatodynia. In: Fitzpatrick JM, Krane RJ eds. *The Prostate.* Edinburgh, London, Melbourne, New York: Churchill Livingstone, 1989: 63–75.
7 Joly-Gouillou ML, Lasry S. Practical recommendations for the drug treatment of bacterial infections of the male genital tract including urethritis, epididymitis and prostatitis. *Drugs* 1999; **57**: 743–50.
8 Madsen PO, Drescher P, Gasser TC. Basis for antibacterial treatment of prostatitis: experimental and clinical pharmacokinetic studies and models. In: Weidner W, Madsen PO, Schiefer HG eds. *Prostatitis.* Berlin, Heidelberg, New York, London, Paris, Tokyo, Hong Kong, Barcelona, Budapest: Springer, 1994: 110–22.

9 Bjerklund-Johansen TE, Grüneberg RN, Guibert J *et al*. The role of antibiotics in the treatment of chronic prostatitis: a consensus statement. *Eur Urol* 1998; **34**: 457–66.

10 Barbalias GA, Nikiforidis G, Liatsikos EN. α-blockers for the treatment of chronic prostatitis in combination with antibiotics. *J Urol* 1998; **159**: 883–7.

11 Weidner W, Ludwig M, Brähler E, Schiefer HG. Outcome of antibiotic therapy with ciprofloxacin in chronic bacterial prostatitis. *Drugs* 1999; **58**(Suppl. 2): 103–106.

12 Nickel JC, Olson ME, Barabas A *et al*. Pathogenesis of chronic bacterial prostatitis in an animal model. *Br J Urol* 1990; **66**: 47–54.

13 Ludwig M, Weidner W. Prostato-urethritis. In: Hofstetter A, ed. *Urogenitale Infektionen*. Berlin, Heidelberg, New York, Barcelona, Hong Kong, London, Maryland, Paris, Singapore, Tokyo: Springer, 1998: 297–319.

14 Krieger JN. Chronic urogenital infections in the man. *Urologe A* 1994; **33**: 196–202.

15 Nickel JC. Prostatitis: evolving management strategies. *Infect Urol* 1999; **26**: 737–51.

16 Nickel JC, Downey J, Johnston B *et al*. Predictors of patient response to antibiotic therapy for the chronic prostatitis/chronic pelvic pain syndrome: a prospective multicenter clinical trial. *J Urol* 2001; **165**; 1539–44.

17 Krieger JN, Riley DE. Bacteria in the chronic prostatitis-chronic pelvic pain syndrome: molecular approaches to critical research questions. *J Urol* 2002; **167**: 2574–83.

18 Shoskes DA, Zeitlin SI. Use of prostatic massage in combination with antibiotics in the treatment of chronic prostatitis. *Prostate Cancer Prostatic Dis* 1999; **2**: 159–62.

19 Mayo ME, Ross SO, Krieger JN. Few patients with "chronic prostatitis" have significant bladder outlet obstruction. *Urology* 1998; **52**: 417–21.

20 de la Rosette JJ, Karthaus HF, van Kerrebroeck PE, *et al*. Research in "prostatitis syndromes": the use of alfuzosin (a new 1-receptor-blocking agent) in patients mainly presenting with micturition complaints of an irritative nature and confirmed urodynamic abnormalities. *Eur Urol* 1992; **22**: 222–7.

21 Persson BE, Ronquist G. Evidence for a mechanistic association between nonbacterial prostatitis and levels of urate and creatinine in expressed prostatic secretions. *J Urol* 1996; **155**: 958-60.

22 Mehik A, Hellström P, Nickel JC *et al*. The chronic prostatitis-chronic pelvic pain syndrome can be characterized by prostatic tissue pressure measurements. *J Urol* 2002; **167**: 137–40.

23 Persson BE, Ronquist G, Ekblom M. Ameliorative effect of allopurinol on nonbacterial prostatitis: a parallel double-blind controlled study. *J Urol* 1996; **155**: 961–4.

24 Nickel JC, Siemens DR, Lundie JR. Allopurinol for prostatitis: where is the evidence? *Lancet* 1996, **347**: 1711.

25 Osborn DE, George JR, Rao PN *et al*. Prostatodynia – physical characteristics and rational management with muscle relaxants. *Br J Urol* 1981; **53**: 621–3.

26 Leskinen M, Lukkarinen O, Marttila T. Effects of finasteride in patients with inflammatory chronic pelvic pain syndrome: a double-blind, placebo-controlled, pilot study. *Urology* 1999; **53**: 502–505.

27 Miller JL, Rothman I, Bavendam TG *et al*. Prostatodynia and interstitial cystitis: one and the same? *Urology* 1995; **45**: 587–90.

28 Nickel JC, Johnston B, Downey J *et al*. Pentosan polysulfate therapy for chronic nonbacterial prostatitis (chronic pelvic pain syndrome category IIIA): a prospective multicenter clinical trial. *Urology* 2000; **56**: 413–17.

29 Satyanarayana K, Shoskes DA. A molecular injury-response model for the understanding of chronic disease. *Mol Med Today* 1999; **3**: 331–4.

30 Shoskes DA, Zeitlin SI, Shahed A *et al*. Quercetin in men with category III chronic prostatitis: a preliminary prospective, double-blind, placebo-controlled trial. *Urology* 1999; **54**: 960–63.

31   Chodirker WB, Tomasi TB. Gamma-globulins; quantitative relationships in human serum and nonvascular fluids. *Science* 1963; **142**: 1080–4.

32   Ludwig M, Schroeder-Printzen I, Schiefer HG *et al.* Immunologische Aspekte der akuten und chronischen Prostatitis. *Aktuelle Urol* 1995; **26**: 221–7.

33   Alexander RB, Ponniah S, Hasday J *et al.* Elevated levels of proinflammatory cytokines in the semen of patients with chronic prostatitis/chronic pelvic pain syndrome. *Urology* 1998; **52**: 744–9.

34   Hochreiter WW, Nadler RB, Koch AE *et al.* Evaluation of the cytokines interleukin 8 and epithelial neutrophil activating peptide 78 as indicators of inflammation in prostatic secretions. *Urology* 2000; **56**: 1025–9.

35   Nadler RB, Koch AE, Calhoun EA *et al.* IL-1β and TNF-α in prostatic secretions are indicators in the evaluation of men with chronic prostatitis. *J Urol* 2000; **164**: 214–18.

36   John H, Barghorn A, Funke G *et al.* Noninflammatory chronic pelvic pain syndrome: immunological study in blood, ejaculate and prostatic tissue. *Eur Urol* 2001; **39**: 72–8.

37   Orhan I, Onur R, Ilhan N *et al.* Seminal plasma cytokine levels in the diagnosis of chronic pelvic pain syndrome. *Int J Urol* 2001; **8**: 495–9.

38   Shahed AR, Shoskes DA. Correlation of β-endorphin and prostaglandin E2 levels in prostatic fluid of patients with chronic prostatitis with diagnosis and treatment response. *J Urol* 2001; **166**: 1738–41.

39   Miller LJ, Fischer KA, Goralnick SJ *et al.* Nerve growth factor and chronic prostatitis/chronic pelvic pain syndrome. *Urology* 2002; **59**: 603–608.

40   Miller LJ, Fischer KA, Goralnick SJ *et al.* Interleukin-10 levels in seminal plasma: implications for chronic prostatitis-chronic pelvic pain syndrome. *J Urol* 2002; **167**: 753–6.

41   Ponniah S, Arah I, Alexander RB. PSA is a candidate self-antigen in autoimmune chronic prostatitis/chronic pelvic pain syndrome. *Prostate* 2000; **44**: 49–54.

42   Rugendorff EW, Weidner W, Ebeling L *et al.* Results of treatment with pollen extract (Cernilton® N) in chronic prostatitis and prostatodynia. *Br J Urol* 1993; **71**: 433–8.

43   Meares EM. Nonbacterial prostatitis and prostatodynia. In: Lepor H, Lawson RK eds. *Prostate Diseases*. Philadelphia, London, Toronto, Montreal, Sydney, Tokyo: Saunders, 1993: 419–24.

44   Nickel JC, Nyberg LM, Hennenfent M. Research guidelines for chronic prostatitis: consensus report from the first National Institutes of Health International Prostatitis Collaborative Network. *Urology* 1999; **54**: 229–33.

45   Socher S, O'Leary MP, Richie JP *et al.* Prevalence of prostatitis in men undergoing biopsy for elevated PSA or abnormal digital rectal exam. *J Urol Suppl* 1996; **155**: 425A.

46   Schatteman PHF, Hoekx L, Wyndaele JJ *et al.* Inflammation in prostate biopsies of men without prostatic malignancy or clinical prostatitis. *Eur Urol* 2000; **37**: 404–12.

47   Letran JL, Brawer MK. Prostate specific antigen and prostatitis. In: Nickel JC, ed. *Textbook of Prostatitis*. Oxford: Isis Medical Media, 1999: 241–4.

48   Potts JM. Prospective identification of National Institutes of Health category IV prostatitis in men with elevated prostate specific antigen. *J Urol* 2000; **164**: 1550–53.

49   Clinical effectiveness group (Association of Genitourinary Medicine and the Medical Society for the study of veneral diseases). National guideline for the treatment of prostatitis. *Sex Transm Infect* 1999; **75**(Suppl. 1): 46–50.

50   Martin DH, Mroczkowski TF, Dalu ZA *et al.* A controlled trial of a single dose of azithromycin for the treatment of chlamydial urethritis and cervicitis. *N Engl J Med* 1992; **327**: 921–5.

51   Stamm WE, Hicks CB, Martin DH *et al.* Azithromycin for empirical treatment of the nongonococcal urethritis syndrome in men. A randomized double-blind study. *JAMA* 1995; **274**: 545–9.

52 Lacquaniti S, Destitto A, Servello C *et al.* Terazosine and tamsulosin in non bacterial prostatitis: a randomized placebo-controlled study. *Arch Ital Urol Androl* 1999; **71**: 283–5.

53 Neal DE, Moon TD. Use of terazosin in prostatodynia and validation of a symptom score questionnaire. *Urology* 1994; **43**: 460–65.

54 Canale D, Turchi P, Giorgi PM *et al.* Treatment of abacterial prostato-vesiculitis with nimesulide. *Drugs* 1993; **46**: 147–50.

55 Karazanashvili G, Managadze L. Prostate-specific antigen (PSA) value change after anti-bacterial therapy of prostate inflammation, as a dignostic method for prostate cancer screening in cases of PSA value within 4–10 ng/ml and nonsuspicious results of digital rectal examination. *Eur Urol* 2001; **39**: 538–43.

56 Bozeman CB, Carver BS, Eastham JA *et al.* Treatment of chronic prostatitis lowers serum prostate specific antigen. *J Urol* 2002; **167**: 1723–6.

57 Neal DE Jr. Treatment of acute prostatitis. In: Nickel JC, ed. *Textbook of Prostatitis*. Oxford: Isis Medical Media, 1999: 279–84.

58 Pust RA, Ackenheil-Koppe HR, Gilbert P *et al.* Clinical efficacy of ofloxacin (Tarivid®) in patients with chronic bacterial prostatitis: preliminary results. *J Chemother* 1989; **1**(Suppl. 4): 869–71.

59 Schaeffer AJ, Darras FS. The efficacy of norfloxacin in the treatment of chronic bacterial prostatitis refractory to trimethoprim–sulfamethoxazole and for carbicilline. *J Urol* 1990; **144**: 690–93.

60 Weidner W, Schiefer HG, Brähler E. Refractory chronic bacterial prostatitis: a reevaluation of ciprofloxacin treatment after a median follow-up of 30 months. *J Urol* 1991; **146**: 350–52.

61 Naber KG, Busch W, Focht J, the German Prostatitis Study Group. Ciprofloxacin in the treatment of chronic bacterial prostatitis: a prospective, non-comparative multicentre clinical trial with long-term follow-up. *Int J Antimicrob Agents* 2000; **14**: 143–9.

62 McNaughton Collins, Fowler FJ, Elliott DB *et al.* Diagnosing and treating chronic prostatitis: do urologists use the four-glass test? *Urology* 2000; **55**: 403–407.

63 Propert KJ, Alexander RB, Nickel JC *et al.* Design of a multicenter randomized clinical trial for chronic prostatitis/chronic pelvic pain syndrome. *Urology* 2002; **59**: 870–76.

64 Bahk JY, Hyun JS, Lee JY *et al.* Concentrations of ofloxacin in canine prostate tissue and prostate fluid after intraprostatic injection of biodegradable sustained-releasing microspheres containing ofloxacin. *J Urol* 2000; **163**: 1560–64.

65 Sahin A, Eiley D, Goldfischer ER *et al.* The in vitro bactericidal effect of microwave energy on bacteria that cause prostatitis. *Urology* 1998; **52**: 411–16.

8: Perioperative Antimicrobial Prophylaxis in Urological Interventions of the Urinary and Male Genital Tract

Kurt G. Naber

Introduction

Almost 50 years after its introduction, perioperative antimicrobial prophylaxis is still controversial. Whereas a clear benefit was established for certain surgical operations especially for those of the categories 'clean-contaminated' and 'contaminated', e.g. elective colonic surgery [1], there is no general consensus on the use of antimicrobial prophylaxis for elective operations of the category 'clean', because studies including enough patients for meaningful statistical analysis are missing. Moreover, the traditional classification of surgical procedures according to Cruse [2] into 'clean', 'clean-contaminated', 'contaminated' and 'dirty' does not adequately describe the risk of infection. Numerous patient's and surgical conditions, such as duration of operation, blood loss, have been demonstrated to correlate with risk of infection [3]. Such risk factors can also lead to infectious complications even in 'clean' operations [4]. However, the significance of each factor is not yet quantified. This is especially true for open operations and endoscopic procedures in urology [5].

Appropriate prospective randomized studies are missing. At present, most studies are poorly designed. The differentiation between therapy and prophylaxis is not clear. Evaluation of risk factors is unsatisfactory, and the terms 'bacteriuria' and 'infection' are used uncritically. In addition, many of these studies lack knowledge of pharmacokinetics and pharmacodynamics of the antimicrobial agents, bacterial pathogenicity and resistance and the role of nosocomial infections. It is thus not surprising that the literature is inconclusive in regard to prophylaxis, showing negative as well as positive results for every kind of urological intervention.

A survey of 320 German urologists revealed controversial opinions about perioperative antimicrobial prophylaxis [6]. It was administered in more than half of the procedures involving the urinary tract, and most urologists did use prophylaxis when opening the intestine. There was, however, little agreement on the choice of antimicrobials and the duration of prophylaxis. Consequently, guidelines for the indication of perioperative prophylaxis in urology are certainly necessary.

In this chapter we present practical recommendations. These recommendations are based on clinical studies, expert opinion and professional consensus. The common principles for perioperative prophylaxis (Table 8.1), a result of a consensus conference of the Paul Ehrlich Society for Chemotherapy [7], were also considered. They also considered the recommendations of other societies, such as Paul Ehrlich Society for Chemotherapy [8], Association Français d'Urologie [9], Swedish–Norwegian Consensus Group [10] and the European Association of Urology [11].

Goals of perioperative antimicrobial prophylaxis

The aim of perioperative prophylaxis is to limit infection related to intervention. However, it can never compensate for poor hygiene and operative technique. Antimicrobial prophylaxis is only one component of infection prevention management. Other important factors should not be neglected, e.g. catheter care, closed drainage system [12].

The end points of perioperative prophylaxis in urology are debatable. It is generally agreed that its main aim in urology is to prevent symptomatic/febrile genitourinary infections, such as acute pyelonephritis, prostatitis, epididymitis and urosepsis, as well as serious wound infections. Should this be extended to include postoperative asymptomatic bacteriuria or even a small wound infection, which could easily be treated on an outpatient

Table 8.1 General aspects of perioperative antimicrobial prophylaxis [7]

Perioperative antimicrobial prophylaxis is an important factor for quality control of operative procedures.

The primary aim of perioperative prophylaxis is to limit postoperative infectious complications. This includes local, e.g. wound infection, as well as systemic infections, e.g. deep respiratory and UTIs.

Perioperative antimicrobial prophylaxis should be adapted to the risk of the individual patient.

The risk of infection starts at the beginning of the operation. Considering the pharmacokinetics of the substance, an effective antimicrobial concentration has to be maintained throughout the whole period at risk.

Too early administration of the antimicrobial is not useful, probably even harmful.

An antimicrobial substance is selected according to the risk for infection (expected pathogens and individual patient's risk) and the regional epidemiology. Of specific interest are secondary infections due to Gram-negative bacteria.

For perioperative antimicrobial prophylaxis only substances that turned out to be effective in controlled clinical studies should be selected.

For the individual patient emergence of resistant pathogens may be of minimal risk, but this is not true for the entire hospital.

---

basis? On the other hand, is prevention of postoperative pneumonia and sepsis also an issue of perioperative prophylaxis? Certainly, perioperative antimicrobial prophylaxis in urology has to go beyond the traditional aim of prophylaxis, which is prevention of wound infections [13].

In transurethral resection (TUR) of the prostate, several controlled studies have shown that the rate of postoperative bacteriuria can be reduced by perioperative prophylaxis. In some studies, this translated into reduction of symptomatic urinary tract infections (UTIs) or prevention of febrile episodes [14–18]. Moreover, since the rate of septic complications is generally below 1%, a prospective study requires large numbers of patients to be recruited to reach statistical power. Until now most of our knowledge on the prevention of urosepsis has come from retrospective studies only [19].

Indications for perioperative antimicrobial prophylaxis

The need for prophylaxis depends not only on the type of intervention but also on the individual risk for each individual patient. Patient's risk factors, such as chronic debility, diabetes mellitus, immunosuppression, increased risk for endocarditis in patients with artificial cardiac valves, have to be considered.

Increased exposure to endogenous bacteria can be expected in procedures that include bowel segments and transrectal biopsy of the prostate and in contaminated tissue. Furthermore, bacterial contamination in the urinary tract is often associated with long-term drainage (e.g. catheter, splints, nephrostoma) or with obstruction due to urolithiasis, tumours, etc. (Table 8.2). In infected stones pretreated with antimicrobials, persistence of pathogens within the stone must be considered even if the preoperative urine is sterile.

In the absence of risk factors and with sterile urine, prophylaxis may not be necessary. However, if the anticipated risk changes during operation (e.g. high blood loss, duration of operation longer than 2–3 h, accidental perforation of the intestine or the urinary tract), intraoperative administration of

Table 8.2 General risk factors

Risk factors due to Patient's condition	Increased bacterial load
Reduced general condition	OP using bowel segments
Metabolic dysfunction, e.g. diabetes mellitus	Transrectal biopsy of the prostate
Immunosuppression	Long-term urinary tract drainage
Special risk, e.g. artificial cardiac valve	Urinary obstruction
Reoperation	

antimicrobials should be considered. In the preoperative work-up of the patient any infection, especially of the urinary tract, should be identified. If an infection is present and the intervention cannot be delayed, antimicrobial therapy should be given on an empirical basis before surgery and continued afterwards, preferably according to sensitivity testing, when it becomes available.

From a microbiological point of view, any perioperative antimicrobial prophylaxis represents a compromise. The desired effect of reducing the bacterial load has to be balanced against the negative consequences, e.g. drug-induced adverse events and possible selection of resistant strains (Fig. 8.1).

Timing and duration of perioperative antimicrobial prophylaxis

Basic studies [20–22] have shown that wound infections are usually prevented by administration of an antimicrobial before contamination takes place. High blood levels are needed at the start of the surgical procedure and therefore timing and dosing are important factors [23]. In clinical practice, the best time for administration is 30–60 min before start of operation, i.e. when anaesthesia is initiated, if the antimicrobial is given intravenously. If intraoperative complications occur, the antimicrobial should be given immediately. This approach has been particularly effective in emergency general surgery [24].

Clinical studies have shown a significant increase of postoperative infections if the single prophylactic dose of any antimicrobial is not given within 2 h before or after the start of the operation [21]. Any antimicrobial given after wound closure will not alter the rate of wound infection. Only the rate of adverse events and the selection pressure for antimicrobial resistance will increase. There are, however, no studies demonstrating specifically such a correlation in endoscopic procedures. Extrapolation of these results, however, seems reasonable.

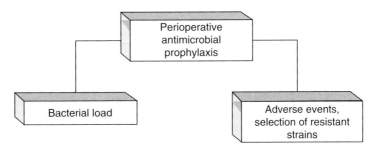

Figure 8.1 Perioperative antimicrobial prophylaxis has to be balanced between reduction of bacterial load on one hand and increase of adverse events and selection of resistant strains on the other hand.

Generally, a single full dose of a suitable antimicrobial will be as effective as multiple dosing. Only in the case of prolonged intervention (> 2.5–3 h) is an additional dose whose size and timing are dictated by the pharmacokinetics required. Antimicrobial prophylaxis should not be continued for more than 24 h [7–11,25–27]. The administration of antimicrobials for more than 1 day is not considered to be prophylaxis, but therapy. This may become necessary in case of severe contamination. Also, interventional therapy becomes necessary.

Choice of antimicrobials

A suitable antimicrobial should be highly effective, well-tolerated and cheap. Its antimicrobial spectrum should include the expected range of normal flora and pathogens usually found at the site of operation and on the surrounding skin and mucous membranes. In patients with preceding antimicrobial therapy, account should be taken of the altered bacterial spectrum and its resistance pattern (Table 8.2).

Broad-spectrum antimicrobials, such as third-generation cephalosporins, acylaminopenicillins plus beta-lactamase inhibitor (BLI) and carbapenems, should only be used sparingly, e.g. if the site of operation is contaminated with multiresistant bacteria. Usually, their administration should be restricted to the treatment of severe infections [25,27]. This applies also to the routine use of vancomycin in prophylaxis, such as in patients on dialysis or with suspected infections caused by venous catheters, because such policy may select vancomycin-resistant enterococci.

The choice of the antimicrobial also depends on its pharmacokinetic properties, and dosage should secure effective tissue levels during the operation. Depending on the antimicrobial's half-life and the duration of the intervention, an additional dose may be indicated. For urological indications it is advisable to choose a drug with high urinary concentrations.

Mode of application

Parenteral and preferably intravenous administration of the antimicrobial is primarily recommended, to reach sufficient tissue concentrations, particularly in an emergency. Oral administration of fluoroquinolone in patients undergoing TUR and transrectal biopsy of the prostate is also successful [18,28]. Oral antimicrobials with high bioavailability should only be administered if intestinal reabsorption is secured. Fluoroquinolones of group 2 or 3, according to the classification of the Paul Ehrlich Society for Chemotherapy [29], are suitable, which also can be used for systemic therapy and are highly excreted by the kidneys. From a pharmacoeconomic aspect, oral application 1–2 h before the procedure is an attractive alternative.

Recommendations according to type of urological interventions

For perioperative antimicrobial prophylaxis, the urological interventions are categorized into open and endoscopic-instrumental operations (including extracorporal shock wave lithotripsy (ESWL)) and diagnostic procedures (Table 8.3). The recommended antimicrobials are shown in Table 8.4.

Urological operations including bowel segments

Intestinal microorganisms are usually responsible for development of postoperative infections after operations that include intestinal segments. The most frequent are *Escherichia coli* and other Enterobacteriaceae, enterococci, anaerobes and streptococci, as well as staphylococci in wound infections. Therefore aminopenicillins combined with BLI and second-generation cephalosporins, in combination with metronidazole, are recommended; correspondingly in high-risk patients, acylaminopenicillins combined with BLI and third-generation cephalosporins.

It is a matter of discussion, but not proved by clinical studies, whether continent pouches or bladder replacements require prolonged postoperative

Table 8.3 Classification of urological operations/interventions

1 Open operations
   - Urinary tract including bowel segments
   - Urinary tract without bowel segments
   - Outside the urinary tract
     Special operations:
     Using implants, e.g. penis and sphincter prosthesis
     Reconstructive genital operations
     Acute operation
     Secondary operation
2 Endoscopic-instrumental operations
   - Prostate
   - Bladder
   - Ureter and kidney
   - Percutaneous litholapaxy
   - Laparoscopic operations
   - Extracorporal shock wave lithotripsy
3 Diagnostic interventions
   - Prostate biopsy
     Transrectal
     Perineal
   - Urethrocystoscopy
   - Ureterorenoscopy
   - Percutaneous pyeloscopy
   - Laparoscopic procedures

Table 8.4 Recommendations for perioperative antimicrobial prophylaxis in urological interventions

Procedure	Most common pathogen(s)	Antimicrobial(s) of choice	Alternative antimicrobial(s)	Remarks
1 Open operations				
Urinary tract including bowel segments	Enterobacteriaceae, enterococci, anaerobes, streptococci, wound infection (straphylococci)	Aminopenicillin + BLI, cephalosporins 2° + metronidazole	In high-risk patients: cephalosporin 3°, acylaminopenicillin + BLI	In all patients
Urinary tract without bowel segments	Enterobacteriaceae, enterococci, wound infection (staphylococci)	Fluoroquinolone,* cephalosporin 2°, aminopenicillin + BLI	In high-risk patients: cephalosporin 3°, acylaminopenicillin + BLI	In patients with increased risk of infection
Implant/prosthesis, penis, sphincter	Staphylococci	Cephalosporin 1°/2°		In all patients
2 reconstructive genital operation	Staphylococci	Cephalosporin 1°/2°		In secondary operations and in patients with increased risk of infection
Other interventions outside of the urinary tract	Staphylococci	Cephalosporin 1°/2°		In patients with increased risk of infection
3 Endoscopic-instrumental operations				
Prostate, bladder, ureter, kidney, incl. percutaneous litholapaxy and ESWL, laparoscopic operations	Enterobacteriaceae, staphylococci, enterococci	fluoroquinolone,* aminopenicillin + BLI, cephalosporin 2°, fosfomycin, trometamol	Co-trimoxazole	In patients with increased risk of infection
4 Diagnostic interventions				
Transrectal biopsy of the prostate (with thick needle)	Enterobacteriaceae, enterococci, anaerobes, streptococci	Fluoroquinolone,* aminopenicillin + BLI, cephalosporin 2°+ metronidazole	Aminoglycoside	In all patients
Perineal biopsy of the prostate, urethrocystoscopy, ureterorenoscopy, percutaneous pyeloscopy, laparoscopic procedures	Enterobacteriaceae, enterococci, staphylococci	Fluoroquinolone, *aminopenicillin + BLI, cephalosporin 2°	Co-trimoxazole	In patients with increased risk of infection

*Fluoroquinolone with sufficient renal excretion; BLI, beta-lactamase inhibitor; ESWL, extracorporal shock wave lithotripsy.

'preventive antimicrobial therapy'. Indwelling catheters and regular irrigation of the colonized intestinal segment (neobladder) with increase of pressure could result in postoperative bacteraemia. Local antimicrobial irrigation is, however, not recommended.

Urological operations without bowel segments

General antimicrobial prophylaxis is not required in open operations without bowel segments. It is necessary only in patients with an increased risk of infection (Table 8.2). The most frequent infecting organism is *E. coli* followed by enterococci, *Proteus* spp. and *Klebsiella* spp. in the urinary tract and staphylococci for wound infections. In case of preceding antimicrobial therapy even for remote infections, selection of resistant bacterial strains and, if the patient is hospitalized for a longer time, the bacterial spectrum of nosocomial pathogens must also be taken into consideration (Table 8.5).

A perioperative antimicrobial regime recommended for prophylaxis according to the expected range of pathogens includes fluoroquinolones with sufficient renal excretion, aminopenicillins with BLI or second-generation cephalosporins. Third-generation cephalosporins or acylaminopenicillins with BLI are available as alternatives for patients with an increased risk of infection, when treated previously with an antimicrobial or with permanent catheter or nephrostomy drainage.

Urological operations outside of the urinary tract

Perioperative antimicrobial prophylaxis is not generally recommended except in long reconstructive operations on the genital area or with implant surgery (artificial urinary sphincter or penile prosthesis). It can be achieved with first- or second-generation cephalosporins, since staphylococcal infection predominates. In elective operations, in which any wound infection may become a serious event, e.g. loss of implant, the patient might be screened preoperatively for methicillin-resistant *Staphylococcus aureus* (MRSA) by a nasal swab.

Table 8.5 Most common pathogens causing nosocomial urinary tract infections	
	Escherichia coli
	Proteus mirabilis
	Enterococci
	Pseudomonas spp.
	Staphylococci
	(Candida spp.)

Endourological operations (including ESWL)

Perioperative prophylaxis is only recommended in cases with increased risk of infection (Table 8.1). Appropriate antimicrobial regimens are fluoroquinolones with sufficient renal excretion, aminopenicillins with BLI, second-generation cephalosporins and cotrimoxazole. Comparative studies of short-term prophylaxis using fluoroquinolones versus cotrimoxazole are not available. Perioperative prophylaxis in patients without risk factors is questionable.

Diagnostic urological interventions

Perioperative antimicrobial prophylaxis, e.g. with an aminopenicillin plus a BLI, a fluoroquinolone with sufficient renal excretion [28,29] or an aminoglycoside [30], is generally recommended only in transrectal prostate biopsy. In other diagnostic procedures of the urinary tract, prophylaxis is only suggested in high-risk patients. A fluoroquinolone or cotrimoxazole is appropriate.

Postoperative drainage of the urinary tract

When continuous urinary drainage is left in place after operation, prolongation of perioperative antimicrobial prophylaxis is not indicated [31]. Asymptomatic bacteriuria has only to be treated before any urinary tract intervention or when the drainage tube is removed. In case of short-term catheterization and persistent asymptomatic bacteriuria in female patients a short-term antimicrobial regimen is sufficient [32].

Pharmacoeconomics

The results of the largest study performed worldwide for control of nosocomial infections (SENIC) have shown that UTIs (42%), followed by wound infections (24%), are the most frequent cause of infective postoperative complications [33]. If these can be prevented, there is obviously great potential for cost reduction in surgery. However, cost-benefit considerations of perioperative antimicrobial prophylaxis have not been fully addressed. One exception is a meta-analysis of eight prospective randomized controlled trials in ESWL, where a 50% reduction of median risk of UTI occurred in patients treated with prophylaxis compared with those not treated (2.1% vs a median risk of 5.7%). This difference was statistically significant ($p = 0.0005$), and the authors calculated a cost benefit for those patients who received prophylaxis [34]. Similar studies, e.g. for TUR of the prostate and of bladder tumours, are missing. Nevertheless, an appreciation of cost saving by perioperative prophylaxis can only be evaluated by suitable studies.

References

1 Clarke IS, Condon RE *et al*. Preoperative oral antimicrobials reduce septic complications of colon operations: results of a prospective, double-blind clinical study. *Ann Surg* 1979; **186**: 251–9.

2 Cruse PJE, Foord R. The epidemiology of wound infection: a 10-year old prospective study of 62,939 wounds. *Surg Clin North Am* 1980; **60**: 27–40.

3 Vogel F, Naber KG, Wacha H, Shah P *et al*. and an expert group of the Paul Ehrlich Society for Chemotherapy. Parenterale Antibiotika bei Erwachsenen. *Chemother J* 1999; **8**: 3–56.

4 Culver DH, Horan TC, Gaynes RP *et al*. Surgical wound infection rates by wound class, operative procedure, and patient risk index. *Am J Med* 1991; **91**(Suppl. 3B): 152S–7S.

5 Knopf H-J, Weib P, Schäfer W, Funke P-J. Nosocomial infections after transurethral prostatectomy. *Eur Urol* 1999; **36**: 207–12.

6 Bruns T, Höchel S, Tauber R. Perioperative Antibiotikaprohylaxe in der operativen Urologie. *Urologe B* 1998; **38**: 269–72.

7 Wacha H, Görtz G, Hell K, Hoyme U *et al*. Standortbestimmung zur Antibiotikaprophylaxe bei chirurgischen Eingriffen. *Zentralbl Chir* 1998; **123**: 1188–90.

8 Naber KG, Hofstetter AG, Brühl P, Bichler KH, Lebert C. Guidelines for the perioperative prophylaxis in urological interventions of the urinary and male genital tract. *Int J Antimicrob Agents* 2001; **17**: 321–6.

9 Société Francaise d'Anesethésie et de Réanimation (SFAR). Recommandations pour la pratique de l'antibioprophylaxie en chirurgie. Actualisation 1999. *Pyrexie* 1999; **3**: 21–30.

10 Swedish–Norwegian Consensus Group. Antimicrobial prophylaxis in surgery: summary of a Swedish–Norwegian consensus conference. *Scand J Infect Dis* 1998; **30**: 547–57.

11 Members of the UTI Working Group: Naber KG, Bergman B, Bishop MC, Bjerklund-Johansen TE, Botto H, Lobel B, Cruz FJ, Selvaggi FP. EAU guidelines for the management of urinary and male genital tract infections. *Eur Urol* 2001; **40**: 576–88.

12 Daschner F, Chiarello LA, Dettenkofer M, Fabry J, Francioli P, Knopf H-J, Mehtar S, Murphy C. Hygiene and infection control of nosocomial catheter-associated urinary tract infection. In: Naber KG, Pechere JC, Kumazawa J, Khoury S, Gerberding JL, Schaeffer AJ, eds. *Nosocomial Health Care Associated Infections in Urology*. Plymouth: Health Publication, Plymbridge Distributors, 2001: 105–18.

13 Larsen EH, Gasser TC, Madsen PO. Antibiotikaprophylaxe bei operativen Eingriffen in der Urologie. *Extracta urologica* 1989; **12**: 340–63.

14 Berry A, Barra HA. Prophylactic antibiotic use in transurethral prostatic resection: a meta-analysis. *J Urol* 2002; **167**: 571–7.

15 Hargreave TB, Hindmarsh JR, Elton R *et al*. Short term prophylaxis with cefotaxime for prostatic surgery. *Br Med J* 1982; **284**: 1008–10.

16 Hargreave TB, Botto H, Rikken GHJM, Hindmarsh JR, Mc Dermott TED, Mjolnerod OK, Petays P, Schalkhäuser K, Stellos A. European collaborative study of antibiotic prophylaxis for transurethral resection of prostate. *Eur Urol* 1993; **23**: 437–43.

17 Raz R, Almog D, Elhanan G, Shental J. The use of ceftriaxon in the prevention of urinary tract infection in patients undergoing transurethral resection of the prostate (TUR-P). *Infection* 1994; **22**: 347–9.

18 Shearman CP, Silverman SH, Johnson M, Young CH, Farrar DJ, Keighley MRB, Burdon DW. Single dose, oral antibiotic cover for transurethral prostatectomy. *Br J Urol* 1988; **62**: 424–38.

19   Del Rio G, Dalet F, Chechile G. Antimicrobial prophylaxis in urologic surgery: does it give some benefit? *Eur Urol* 1993; **24**: 305–11.

20   Burke JF. The effective period of preventive antibiotic action in experimental incisions and dermal lesions. *Surgery* 1961; **50**: 161–8.

21   Classen DC, Evans RS, Pestotink SL, Horn SD, Menlove RL, Burke JP. The timing of prophylactic administration of antibiotics and the risk of surgical wound infection. *N Engl J Med* 1992; **326**: 281–6.

22   Miles AA, Miles EM, Burke J. The value and duration of defense reactions of the skin to the primary lodgement of bacteria. *Br J Exp Pathol* 1957; **38**: 79–96.

23   Bergamini TM, Polk HC Jr. The importance of tissue antibiotic activity in the prevention of operative wound infection. *J Antimicrob Chemother* 1998; **23**: 301–13.

24   Bates T, Siller G, Crathern BC, Bradley SP, Zlotnik RD, Couch C, James RDG, Kaye CM. Timing of prophylactic antibiotics in abdominal surgery: trial of a pre-operative versus an intraoperative first dose. *Br J Surg* 1989; **76**: 52–6.

25   ASHP Commission on Therapeutics. ASHP therapeutic guidelines on antimicrobial prophylaxis in surgery. *Clin Pharm* 1992; **11**: 483–513.

26   Dellinger EP, Gross PA *et al.* Quality standard for antimicrobial prophylaxis in surgical procedures. *Infect Control Hosp Epidemiol* 1994; **15**: 182–8.

27   DGKH. Empfehlungen der DGKH zur perioperativen Antibiotikaprophylaxe. *Hyg Med* 1994; **19**: 213–22.

28   Kapoor DA, Klimberg IW, Malek GH, Wegenke JD, Cox CE, Patterson AL, Graham E, Echols RM, Whalen E, Kowalsky SF. Single-dose oral ciprofloxacin versus placebo for prophylaxis during transrectal prostate biopsy. *Urology* 1998; **52**: 552–8.

29   Naber KG, Adam D. Classification of fluoroquinolones. *Int J Antimicrob Agents* 1998; **10**: 255–7.

30   Rodriguez LV, Terris MK. Risks and complications of transrectal ultrasound biopsy. *Curr Opin Urol* 2000; **10**: 111–16.

31   Martius J, Brühl P, Dettenkofer M, Hartenauer U *et al.* Empfehlungen zur Prävention und Kontrolle Katheter-assoziierter Harnwegsinfektionen. *Bundesgesundheitsbl – Gesundheitsforsch – Gesundheitsschutz* 1999; **42**: 806–809.

32   Harding GKM, Nicolle LE, Ronald AR, Psiksaitis JK *et al.* How long should catheter-acquired urinary tract infection in women be treated? *Ann Intern Med* 1991; **1**(14): 713–19.

33   SENIC. NNIS National Infections Surveillance Report. NNIS-report, data summary from October 1986 – April 1996, issued May 1996. *Am J Infect Control* 2000; **24**: 380–88.

34   Pearle MS, Roehrborn CG. Antimicrobial prophylaxis prior to shock wave lithotripsy in patients with sterile urine before treatment: a meta-analysis and cost-effectiveness analysis. *Urology* 1997; **49**: 679–86.

9: Candiduria

Jack D. Sobel

Introduction

Since the 1980s, there has been a marked increase in opportunistic fungal pathogens involving the urinary tract, of which *Candida* species are the most prevalent [1–5]. The kidney and the urinary tract become infected as a result of haematogenous spread or from an ascending infection, usually in the presence of urinary obstruction. *Candida* species are common causes of ascending infection in catheterized and obstructed urinary tracts, particularly in diabetics. Patients receiving immunosuppression therapy for renal transplantation are at risk for invasive fungal urinary tract infection (UTI) caused by *Candida*, Aspergillus and Cryptococcus species. The acquired immunodeficiency syndrome (AIDS) is associated with mucosal *Candida* infections but not with candiduria; however, disseminated histoplasmosis and cryptococcosis, both common complications of AIDS, frequently involve the urinary tract.

Candida species are the main fungal species commonly associated with urethritis, cystitis and pyelonephritis. Nevertheless, many species of fungi can cause prostatitis, epididymitis, chronic bladder inflammation or ulceration, and ureteric obstruction. In the absence of obstruction, *Candida* infections rarely cause renal insufficiency. Fungal infection should always be considered in the differential diagnosis of filling defects in the collecting system.

Epidemiology

Candida frequently exists as saprophytes on the external genitalia or urethra; however, yeast in measurable quantities are found in < 1% of clean voided urine specimens. *Candida* infections currently account for 5% of urine isolates in the general hospital and 10% of positive urinary cultures in tertiary care centres [3]. Candiduria is especially common in the intensive care unit (ICU), and may represent the most common urinary infection in surgical ICUs [4]. Presently, 10–15% of nosocomial UTIs are caused by *Candida* species [5–7]. Platt *et al.* showed that 26.5% of all urinary infections related to indwelling catheters were due to fungi [2]. Rivett *et al.* found that 2% of urine specimens submitted to a hospital microbiology laboratory were positive for yeast, versus 11% in the leukaemia and bone marrow transplantation unit from the same hospital [3]. Nosocomial candidiasis is also common in the neonatal and paediatric ICU [6]. Most positive cultures are isolated or transient and represent colonization rather than true infection; however, candiduria may lead to symptomatic UTI and/or fungaemia.

Microbiology

Candida albicans is the most common fungal species isolated from the urine and in one study was found in 446 (52%) of 861 patients with funguria [4]. *Candida glabrata* accounts for 25–35% of infections whereas 8–28% of infections are due to *Candida tropicalis*, *Candida krusei* and *Candida parapsilosis* (Table 9.1) [4,7,8]. Unusual species are common in hospitalized patients, especially diabetics, with chronic indwelling bladder catheters. Mixed infections caused by more than one *Candida* species are not infrequent, as is concomitant bacteriuria.

Pathogenesis

Candida infections of the urinary tract generally occur in the presence of predisposing factors or in immunocompromised hosts (Table 9.2) [4,9]. Most infections are associated with the use of indwelling urinary devices including Foley catheters, internal stents and percutaneous nephrostomy tubes. Diabetics have an increased overall risk of UTI for both bacterial and fungal infection [2,4]. *Candida* growth in urine is enhanced when urinary levels of glucose exceed 150 mg/dl. Diabetic females have higher perineal and periurethral *Candida* colonization rates. Diabetics also have impaired phagocytic and fungicidal activity of neutrophils; however, the dominant predisposing factor to candiduria is increased instrumentation, urinary stasis and obstruction secondary to autonomic neuropathy.

Yeast species	Number (%) of patients
Candida albicans	446 (51.8)
Candida glabrata	134 (15.6)
Candida tropicalis	68 (7.9)
Candida parapsilosis	35 (4.1)
Candida krusei	9 (1)
Others	20 (2.3)
Undetermined	184 (21.4)

Table 9.1 Initial yeast isolates from urine of 8651 patients with funguria*

*Kauffman *et al.* [4].

Table 9.2 Risk factors for *Candida* UTI

	Route	Risk factors
Renal candidiasis	Haematogenous (anterograde)	Neutropenia (prolonged), intravascular drug use, burns, recent surgery (abdominal thoracic), systemic infection
Candida lower UTI	Ascending (retrograde)	Foley catheter, female gender, extremes of age, instrumentation, diabetes mellitus, obstruction/stasis, recent antibacterial therapy, recent bacterial UTI, urinary stent, nephrostomy tube, renal transplantation
Candida pyelonephritis	Ascending	Diabetes, obstruction/stasis, instrumentation, postoperative, nephrostomy tube, ureteral stent, nephrolithiasis

Antibiotic therapy has a major role in predisposing to candiduria. No antibiotic appears exempt from this complication, although there is higher risk either with prolonged use or with broad-spectrum agents. By suppressing susceptible endogenous bacterial flora in the gastrointestinal and lower genital tract, antibiotic use results in the emergence of fungi colonizing these epithelial surfaces with ready access to the urinary tract especially in the presence of indwelling bladder catheters.

Most lower UTIs are caused by genital or perineal colonization with retrograde infection from an indwelling catheter. The upper urinary tract may rarely become involved via ascending infection and then usually only in the presence of urinary obstruction, reflux or diabetes.

The majority of cases of renal candidiasis occur not as a result of ascending spread from the lower urinary tract but as a consequence of haematogenous seeding of the renal parenchyma. *Candida* species express a tropism for the kidney. An autopsy study performed by Lehner documented that 90% of the patients dying with disseminated candidiasis had renal involvement, although renal infection (candidiasis) may occur as an isolated site of metastatic spread especially following transient candidemia [10]. Autopsy studies demonstrated multiple abscesses in the renal interstitium, glomeruli and peritubular vessels, with not infrequent papillary necrosis and, rarely, complicating emphysematous pyelonephritis.

Clinical features

Most patients with candiduria are asymptomatic. Patients who have an indwelling bladder catheter most often are colonized rather than infected with a *Candida* species. Hospitalized candiduric patients with constitutional or systemic symptoms usually have another cause for their symptoms.

However, patients with *Candida* cystitis may present with frequency, dysuria, urgency, haematuria and pyuria. Cystoscopy reveals soft, pearly white, slightly elevated patches that resemble oral thrush, as well as hyperaemia and inflammation of the bladder mucosa. Most symptomatic patients with *Candida* cystitis are not catheterized and the converse also applies.

Ascending infection, although rare, may result in *Candida* pyelonephritis characterized by fever, leucocytosis, rigors and costovertebral angle tenderness. Ultrasonography and computed tomography (CT) scanning are useful in diagnosing an intrarenal and perinephric abscess. Excretory urography may reveal ureteropelvic fungus balls with or without accompanying papillary necrosis. Ascending infection with *Candida* species uncommonly causes candidemia, with only 3–10% of episodes of candidemia being secondary to candiduria [11]. When candidemia occurs it invariably complicates anatomic obstruction, manipulation or a urologic procedure.

Fungal bezoars may develop anywhere in the urinary drainage system but most commonly are found in the pelvis or upper ureters. Fungal balls are rare and their presence is suggested by signs of ureteral obstruction associated with candiduria. When bilateral, they may induce obstruction sufficient to cause azotaemia. Obstruction may be intermittent or passage of the fungal balls may result in renal colic or the passage of 'soft' stones. Excretory urography or retrograde pyelography reveals a filling defect in the collecting system. Fungal balls in the urinary tract have also been described with Aspergillus, Penicillium species and zygomycetes.

Renal candidiasis secondary to haematogenous spread represents a systemic infection usually accompanied by fever and other constitutional manifestations of sepsis. Positive blood cultures may be obtained; however, often when the diagnosis of renal candidiasis is considered, blood cultures are no longer positive, causing difficulty in diagnosis. Manifestations of disseminated candidiasis may include maculopapular skin rash and endophthalmitis. Most patients with candiduria secondary to renal candidiasis are febrile but lack other clinical manifestations that indicate renal involvement other than variable reduction in renal function. Accordingly, finding candiduria may be the only clue to the diagnosis of invasive and disseminated candidiasis [12].

Diagnosis

Isolation of *Candida* species from a urine sample may represent contamination, vulvovestibular or catheter colonization, or a superficial/deep infection of the lower or upper urinary tract. Contamination of the sample is common in women with vulvovaginal colonization. Contamination can usually be excluded by repeating the urine culture, with special attention to proper collection techniques. Two consecutive positive isolates of *Candida* are essential before initiating antifungal therapy. Rarely, in hospitalized female patients, a bladder urine sample obtained with a straight catheter is necessary to determine the source.

Differentiating infection from colonization of the urinary tract is difficult, if not impossible, especially in patients with catheters [8]. Clinical features are not specific, and in critically ill patients in ICUs, fever and leucocytosis may have other sources. The presence of pyuria in catheterized patients does not differentiate infection from colonization, as an indwelling catheter may itself lead to pyuria from mechanical irritation of bladder mucosa and because of concomitant bacteriuria. Quantitative urine colony counts are also not of value in the patient with an indwelling catheter. Fungal morphology (such as the presence of hyphae) is only helpful if hyphae or pseudohyphae are found within hyaline or granular casts.

In patients without catheters, there is greater likelihood for true infection in the presence of candiduria, particularly if urinary counts are > 10 000–15 000 cells/ml urine. However, renal candidiasis has rarely been reported with a colony count of > 10^3 cells/ml. Therefore, considerable overlap occurs and quantitative cultures are not the final determinant in therapeutic decision-making; similarly, negative urine cultures cannot be used to exclude renal candidiasis.

After candiduria is deemed to represent infection, the challenge to the clinician is to localize the anatomic level of infection. Localization is critical in the management of candiduria. No useful test to differentiate *Candida* invasion of kidneys from the frequent lower tract *Candida* infection exists, other than the rare detection of *Candida* hyphae or pseudohyphae within casts. Quantitative cultures, fungal morphology on microscopy and pyuria also have little value in localizing infection. Non-specific evidence of upper UTI is suggested by declining renal function, constitutional features, and radiographic findings on CT scans and ultrasonography. Serologic tests for *Candida* as a marker for parenchymal invasion remain insensitive. A newly introduced blood test (Fungitel[R]) that detects serum fungal glucan may be useful. A 5-day bladder irrigation with amphotericin B solution (50–100 mg/L 5% dextrose in water) may be effective in establishing the source of candiduria in that persistent postirrigation candiduria is indicative of fungal infection originating above the bladder. This implies the need for further investigation and raises the suspicion of renal candidiasis. Unfortunately, the lengthy nature of the conventional amphotericin B irrigation test excludes its utility in febrile, critically ill patients with candiduria. A 3-h rapid bladder irrigation test using amphotericin B at 200 mg/ml has been recommended based upon *in vitro* studies but has yet to be shown reliable in patients [13].

Treatment of candiduria (Table 9.3)

ASYMPTOMATIC CANDIDURIA

Asymptomatic colonization with *Candida* is the most common syndrome associated with candiduria and requires no therapy. The candiduria is often transient and, even if persistent, uncommonly results in serious morbidity. The risk of invasive complications is also small [4,11].

In a prospective, multicentre placebo-controlled study, Sobel *et al.* [14] found that asymptomatic candiduria resolved with urinary catheter elimination in ∼ 41% of hospitalized, catheterized patients. After changing a catheter, untreated candiduria resolved in 20% of patients. Storfer *et al.* [15] found a similar rate of resolution of untreated candiduria.

While antifungal therapy, either with systemic amphotericin B or fluconazole or with local amphotericin B irrigation, can eliminate candiduria in catheterized patients [5,16,17] there is no evidence that patients benefit from therapy. Furthermore, relapse is frequent. For example, Sobel *et al.* [14] reported that fluconazole treatment resulted in high short-term rates of eradication of *Candida* from the urine, but 2 weeks after therapy was discontinued the frequency of candiduria was similar in the fluconazole and placebo groups. Interestingly, *C. glabrata* responded equally well to

Table 9.3 Treatment of candiduria

Condition	First-line treatment	Second-line treatment
Asymptomatic candiduria	Rarely requires treatment; modify risk factors, remove catheter	*Fluconazole 200 mg/day orally for 7–14 days if elected to treat (see text) AmB bladder irrigation (50 mg/L) for 5 days or AmB IV 0.3 mg/kg single dose or oral flucytosine 150 mg/kg/day for 7–14 days (qid)
Symptomatic *Candida* cystitis†	Fluconazole, 200 mg/day orally for 7–14 days	
Ascending pyelonephritis	Surgical drainage plus prolonged therapy (2–6 weeks) with fluconazole 6 mg/kg/day, AmB IV > 0.6 mg/kg/day or caspofungin 50 mg/day	
Renal candidiasis (haematogenous)	Prolonged therapy (2–6 weeks) with fluconazole 6 mg/kg/day, AmB > 0.6 mg/kg/day or caspofungin 50 mg/day	

AmB, amphotericin B; IV, intravenous.
*Low birth weight infant, renal transplant patient, febrile neutropenia, preoperative urology.
†Selection for *C. albicans*. For non-albican *Candida* species use second-line treatment.

fluconazole as *C. albicans* despite having higher mean inhibitory concentrations (MICs) to fluconazole. This may be due to the high concentrations (10-fold that of serum) that fluconazole achieves in the urine.

Persistent asymptomatic candiduria in patients without catheters should be investigated for upper tract disease since the likelihood of obstruction or stasis is relatively high. Persistent asymptomatic candiduria in catheterized low birth weight infants and in the afebrile neutropenic patient may also require antifungal therapy and investigation to exclude the possibility of renal or systemic involvement. Candiduria should be considered a complicated UTI; hence when treatment is occasionally indicated, as described below, therapy should not be of short duration or of low dose but require 10–14 days.

The management of asymptomatic candiduria in the renal transplant patient is particularly perplexing. Many of the patients are diabetic, are receiving perioperative antibiotics and immunosuppressive agents and/or have Foley catheters and intraoperative ureterocystic stent placement. The risk of ascending infection is high given the stent, glycosuria, short ureter and frequent reflux. Nevertheless, parenchymal invasion of the graft and candidemia is rare in the absence of obstruction. It has been considered reasonable in the presence of asymptomatic infection to attempt eradication of candiduria, but many experts prefer to observe these candiduric patients until all foreign bodies are removed. A recent large retrospective study of renal transplant recipients found that treatment of asymptomatic posttransplant candiduria had no effect on morbidity and survival of patients, accordingly routine therapy does not appear justified [18]. When fever and sepsis due to invasive candidiasis supervenes, antifungal therapy is justified, the choice of which is influenced by selecting non-nephrotoxic agents in the presence of a valued graft and recognizing that azole agents may interact with immunosuppressive agents. Fluconazole may raise the level of cyclosporin or tacrolimus and will indirectly cause an elevation in the creatinine.

Patients with asymptomatic candiduria in whom urologic instrumentation or surgery is planned should have the candiduria eliminated or suppressed before and during the procedure in order to avoid the risk of invasive candidiasis and candidemia. Successful elimination can be achieved through amphotericin B or miconazole bladder irrigation, or with systemic therapy utilizing amphotericin B, flucytosine or fluconazole.

CANDIDA CYSTITIS

Symptomatic cystitis requires treatment with either amphotericin B bladder instillation (50 mg/L) or systemic therapy, utilizing intravenous amphotericin B, flucytosine or fluconazole [5–13,16,17,19]. The latter would be preferable in the non-catheterized subject. In contrast to fluconazole in which 80% of the drug is excreted unchanged in the urine, both ketoconazole and itraconazole are poorly excreted in the urine and should not be used. Single-dose intravenous amphotericin B 0.3 mg/kg has also been shown to be useful in the treatment of lower urinary tract candidiasis, with therapeutic urine concentrations continuing for a considerable time after the administration of the single dose of amphotericin B [20]. Amphotericin B or flucytosine orally may be preferable for resistant fungal species. Most patients without indwelling catheters are conveniently effectively managed with oral fluconazole, although failure with *C. glabrata* and *C. krusei* infection are reported [21,22].

Ascending pyelonephritis and *Candida* urosepsis

Invasive upper tract infections require systemic antifungal therapy as well as immediate investigation and visualization of the urinary drainage system to exclude urinary obstruction, papillary necrosis and fungus ball formation [23]. The most widely accepted therapy traditionally has been intravenous amphotericin B 0.6 mg/kg daily. Duration of therapy depends upon the severity of infection, presence of candidemia and response to therapy, in general 14 days after resolution of candidemia. Several alternatives to treatment with amphotericin B now exist. Systemic therapy with fluconazole 6 mg/kg daily (intravenous or oral) offers an effective and less toxic therapy [12]. Since fluconazole is excreted unchanged into the urine, coexistent severe renal failure may frequently result in subtherapeutic urinary concentrations of fluconazole. Accordingly, systemic doses of fluconazole should not be reduced in renal failure and postrenal candiduria [14]. The echinocandin class, e.g. caspofungin 50 mg IV/day, now offers a safer broad-spectrum alternative to amphotericin B, caspofungin is not nephrotoxic and requires no dose adjustments even with advanced renal failure. Accordingly, while it is reasonable to initiate antifungal therapy for *C. albicans* urosepsis with fluconazole, the presence of less susceptible species (*C. glabrata, C. krusei*) or lack of success with fluconazole should result in early, timely switch to caspofungin [21]. Many patients have renal insufficiency, accordingly it is tempting to use the less nephrotoxic lipid formulations of amphotericin B that are currently available. However, in spite of their clinical record of at least equivalent efficacy compared with amphotericin B desoxycholate, the very physicochemical structure that protects the kidney from the toxic effects of amphotericin B may impair their urinary excretions [24].

Infection refractory to medical management should be treated surgically with drainage, or in cases of a nonviable kidney, nephrectomy. An obstructed kidney with hydronephrosis requires a percutaneous nephrostomy. The management of ureteral fungal balls depends upon the extent, site and severity of infection. In some patients, bezoars spontaneously lyse or become dislodged during placement of ureteral stents [23]. In many patients, upper tract external drainage via a nephrostomy tube must be combined with local amphotericin B or fluconazole irrigation. Occasionally, the fungal bezoars must be removed surgically.

Renal and disseminated candidiasis

Management of renal candidiasis secondary to haematogenous spread is essentially that of systemic candidiasis, including intravenous amphotericin B 0.6 mg/kg daily or intravenous fluconazole 400 mg daily [25]. Dosage modifications of fluconazole may be necessary in the presence of severe azotemia. Prognosis depends upon correction of the underlying factors, i.e. resolution of neutropenia or removal of the intravascular catheters implicated. Systemic candidiasis requires prolonged therapy over 4–6 weeks. Lipid formulations of amphotericin B, although less nephrotoxic than the standard desoxycholate form, have not been shown to be of superior efficacy.

References

1   Wise GJ, Silver DA. Fungal infections of the genitourinary system. *J Urol* 1993; **149**: 1377–88.
2   Platt R, Polk BT, Murdock B *et al*. Risk factors for nosocomial urinary tract infection. *Am J Epidemiol* 1986; **124**: 977.
3   Rivett AG, Perry JA, Cohen J. Urinary candidiasis: a prospective study in hospitalized patients. *Urol Res* 1986; **14**: 183–6.
4   Kauffman CA, Vazquez JA, Sobel JD *et al*. Prospective multicenter surveillance study of funguria in hospitalized patients. *Clin Infect Dis* 2000; **30**: 14–18.
5   Jacobs LG, Skidmore EA, Freeman K *et al*. Oral fluconazole compared with amphotericin B bladder irrigation for fungal urinary tract infections in the elderly. *Clin Infect Dis* 1996; **22**: 30–35.
6   Phillips JR, Karlowicz MG. Prevalence of *Candida* species in hospital-acquired urinary tract infections in a neonatal intensive care unit. *Pediatr Infect Dis J* 1997; **16**: 190–94.
7   Febre N, Silva V, Medeiros EA *et al*. Microbiological characteristics of yeasts isolated from urinary tracts of intensive care unit patients undergoing urinary catheterization. *J Clin Microbiol* 1999; **37**: 1584–6.
8   Kozinn PJ, Taschdjian CL, Goldberg PK *et al*. Advances in the diagnosis of renal candidiasis. *J Urol* 1978; **119**: 184–7.
9   Harris AD, Castro J, Sheppard DC *et al*. Risk factors for nosocomial candiduria due to *Candida glabrata* and *Candida albicans*. *Clin Infect Dis* 1999; **29**: 926–8.
10 Lehner T. Systemic candidiasis and renal involvement. *Lancet* 1964; **1**: 1414–16.
11 Ang BSP, Telenti A, King B *et al*. Candidemia from a urinary tract source: microbiological aspects and clinical significance. *Clin Infect Dis* 1993; **17**: 622–6.

12 Nassoura Z, Ivatury RR, Simon RJ *et al.* Candiduria as an early marker of disseminated infection in critically ill surgical patients: the role of fluconazole therapy. *J Trauma* 1995; **35**: 290–95.

13 Fong LW, Cheng PC, Hinton NA. Fungicidal effects of amphotericin B in urine: in vitro study to assess feasibility of bladder washout for localization of site of candiduria. *Antimicrob Agents Chemother* 1991; **35**: 1856–9.

14 Sobel JD, Kauffman CA, McKinsey D *et al.* Candiduria – a randomized double-blind study of treatment with fluconazole and placebo. *Clin Infect Dis.* 2000; **30**: 19–24.

15 Storfer SP, Medoff G, Fraser VJ *et al.* Candiduria: retrospective review in hospitalized patients. *Infect Dis Clin Pract* 1994; **3**: 23–9.

16 Fan-Havard P, O'Donovan C, Smith SM *et al.* Oral fluconazole versus amphotericin B bladder irrigation for treatment of candidal funguria. *Clin Infect Dis* 1995; **21**: 960–65.

17 Leu HS, Huancy CT. Clearance of funguria with short course antifungal regimens: a prospective randomized controlled study. *Clin Infect Dis* 1995; **20**: 1152–7.

18 Safdar N, Slattery WR, Knasinski V, Gangnon RE, Li Z, Pirsch JD, Andes D. Predictors and outcomes of candiduria in renal transplant recipients. *Clin Infect Dis* 2005; **40**: 1413.

19 Wong-Beringer A, Jacobs RA, Guglielmo BJ. Treatment of funguria. A critical review. *J Am Med Assoc* 1992; **267**: 2780–85.

20 Fisher JF, Hicks BC, Dipiro JT *et al.* Efficacy of a single intravenous dose of amphotericin B in urinary tract infections caused by *Candida. J Infect Dis* 1987; **156**: 685–7.

21 Wise GJ, Lajeune JG, Goldman W *et al.* Candida infections of the genitourinary system. Limitations of fluconazole monotherapy. *Infect Urol* 2001; **14**: 87–93.

22 Ansari SH, Levin MH, Lipshitz S. Fluconazole treatment in *Torulopsis glabrata* upper urinary tract infection causing ureteral obstruction. *J Urol* 1995; **154**: 1870.

23 Irby PB, Stoller MI, McAninch JW. Fungal bezoars of the upper urinary tract. *J Urol* 1990; **143**: 447–51.

24 Agustin J, Lacson S, Raffalli J *et al.* Failure of a lipid amphotericin B preparation to eradicate candiduria: preliminary findings based on three cases. *Clin Infect Dis* 1999; **29**: 686–7.

25 Pappas PG, Rex JH, Sobel JD, Filler SG, Dismukes WE, Walsh TJ, Edwards JE; Infectious Diseases Society of America. Guidelines for treatment of candidiasis. *Clin Infect Dis* 2004; **38**: 161–89.

Part 3
Urological Oncology

10: Pharmacotherapy in the Management of Prostate Cancer

Jeetesh Bhardwa & Roger S. Kirby

Prostate cancer is now the second leading cause of death due to cancer in men. Prostate cancer is usually classified as being early/localized (organ confined), locally advanced, metastatic or hormone-relapsed. The management of prostate cancer depends largely upon the stage and the Gleason grade of the tumour, as well as the patient's general medical condition and treatment preference. Surgical intervention is usually reserved for (early) localized prostate cancer, which is deemed to be confined to the prostate capsule. In the more advanced cases surgery is only used for performing channel transurethral resection of prostate (TURP) to relieve severe lower urinary tract symptoms (LUTSs).

The management of prostate cancer is sometimes controversial, not least as the diagnosis of localized or locally advanced prostate cancer is often difficult to establish precisely. Current modalities for diagnosing prostate cancer include prostate-specific antigen (PSA), digital rectal examination (DRE), transrectal rectal ultrasound scan (TRUS) and computerized tomography (CT)/ magnetic resonance imaging (MRI). Often tumours thought to be localized (organ-confined) on the basis of these tests are upgraded to locally advanced when the pathologist receives the specimen after a radical prostatectomy.

The mainstay of pharmacotherapy of prostate cancer is androgen ablation either with luteinizing hormone-releasing hormone (LHRH) analogues and/ or antiandrogens. When the efficacy of this approach begins to wane, presumably as a result of the clonal selection of androgen-independent cells, the use of taxanes as chemotherapy may be indicated in selected patients. This clinical condition is termed as hormone-relapsed prostate cancer (HRPC).

Bisphosphonates have also been shown to be beneficial in delaying skeletal-related events, such as pathological fractures and spinal cord compression, but do not prolong overall survival. They may also have a place in reducing the osteoporotic effects of androgen deprivation.

Chemoprevention of prostate cancer

Before discussing the options for treatment of the various stages of established prostate cancer it is pertinent to consider briefly the various methods of chemoprevention of prostate cancer that are currently available. While there

161

are genetic and environmental factors that explain the wide variation in the prevalence of prostate cancer in various countries and racial groups, there are some ways that prostate cancer may be prevented or delayed from progression.

Limited evidence currently exists for the role of vitamin E and selenium as chemopreventive agents for prostate cancer; however, many patients use them. A long-term randomized study, known as Selenium and Vitamin E Cancer Prevention Trial (SELECT) is currently evaluating their efficacy. As yet no results are available. The recommended dose for selenium is 200 μg/day. The recommended dose for vitamin E has just been reduced to 150 IU/day because of possible cardiovascular effects of higher doses.

5 Alpha-reductase inhibitors

In the prostate cancer prevention trial (PCPT) 18 882 men 55 years of age or older with a normal DRE and a PSA level of 3.0 ng/ml were randomly assigned to treatment with finasteride (5 mg/day) or placebo for 7 years. Prostate cancer was detected in 803 of the 4368 men in the finasteride group and 1147 of the 4692 men in the placebo group (18.4% vs 24.8%). The prevalence of prostate cancer was reduced by 6.4% (HR = 0.75), from 24.8% to 18.4% in those taking finasteride compared with placebo [1].

Tumours of Gleason grade 7, 8, 9 or 10 were more common in the finasteride group (37.0%) than in the placebo group (22.2%). It was concluded that finasteride prevents or delays the appearance of prostate cancer, but this possible benefit and a reduced risk of urinary problems must be weighed against sexual side-effects and the moderately increased risk of high-grade prostate cancer [2].

The dual 5-α-reductase inhibitor dutasteride is being evaluated in a similar activity in the Reduction by Dutasteride of Prostate Cancer Events (REDUCE) study but no results are available as yet. As a consequence, 5-α-reductase inhibitors are not yet recommended as chemopreventative agents.

Drugs used in the treatment of prostate cancer

Before the various stages of prostate cancer and the drugs that might be used and the evidence for them are discussed, it is relevant to outline the various types of hormone therapy that are used in the treatment of prostate cancer.

Hormone therapy

LHRH ANALOGUES

LHRH analogues are as effective as orchidectomy at suppressing testosterone levels. However, they cause initial stimulation followed by depression of luteinizing hormone release by the pituitary. During the initial stage, lasting up to 2 weeks after the LHRH analogues are commenced, the increased testosterone production and higher circulating levels may be associated with a brief progression of prostate cancer and it may lead to a 'tumour flare'. In susceptible patients this may manifest itself with spinal cord compression, ureteric obstruction and worsening of renal failure and increased bone pain. Therefore this period of 2–4 weeks is usually covered with the administration of an antiandrogen. The antiandrogen treatment is started 3–5 days before the administration of LHRH analogues and continued for up to 3–4 weeks. There are various LHRH analogues currently available in the market including:

• buserelin (Suprefact®) initially given as a subcutaneous injection three times daily for 7 days and then intranasally 6 times a day;
• goserelin (Zoladex®) is available as a 1-or 3-monthly (Zoladex LA®) depot injection;
• leuprorelin (Prostap® SR or Prostap®3, which are available as 1-or 3-monthly injections, respectively);
• triptorelin (De-capeptyl® SR) available as a once-monthly injection;
• LHRH agonists, which should avoid the 'flare phenomenon', are currently under development, but have not been approved for clinical use.

Nonsteroidal antiandrogens

Flutamide and bicalutamide (Casodex®) are the most commonly prescribed antiandrogens. They are mainly used to treat advanced prostate cancer or as adjuvant therapy. They may, however, also be used as monotherapy, as discussed in the relevant sections below.

Steroidal antiandrogen

Cyproterone acetate is the most commonly used steroidal antiandrogen in the management of prostate cancer. It can also be used in the management of hot flushes following treatment with LHRH analogues.

Unwanted effects of androgen ablation

Common unwanted effects of hormone therapy include hot flushes, loss of libido or erectile dysfunction, weight gain, painful gynaecomastia, osteoporosis fatigue/tiredness and much less frequently reduced cognitive functioning. The antiandrogen bicalutamide has a less profound negative impact on sexual function than LHRH analogues. Both steroidal and nonsteroidal antiandrogens should be used with caution in patients with hepatic dysfunction and periodic liver function tests should be carried out. Cyproterone acetate used in the long term has been associated with the development of hepatoma, as a consequence long-term use is now discouraged.

Management of localized prostate cancer

Patients with clinically localized prostate cancer are generally offered either active surveillance or radical treatment, depending on their general condition and own preferences. Standard treatments for localized prostate cancer include radical surgery, radiation therapy (external beam or brachytherapy with and without androgen ablation) or active surveillance, which is also termed watchful waiting. There is a lack of randomized controlled trials comparing the various treatments for localized prostate cancer and hence results obtained from trials of other stages of prostate cancer are often extrapolated to localized prostate cancer. Randomized trials have shown a survival benefit for patients with locally advanced prostate cancer receiving hormone therapy plus radiotherapy compared with radiotherapy alone [3,4] and this observation has sometimes been applied to patients with localized prostate cancer.

Treatment options in localized prostate cancer

WATCHFUL WAITING

Current evidence suggests that patients managed by watchful waiting for more than 15 years often sustain eventual disease progression [5]. Although many prostate cancers diagnosed at an early stage have an indolent course, local tumour progression and aggressive metastatic disease may develop in the long term. These findings support early radical treatment, especially for patients with an estimated life expectancy exceeding 15 years. This is particularly the case as mortality from other causes continues to fall due to improved medical care.

HORMONE THERAPY

Hormone therapy alone is not generally used in the treatment of localized prostate cancer, instead it is reserved for the more advanced forms of prostate cancer. However, it may be used in combination with other forms of treatment to manage localized prostate cancer as adjuvant or neoadjuvant to radiotherapy or radical surgery.

RADICAL PROSTATECTOMY PRECEDED BY HORMONE THERAPY

Neoadjuvant hormone therapy in the form of 3 months of flutamide and leuprorelin before radical prostatectomy in patients with localized prostate cancer reduced the likelihood of cancer at the surgical margins by 30% and of capsular penetration by 31% [6]. A 5-year follow-up of these patients however did not reveal a difference in the recurrence rate [7]. Although neoadjuvant hormone therapy reduced prostate volume and increases the likelihood of organ-confined disease it is uncertain whether it improves clinical outcome [8].

RADICAL PROSTATECTOMY AND NEOADJUVANT CHEMOTHERAPY

Patients in the Cancer and Leukemia Group B 90203 study (CALGB 90203) have been randomized to receive neoadjuvant therapy in the form of estramustine and docetaxel followed by radical prostatectomy or radical prostatectomy alone [9]. The purpose of this ongoing study is to determine which of two treatment strategies is superior in treating men with high-risk, clinically localized adenocarcinoma of the prostate (stage T1 to T3a NX M0). The primary study end point is to determine if early systemic treatment with neoadjuvant estramustine and docetaxel before radical prostatectomy in patients with high-risk prostate cancer will decrease 5-year recurrence rates when compared with radical prostatectomy alone. The results of this study are awaited.

Neoadjuvant chemotherapy has several theoretical advantages. The first is to provide early systemic therapy for undetectable micrometastasis, the second to reduce locally advanced tumours (as a proportion of tumours thought to be localized preoperatively are subsequently upgraded) to provide clearer surgical margins.

RADIOTHERAPY PLUS ANDROGEN ABLATION

Adding 2 months of neoadjuvant androgen ablation along with conformal radiotherapy to patients with high-risk localized prostate cancer (PSA > 10 and Gleason score $\geq$ 7) increased overall survival at 5 years by 10–88% [10]. The differences in survival were not significant for low-risk patients although a slight reduction in recurrence rates has been reported with intermediate-risk prostate cancers [4]. Several Radiation Therapy Oncology Group and European Organization for Research and Treatment of Cancer trials have determined that androgen ablation, when combined with external radiation, yields improved disease-specific survival and increased time to recurrence in patients with locally advanced or high-grade prostate cancer (Fig. 10.1). The advantage of this approach in patients with early disease remains to be determined, but it could offer significant advantages when used in younger patients with significant longevity (> 20 years).

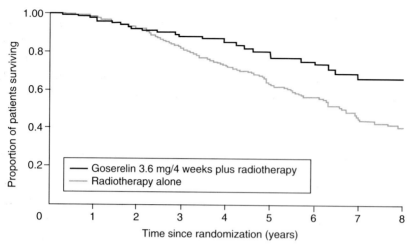

HR 0.51; 95% CI 0.36, 0.73; $p < 0.0001$

Figure 10.1 Kaplan–Meier curve of overall survival in patients with locally advanced prostate cancer who have received goserelin adjuvant to radiotherapy or radiotherapy alone as part of the European Organization of Research and Treatment of Cancer (EORTC) study number 22 863 ($n = 412$) [4].

Management of locally advanced prostate cancer

Hormone therapy alone is generally employed for unfit patients with localized prostate cancer, a life expectancy of < 10 years and a Gleason score of > 4, or for large, locally advanced disease in patients with a life expectancy of < 10 years and a PSA level of > 25 ng/ml.

Hormone therapy in the treatment of locally advanced prostate cancer

BICALUTAMIDE

Bicalutamide is a nonsteroidal pure antiandrogen usually given at a dosage of 150 mg once daily as monotherapy for the treatment of early (localized or locally advanced) nonmetastatic prostate cancer. It is also used at a dosage of 50 mg once daily in combination with a LHRH analogue or surgical castration for the treatment of advanced prostate cancer.

Bicalutamide is slowly absorbed after oral administration, but absorption is unaffected by food. It has a long plasma elimination half-life (1 week) and accumulates about tenfold in plasma during daily administration.

Daily administration of bicalutamide increases circulating levels of gonadotrophins and sex hormones; although testosterone may increase by up to 80%, concentrations in most patients remain within the normal range.

Bicalutamide produces a dose-related decrease in PSA at dosages of 50–150 mg/day.

Treatment options in locally advanced prostate cancer

ANDROGEN ABLATION ALONE

Bicalutamide 150 mg is indicated as an alternative to castration for patients with locally advanced prostate cancer, either alone or as an adjuvant therapy; it is no longer approved in patients with localized disease who would normally be managed by observation, i.e. patients with a life expectancy of less than 10 years. The latest results from the Early Prostate Cancer (EPC) programme have shown that the greatest progression-free survival benefits for this treatment are in patients with locally advanced disease. As such patients are at significant risk of disease progression, any additional therapies that can reduce this risk, with minimal effects on lifestyle, are important [11].

In one randomized controlled trial adding 150 mg bicalutamide to standard care (i.e. radical prostatectomy, radiotherapy or watchful waiting) resulted in improved survival in men with locally advanced prostate cancer (HR 0.68, 95% CI 0.50–0.92), while the greatest increase in progression-free survival was for patients with locally advanced prostate cancer who were treated with bicalutamide alone (HR 0.40, 95% CI 0.31–0.52) [12]. Since 81% of the trial population were untreated before entry and would otherwise probably have undergone watchful waiting, the findings largely reflect the results of immediate hormone therapy versus watchful waiting.

HORMONES PLUS RADIOTHERAPY

The standard care for patients with locally advanced disease is often external-beam radiotherapy and, in this setting, the EPC programme data show that adding bicalutamide 150 mg as adjuvant therapy significantly reduces the risk of disease progression (HR 0.58; $p = 0.0035$) [13]. This does have the disadvantage of the unwanted effects of antiandrogens, as outlined above. Tender gynaecomastia, tiredness and hot flushes are a particular problem and in the longer term, osteoporosis.

HORMONES AFTER RADICAL SURGERY

Many patients with clinically localized disease who have had a radical prostatectomy are restaged by the pathologist to pT3, i.e. locally advanced disease. Adjuvant bicalutamide 150 mg significantly reduced the risk of disease progression in such patients (HR 0.71; $p = 0.0034$) [14]. Bicalutamide 150 mg also showed a significant risk reduction in terms of disease progression

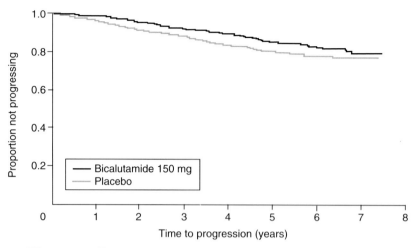

HR 0.71; 95% CI 0.57, 0.89; $p = 0.0034$
Bicalutamide 150 mg events = 136 (15.6%)
Placebo events = 170 (20.0%)

Figure 10.2 Kaplan–Meier curve of progression-free survival in patients with locally advanced disease (T3-4, an N or T1-2, pN+) in the radical prostatectomy subgroup of the ongoing Early Prostate Cancer (EPC) programme [11].

compared with observation alone (HR 0.53, $p < 0.001$) [15] but again at a cost of gynaecomastia and nipple tenderness. Figure 10.2 demonstrates the impact of bicalutamide in reducing the risk of objective progression in patients with nonmetastatic prostate cancer treated by radical prostatectomy.

EARLY HORMONES VERSUS DELAYED ANDROGEN ABLATION

Many conflicting data have been published comparing immediate versus delayed hormone treatment [16,17]. Many recent randomized trials suggest that immediate hormone treatment is better than delayed. Hormone treatment has been used either alone or after surgery [18,19]. Furthermore, the patients' requests and expectations often favour early hormone treatment [20]. However, some problems have been identified in the early (medical) castration approach, including decreased quality of life (especially from depression, decrease in libido, impotence and fatigue), reduced cognitive functioning and an increased risk of osteoporosis.

INTERMITTENT VERSUS DELAYED HORMONE THERAPY

Intermittent therapy has been advocated on the basis that androgens are required for cell differentiation, while apoptosis secondary to androgen withdrawal mainly occurs in differentiated cells. For intermittent versus continuous therapy, one preliminary study showed an early progression-free survival benefit of intermittent treatment in M0 patients only [21]. This approach seems to work best in those patients with relatively differentiated lesions (Gleason $\leq$ 7), a low PSA level and a low PSA nadir during castration, after an 8-month medical castration period [22].

MAXIMUM ANDROGEN BLOCKADE

Maximum androgen blockade (MAB) did not seem to be of any significant advantage in locally advanced disease when goserelin was combined with cyproterone acetate [23]. However, a survival advantage was demonstrated for patients receiving prolonged MAB greater than 120 days when an LHRH analogue was combined with a nonsteroidal antiandrogen. Patients who received 120 days or more of MAB therapy (median survival 1035 days vs 302 days for less than 120 days of therapy). This result was confirmed in the patients who lived at least 2 years, in whom the median survival time was increased by 35% [24].

This treatment approach however remains controversial mainly due to conflicting reports about its usefulness in improving overall survival and reducing progression and the increased side-effects. Moreover, health economics arguments point to the increasing cost of drugs administered.

Management of metastatic prostate cancer

Significant numbers of men present with advanced disease or to develop advanced disease at some time after treatment for their local disease. The mainstay of systemic therapy for prostate cancer has been hormone therapy for many years. Orchidectomy and estrogens were the initial hormone therapies used. Over the past several years a number of agents have been shown to produce similar rates of disease control with improved tolerability profiles. The LHRH agonists are the most frequently used hormonal agents in prostate cancer. Antiandrogens have also been used as single agents, or in combination with LHRH agonists. As mentioned, LHRH antagonists have recently been introduced but are yet to be approved by regulatory authorities.

Hormone-relapsed prostate cancer

Although many men with prostate cancer may be cured by radical treatment, many hundreds of thousands of men worldwide (40 000 in the USA alone) die annually due to prostate cancer [25]. Treatment for hormone-resistant prostate cancer is traditionally palliative and expected survival is 6–12 months [26]. Bone pain can be palliated with radiotherapy but this offers no survival advantage. A number of combination therapies have been tried in an attempt to manage hormone-resistant prostate cancer and improve its outcome in both palliation end points and try and improve survival figures.

Pharmacotherapy in hormone-relapsed prostate cancer

HYDROCORTISONE WITH OR WITHOUT MITOXANTRONE

The above combination was evaluated by the Cancer and Leukaemia group B 9182 study in a randomized controlled trial. Mitoxantrone is an anthracenedione that has activity in a variety of malignancies including prostate cancer. It is well suited to use in the often-frail men with advanced prostate cancer because of its relatively modest toxicity. Although there was a delay in time to treatment failure and disease progression in favour of mitoxantrone and hydrocortisone there was no difference in overall survival: 12.3 months for mitoxantrone and hydrocortisone versus 12.6 months for hydrocortisone alone [27].

PREDNISOLONE WITH OR WITHOUT MITOXANTRONE

In a randomized controlled study 120 men were randomly assigned to receive either prednisolone alone or in combination with mitoxantrone. We concluded that there was a 50% or greater decrease in PSA levels in the mitoxantrone plus prednisone group compared with the prednisone alone group; time to treatment failure was also prolonged in the mitoxantrone plus prednisolone group (8.1 months compared with 4.1 months). However, there was no difference in survival in the two groups at 23 and 19 months, respectively. Death was mainly due to disease progression [28].

DOCETAXEL

Docetaxel is a member of a group of drugs termed taxanes. It is given by intravenous infusion. Docetaxel phosphorylates Bcl-2 *in vitro*, leading to its inactivation and eventually to cell death by apoptosis [29]. There have been recent papers that have compared docetaxel and mitoxantrone in combination with prednisolone and others comparing docetaxel and estramustine as a combination with mitoxantrone and prednisolone as a combination.

DOCETAXEL + PREDNISOLONE VERSUS MITOXANTRONE + PREDNISOLONE

In a recent randomized controlled trial comparing docetaxel in combination with prednisolone to mitoxantrone in combination with prednisolone. The median survival was 16.5 months in the group given mitoxantrone, while it was 18.9 months in the group given docetaxel every 3 weeks [30]. Serum PSA dropped by half in 32% of patients on mitoxantrone compared with 45% of the patients on docetaxel (Fig. 10.3). As a result docetaxel is considered to be superior to mitoxantrone in hormone-resistant prostate cancer, and is now becoming the standard of care in this situation.

DOCETAXEL + ESTRAMUSTINE VERSUS MITOXANTRONE + PREDNISOLONE

Trials of docetaxel and estramustine have shown PSA responses (defined as a PSA reduction of 50%) in 80% of patients [31]. Combining docetaxel with estramustine improves the median survival by 2 months as compared with mitoxantrone and prednisolone in patients with HRPC – 17.5 months versus 15.6 months. The median time to progression was 6.3 months in the group given docetaxel and estramustine compared with 3.2 months in the group given mitoxantrone and prednisolone, while the serum PSA dropped by half in 50% and 27% of patients, respectively [32].

This approach of combining docetaxel and estramustine in patients with hormone-resistant prostate cancer holds out hope for the treatment of this group of patients who have historically been considered to have a poor prognosis.

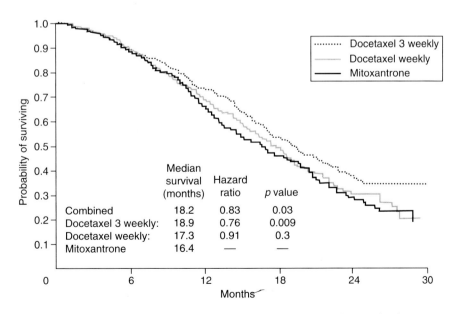

Figure 10.3 Docetaxel versus mitoxantrone. Docetaxel increases overall survival in hormone-relapsed prostate cancer (HRPC) by several months [32].

BISPHOSPHONATES

Bone is a preferred site for prostate cancer metastases, which occur in more than 80% of men with advanced disease [33]. In addition to bone metastases, bone loss resulting from previous orchidectomy or hormone therapies that lower or block androgen activity contribute to an increased risk of fracture, pain and other skeletal complications [34].

As well as being a major cause of morbidity it has now been shown that skeletal fractures correlate negatively with overall survival in men with prostate cancer and are an independent and adverse predictor of survival [35]. It is therefore important that skeletal fractures and skeletal morbidity are kept at a minimum. Bisphosphonates seem a promising way ahead in this respect.

Biochemical and histomorphometric studies indicate that osteolysis (excessive bone destruction) is present in prostate cancer metastases despite the sclerotic appearance on X-rays. In this respect, bisphosphonates, which are pyrophosphate analogues that block osteolysis, may be useful for the treatment of patients with osteoblastic metastases as well as those with osteolytic metastases.

Zoledronic acid is a new nitrogen-containing bisphosphonate that has been evaluated in patients with metastatic HRPC. It has previously been shown to be at least as effective as pamidronate 90-mg infusion in reducing skeletal complications in patients with myeloma or breast cancer [36].

In a randomized controlled trial zoledronic acid (4 mg) was evaluated against a placebo in patients with metastatic HRPC. A greater proportion of patients who received placebo had skeletal-related events than those who received zoledronic acid at 4 mg (44.2% vs 33.2%; difference $= -11.0\%$, $p = 0.021$). Median time to first skeletal-related event was 321 days for patients who received placebo and was (considered as) 420 days for patients who received zoledronic acid at 4 mg ($p = .011$ vs placebo). Zoledronic acid 4 mg given as a 15-min infusion was well tolerated (Fig. 10.4).

Conclusions

Pharmacotherapy for prostate cancer has recently undergone a number of significant advances. The use of the antiandrogen bicalutamide appears to significantly reduce the risk of objective progression in men with locally advanced prostate cancer, albeit at the price of significant gynaecomastia. This, however, may be avoided by breast irradiation or the use of tamoxifen. Bicalutamide has a lesser impact on sexual function than LHRH analogues but is not as effective in the management of metastatic disease Hormone therapy remains the mainstay for advanced disease, but when relapse occurs the use of the taxane docetaxel appears to improve overall survival by

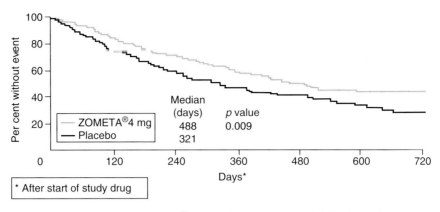

Figure 10.4 Zoledronic acid (Zometa™) delays the time to onset of skeletal complications by a mean of 5 months [36].

several months and sometimes more. Recent data suggest that the bisphosphonate zoledronic acid delays the risk of skeletal-related events by around 5 months. Much work remains to be done to improve outcomes from pharmacotherapy and to reduce unwanted side-effects, but as a result of these advances the outlook for the many men with prostate cancer has improved significantly.

References

1 Klein EA, Thompson IM. Update on chemoprevention of prostate cancer. *Curr opin Urol* 2004; **14**(3): 143–9.

2 Thompson IM, Goodman P, Tangen C *et al*. The influence of finasteride on the development of prostate cancer. *N Engl J Med* 2003; **349**(3): 215–24.

3 Pliepich MV *et al*. Phase III radiation therapy oncology group (RTOG) trial 86-10 of androgen deprivation adjuvant to definitive radiotherapy in locally advanced carcinoma of the prostate. *Int J Radiat Oncol Biol Phys* 2001; **50**: 1243–52.

4 Bolla M *et al*. Improved survival in patients with locally advanced prostate cancer treated with radiotherapy and goserelin. *N Engl J Med* 1997; **337**: 295–300.

5 Johansson JE, Andren O, Andersson SO *et al*. Natural history of early, localized prostate cancer. *J Am Med Assoc* 2004; **291**: 2713–19.

6 Soloway MS *et al*. Randomized prospective study comparing radical prostatectomy alone versus radical prostatectomy preceded by androgen blockade in clinical stage B2 (T2bN× M0) prostate cancer. *J Urol* 1995; **154**: 424–8.

7 Soloway MS *et al*. Neoadjuvant androgen ablation before radical prostatectomy in cT2bN ×M0 prostate cancer: 5 year results. *J Urol* 2002; **167**: 112–16.

8 Lorente JA *et al*. A longer duration of neo adjuvant combined androgen blockade prior to radical prostatectomy may lead to lower tumor volume of localised prostate cancer. *Eur Urol* 2003; **43**: 119–23.

9 Eastham JA, Kelly WK, Grossfeld GD *et al*. Cancer and Leukemia Group B (CALGB) 90203: a randomized phase 3 study of radical prostatectomy alone versus estramustine and docetaxel before radical prostatectomy for patients with high-risk localized disease. *Urology* 2003; **62**(Suppl. 1): 55–62.

10 D'Amico V *et al*. 6-month androgen suppression plus radiation therapy versus radiation therapy alone for patients with clinically localised prostate cancer. A randomised controlled trial. *J Am Med Assoc* 2004; **292**: 821–7.

11 See WA, Iversen P, McLeod DG *et al*. Bicalutamide 150 mg in addition to standard care significantly improves prostate-specific antigen progression-free survival in patients with early, non-metastatic prostate cancer: median 5.4 years' follow-up. *J Urol* 2004; **171**(Suppl.): 280–81, A1062.

12 Iversen P, Johansson JE, Lodding P *et al*. Bicalutamide (150 mg) versus placebo as immediate therapy alone or as adjuvant to therapy with curative intent for early nonmetastatic prostate cancer: 5.3-year median followup from the Scandinavian Prostate Cancer Group Study Number 6. *J Urol* 2004; **172** (5 Pt 1): 1871–6.

13 McLeod D, Iversen P, See W *et al*. Bicalutamide ('Casodex') 150 mg as adjuvant to radiotherapy significantly improves progression-free survival in early non-metastatic prostate cancer: results from the bicalutamide early prostate cancer programme after a median 5.4 years' follow-up. *Eur Urol* 2004; **3**(48): A182.

14 Wirth M, Iversen P, McLeod D *et al*. On behalf of the 'Casodex' Early Prostate Cancer Trialists' Group. Bicalutamide ('Casodex') 150 mg as adjuvant to radical prostatectomy significantly increases progression-free survival in patients with early non-metastatic prostate cancer: analysis at a median follow-up of 5.4 years. *Eur Urol* 2004; **3**(48)(Suppl.): A181.

15 Iversen P, McLeod D, See W *et al*. Bicalutamide ('Casodex') 150 mg in addition to watchful waiting in patients with early non-metastatic prostate cancer: updated analysis at a median 5.4 years' follow-up. *Eur Urol* 2004; **3**(47)(Suppl.): A180.

16 Byar DP, Corle DK. Hormone therapy for prostate cancer: results of the Veterans Administration Cooperative Urological Research Group studies. *NCI Monogr* 1988; **7**: 165–70.

17 The Medical Research Council Prostate Cancer Working Party Investigators Group. Immediate versus deferred treatment for advanced prostatic cancer: initial results of the Medical Research Council Trial. *Br J Urol* 1997; **79**: 235–46.

18 Schröder FH, Kurth KH, Fossa SD *et al*. Early versus delayed endocrine treatment in pN1–3M0 prostate cancer without local treatment of the primary tumor. Results of EORTC 30846 – a phase III study. *J Urol* 2003; **169**: 398.

19 Messing EM, Manola J, Sarosdy M, Wilding G, Crawford ED, Trump D. Immediate hormonal therapy compared with observation after radical prostatectomy and pelvic lymphadenectomy in men with node-positive prostate cancer. *N Engl J Med* 1999; **341**: 1781–8.

20 Soloway MS. Timing of androgen deprivation for prostate cancer: benefits versus side effects – a patient-physician dialogue. *Urology* 2002; **60**: 735–7.

21 Waltregny D, Boca P, Nicolas H *et al*. Intermittent versus continuous total androgen blockade in the treatment of patients with advanced hormone-naive prostate cancer: results of a randomized prospective multicenter clinical trial. *J Urol* 2002; **167**: 175.

22 Strum SB, Scholz MC, McDermed JE. Intermittent androgen deprivation in prostate cancer patients: factors predictive of prolonged time off therapy. *Oncologist* 2000; **5**: 45–52.

23 Thorpe SC, Azmatullah S, Fellows GJ, Gingell JC, O'Boyle PJ. A prospective, randomised study to compare goserelin acetate (Zoladex) versus cyproterone acetate (Cyprostat) versus a combination of the two in the treatment of metastatic prostatic carcinoma. *Eur Urol* 1996; **29**: 47–54.

24 Sarosdy MF, Schellhammer PF, Johnson R *et al*. Does prolonged combined androgen blockade have survival benefits over short-term combined androgen blockade therapy? *Urology* 2000; **55**(3): 391–5.

25 Landis SH, Murray T, Bolden S *et al*. Cancer statistics. 1998. *California Cancer J Clin* 1998; **1**: 6–29.

26 Smith DC *et al*. Chemotherapy for hormone refractory prostate cancer. *Urol Clin North Am* 1999; **26**: 323.

27 Kantoff PW, Halabi S, Conaway M *et al*. Hydrocortisone with or without mitoxantrone in men with hormone refractory prostate cancer: results of the Cancer and Leukaemia group B 9182 study. *J Clin Oncol* 1999; **17**: 2506–13.

28 Berry W, Dakhil S, Modiano M *et al*. Phase III study of mitoxantrone plus low dose prednisolone versus low dose prednisolone alone in patients with asymptomatic hormone refractory prostate cancer. *J Urol* 2002; **168**: 2439–3.

29 Haldar S, Chintapaali J, Croce CM *et al*. Taxol induces Bcl-2 phosphorylation and death of prostate cancer cells. *Cancer Res* 1996; **56**: 1253–5.

30 Tannock IF, de Wit R, Berry WR *et al*. Docetaxel plus prednisone or mitoxantrone plus prednisone for advanced prostate cancer. *N Engl J Med* 2004; **351**(15): 1502–12.

31 Savarese DM, Halabi S, Hars V *et al*. Phase II study of docetaxel, estramustine and low dose hydrocortisone in men with hormone refractory prostate cancer: a final report of CALGB 9780. *J Clin Oncol* 2001; **19**: 2509–16.

32 Petrylak DP, Tangen CM, Hussain MHA. Docetaxel and estramustine compared with mitoxantrone and prednisone for advanced refractory prostate cancer. *N Engl J Med* 2004; **351**(15): 1513–20.

33 Carlin BI, Andriole GL. The natural history, skeletal complications, and management of bone metastases in patients with prostate carcinoma. *Cancer* 2000; **88**: 2989–94.

34 Townsend MF, Sanders WH, Northway RO, Graham SD Jr. Bone fractures associated with luteinizing hormone-releasing hormone agonists used in the treatment of prostate carcinoma. *Cancer* 1997; **79**: 545–50.

35 Oefelein MG, Ricchiuiti V, Conrad W *et al*. Skeletal fractures negatively correlate with overall survival in men with prostate cancer. *J Urol* 2002; **1687**: 1005–1007.

36 Rosen LS, Gordon D, Antonio BS, Kaminski M, Howell A, Belch A *et al*. Zoledronic acid versus pamidronate in the treatment of skeletal metastases in patients with breast cancer or osteolytic lesions of multiple myeloma: a phase III, double-blind, comparative trial. *Cancer J* 2001; **7**: 377–87.

11: Drugs in Superficial Bladder Cancer

Peter Whelan

Introduction

Since the introduction of thiotepa as an intravesical agent by Swinney *et al.* [1] in 1961, drugs have been used in patients with superficial bladder cancer to try and both reduce the recurrence rate and prevent progression of superficial disease to invasive bladder cancer. Whilst new agents have been introduced as intravesical therapies and there is a greater understanding both of the progress of superficial disease and of the action of these agents on superficial bladder cancer since that time, optimal therapy, optimal timing and an optimal agent still remain to be definitively identified.

Rationale for intravesical therapy

Because even patients with well-differentiated superficial bladder tumours have a high recurrence rate of the order of 70% and because with the risk of recurrence the possibility of both progression of stage and grade can occur, the elimination of superficial disease is essential. Although the rate of progression, at possibly 20% overall, is smallest in the pTa G1 lesion (at 2–3%) and greatest in the pT1 G3 lesion, at possibly 40%, the treatment of muscle-invasive disease carries both a significant morbidity and a mortality and even in patients having early aggressive therapy 5-year survivals are little better than at 50%.

Intravesical chemotherapy has been utilized both prophylactically (once the initial superficial lesions have been extirpated) and therapeutically in order to remove both clinical and subclinical areas of tumour.

Although there is a decided association with increasing grade and stage from Ta G1 to T1 G3 as to the risks of progression, clinical trials in superficial bladder cancer have demonstrated that other prognostic factors have a role and are independent predictors of disease progression. These include [2,3]

1 multiplicity of tumours;
2 a rapid recurrence rate;
3 T1 or associated carcinoma in situ (CIS);
4 a grade 3 tumour with adjacent dysplasia or CIS;

5 a positive urine cytology in the absence of overt lesions within the bladder;
6 a positive urethral biopsy;
7 initial large tumour size.

All the above are independent factors both for increased chance of recurrence and for disease progression.

During the last 20 years an attempt at a more systematic approach, based on the results of clinical trials, has been made in the utilization of intravesical cancer therapy of the bladder, but as will be demonstrated in discussion of individual agents that have been used, most of this has evolved by serendipity rather than a rigorous dose-ranging regime, with due attention paid to the pharmacological concepts of optimizing drug therapy. Historically, this has occurred because of the excellent response that early papers have demonstrated with intravesical regimes of both chemotherapy and immunotherapy. Surprisingly, very little clinical attention has been paid to factors that need to be utilized in systemic chemotherapeutic regimes and are known to be capable of altering the cytotoxic effect of chemotherapeutic or immunotherapeutic regimes (such as the effect on the molecular weight of the compound, lipophilicity, optimum pH in which it is utilized, osmolality, dose concentration, dose volumes and the frequency and timing of installations). In only comparatively recent times have attempts been made to control some of the above factors and trials have looked at different dosing regimes, although very frequently only in phase II studies [4–8].

Simple factors such as the optimal time for an agent to be left in the bladder have tended to be judged by the initial reported studies, which probably from convenience have used only 1 or 2 h. There are little or no studies that have investigated whether the control of intravesical recurrence of bladder tumours has any bearing on the inevitable dilution effect that occurs the longer the agent is retained in the bladder and, although most regimes recommend that patients attempt to bring the whole of the bladder into contact with the intravesical agent by rotating themselves through 360° no studies demonstrated whether this actually has the desired effect.

In this chapter the currently available agents for intravesical treatment of superficial bladder cancer are discussed. In the past, attempts have been made to use systemic therapy and small studies using methotrexate and retinoids as oral preparations have failed because of drug toxicity and, in essence, 100% noncompliance by the patients. The difficulty with oral preparations is that in almost all cases, except the odd patient with CIS who has superficial bladder cancer, there are no symptoms and any agent that gives rise to problems exemplified by the above two agents will be rapidly discarded [9].

The role of immunotherapy will be investigated by looking at the possible utilization of other biological response modifiers and the role of photodynamic therapy in superficial bladder cancer and finally by discussing possible novel therapies that can be utilized.

Intravesical chemotherapeutic agents

Thiotepa (triethylene thiophosphoramide)

Thiotepa was first used for intravesical therapy of superficial bladder cancer by Jones and Swinney [1]. It is an alkalizing agent that acts by cross-linking nuclear acids and proteins. It has generally been administered at a dose of 1 mg/ml in either 30 mg in a 30-ml bolus or 60 mg in a 60-ml bolus, with the drug being retained for 2 h. A variety of regimens, including weekly × 6–8 followed by monthly for a year, were frequently used in the 1970s and the early 1980s. It produces complete response rates in approximately 35% of cases and partial remission rates in a further 25% [10] which is somewhat less than other intravesical chemotherapeutic agents. It has also been utilized as a prophylactic agent, with a marked reduction of recurrence rate of 25% over the next 2 years compared with untreated tumours [11].

Because of its low molecular rate (198 Da) thiotepa may readily be absorbed through the bladder wall and can cause marrow suppression in 50–20% of patients. Although it is still utilized occasionally as an active agent, because of its potential toxicity its utilization has tended to fall compared with both other intravesical chemotherapeutic agents and immunotherapeutic agents such as bacille Calmette–Guérin (BCG). There is no evidence that thiotepa prevents progression of superficial disease.

Adriamycin (doxorubicin hydrochloride)

Adriamycin was isolated in 1963 by aerobic fermentation of *Streptomyces peucetius*, a variant of *S. caesius* as an anti-neoplastic antibiotic agent. Chemically, it is an anthracycline excerpting its cytostatic activity through binding specifically with DNA by intercalation between adjacent-based pairs of the double helix, thus interrupting DNA synthesis and also protein synthesis [12] The utilization of this agent intravesically showed complete response compared with transurethral resection (TUR) alone, which ranged between 5% and 39% [13] and its benefits when used in a prophylactic fashion in a reduction of recurrence rate between 20% and 40% compared with TUR alone [2, 11]. From the present available data we can see that for patients with low and intermediate risk superficial bladder tumours [3] the recurrence rate with Adriamycin compared with BCG is lower [14, 15], but in high-risk tumours BCG is superior in reducing the recurrence rate.

Adriamycin has largely been superseded by epirubicin both in its systemic activity in other cancers and in the treatment of superficial bladder disease, but the drug can still be used safely because of its relatively high molecular weight with minimal systemic toxicity.

Epirubicin

Epirubicin differs from doxorubicin by the epimerization of the hydroxyl group at position 4 of the amino acids [16]. It was developed with a view to enhancing the therapeutic activity and has had a significant decrease in side-effects when given parentally as compared with doxorubicin. Its dose, however, not dissimilarly to Adriamycin, has a series of local toxicity profiles and in studies using epirubicin up to 30% of patients are discontinued intravesical treatment because of local toxicity. A significant paper showing the utility of intravesical agents overall was that of Oosterlinck *et al.* [17], which demonstrated that a single installation of 80 mg of epirubicin in all grades (low, intermediate and high risk superficial bladder cancer) produced a 50% reduction in recurrence. Figures were confirmed by the Medical Research Council (MRC) in a series of studies utilizing thiotepa and epirubicin and mitomycin C.

A single installation of a chemotherapeutic agent (either epirubicin or mitomycin C), given within 24 h of resection of the superficial bladder cancer, has this persistent and forecastable benefit and should be considered standard therapy.

Mitomycin C

Mitomycin C is an antibiotic chemotherapeutic agent that acts by inhibition of DNA synthesis. It has a high molecular weight of 334 Da, such that there is little in the way of systemic absorption from the bladder. In 1975, Mishina *et al.* [18] reported the results of a 7-year-long phase II trial using intravesical mitomycin C for superficial bladder cancer. Fifty patients received 20 mg of mitomycin C and 20 ml of saline, which they retained for an average of 3 h, but they were asked to retain it for as long as possible. Patients received three installations per week for 7 weeks, and complete response was achieved in 44% of patients and partial responses in a further 16%. This demonstrated that mitomycin C alone could eradicate tumours from the bladder without preliminary resection.

In 1983, Harrison *et al.* [19] validated this study in 23 patients utilizing the same intensive regime, although the duration of installation was limited to 1 h but with an overall response rate of 77%. It has already been confirmed that a single installation following transurethral resection of prostate (TURP), mitomycin C has the same benefit as epirubicin. Because of the proven efficacy of mitomycin C, in patients debilitated by general medical problems such as severe cardiac or respiratory disease, which are exacerbated by bleeding from superficial bladder lesions thus rendering the patient unfit for an anaesthetic and surgery, naturalisation of the Mishima regimen with mitomycin C at either the 20 or 40 mg in 40 mls dose can often stop the bleeding and allow time for the patient to become fitter before resection and additional therapy can be given.

SIDE-EFFECTS

Because of its relatively large molecular size specific side-effects are small but do include chemical cystitis with associated pain and haematuria. A specific effect relating only to mitomycin usage is contact dermatitis, which is frequently on the hands and around the genitalia and occasionally on the feet. A systematic review of the literature suggests that approximately 9% of patients developed these skin reactions and this is a contraindication given that there are alternatives to further usage of mitomycin C [20].

Mitoxzantrone

This agent is chemically related to doxorubicin and has been shown to be useful with relatively few installations in a phase II study [21]. It has an effect equivalent to epirubicin or mitomycin but needs only half the number of installations. It is a useful second-line agent in patients who have persistent superficial disease, are intolerant of BCG or who find it burdensome to come and have intravesical installations on a weekly basis.

Valrubicin

This is a semi-synthetic analogue of the antibiotic Adriamycin. It is highly lipophilic and installations at a dose of 800 mg and 13.3% ethanol have shown good efficacy levels, as described by Newling *et al.* [22]. Fifty-four per cent of patients had a complete response after six installations, confirmed by review cystoscopy at 3 months. This again is a useful second-line agent but has no proven benefits or superiority over the longer-established mitomycin C or epirubicin.

Immunotherapy

Bacille Calmette–Guérin

Morales *et al.* [23] first reported the benefits of intravesical BCG using six weekly installations of approximately 10^9 cultures. This six-dose installation became the standard regimen although it appears chance alone gave Morales the opportunity to use six installations. A 60% response rate in papillary disease was reported and this has been consistently confirmed [13]. Although useful in papillary disease, its greatest benefit is in the treatment of primary CIS, an uncommon disease in this form although appearing much more commonly associated with aggressive papillary tumours as secondary CIS. In the pure disease, as reported by Herr *et al.*, in excess of 70% response rates are achieved but longer follow-ups have shown that there is a late relapse rate [24] and lifelong follow-up in patients who have achieved a response is mandatory [25–28].

Although effective BCG is associated with a high incidence of both local and systemic side-effects including mortality, much of this appeared to be in the early days of its usage when it was instilled early into bladders in which resections had occurred and undoubtedly there was a systemic absorption that gave rise to BCGosis. After enforcement of a policy of requiring a minimum 2-week delay between resection and the initiation of intravesical BCG therapy, the rate of side-effects and especially the serious systemic side-effects have significantly reduced, although local toxic side-effects remain [29].

The second innovation has been the suggestion that maintenance, i.e. continuing top-up BCG advocated by Lamm, has a better overall efficiency than just a single course. In Lamm's original discussion two to three additional top-up doses of BCG are used every 3–6 months over an 18/24-month period and there is some evidence that this regimen although difficult and susceptible to a high dropout rate of patients does seem to have some effect in limiting progression of the disease to invasive disease. The comparative benefits of BCG versus intravesical chemotherapeutic agents have been the subject of several studies and are discussed below [24].

Interferon-alpha

It is a naturally occurring biological protein with both antiviral and antiprolific properties. Toxicity appears to be limited to mild flu-like symptoms and most studies of interferon have been with interferon-alpha in phase I and II, mostly in CIS. Although its use as a prophylactic agent has been reported with some benefits, its utility has not been demonstrated almost certainly because of the difficulty in obtaining it as an agent and the ready accessibility and utility of BCG [30]. The use of interferon alpha in combination with BCG and also with mitomycin C has been explored with benefit in small phase II studies [31,32]

Keyhole limpet haemocyanin

Keyhole limpet haemocyanin (KLH) is a protein of the mollusc *Megathura crenulata* and is a highly immunogenic protein. It was used for many years as an experimental antigen in the study of delayed hypersensitivity Olsson first noted a marked reduction in papillary tumour recurrence among patients that had been immunized with subcutaneous KLH and he then performed a small prospective trial confirming the apparent anti-tumour effect of KLH in 1972 and 1974, and in 1988 Jurinic showed its benefits in a small randomized trial, with a recurrence rate of only 14% in the KLH arm compared with 39% in the mitomycin C arm [33,34].

It has been this author's frustrating experience that this agent has been virtually unobtainable for further studies in intravesical chemotherapy. Concluding from both the original work of Olsson *et al.* [35] and the one small trial it is at least equivalent to BCG and probably more effective with less side-effects and yet remains frustratingly unavailable. It is an agent about which future comparative studies should and must be made.

Photodynamic therapy

Photodynamic therapy (PDT) is a treatment that uses a photosensitizing drug that when activated by light in the presence of oxygen produces local cell death. Focal light PDT was first described in the bladder in 1976 [36] with whole-bladder wall laser PDT following in 1984. Since then more than 350 patients with superficial bladder cancer have been treated and most of the reported series, however, have been those with CIS. Whilst the remaining patients have had multiple recurrent Ta T1 disease, 3-month response rates in these small numbers, ranging from 33% to 100% and importantly a 50% response rate in patients with previously resistant CIS and papillary disease, have been encouraging. The clinical acceptance of photodynamic therapy has been limited by its complexity and the reported adverse side-effects. These are usually related to the porphyrins that have led to skin photosensitization and this has meant that patients have had to stay out of sunlight for many weeks following this treatment. There have also been serious local effects including bladder fibrosis and associated contracture in more than 10% of reported patients [37,38].

It was felt that these problems were inherent with the early systemically administered photosensitizers, which have typically been porforin or haematoporphyrin derivatives that were slowly metabolized and were associated with poor tumour to detrusor selectivity and that resulted in PDT damage to the bladder muscle. Although careful light dissymmetry could alleviate bladder contractory completely it was claimed that this added a further level of complexity to the delivery of this therapy.

Recently a new 'second generation' intravesically delivered photosensitizer 5-amino levulinic acid (ALA) has enabled a re-evaluation of PDT for superficial bladder transitional cell carcinoma (TCC). Preclinical studies have shown that there is active uptake of the metabolite of ALA within the urothelium and TCC but virtually none within the detrusor. In addition, patients have not been troubled in the small group of patients hitherto studied with photosensitivity because of the rapid metabolization of ALA [39,40].

The treatment is still complex, requiring a special laser light delivery source and the utilization of graded intravesical dosing but a recent article [41] suggests that these second-generation photodynamic therapy agents can be given intravesically under a local anaesthetic. This may make them more useful and acceptable to patients.

Comparisons of intravesical chemo- and immunotherapy [29]

When direct studies comparing the utility of intravesical chemotherapy or of immunotherapy have been used different results were apparent. The studies of Lamm have shown a clear superiority of BCG over Adriamycin and appear to do the same for mitomycin C only at a relatively low dosage. However, Witjes *et al.* [42] in a well-constructed study using BCG RIV (the Dutch-produced BCG strain) against mitomycin found no difference between the two agents both in recurrence rate and in short-term progression rates. It remains contentious whether any form of intravesical therapy has the ability to prevent progressive disease. Certainly the longer-term follow-up of even those patients with complete responses to both BCG and mitomycin tends to suggest that the bladder is always at risk of superficial bladder cancer and that long-term progression can occur after either type of therapy.

Novel therapies

The initial goal of intravesical treatment was to reduce recurrence rates and the currently used agents discussed in this chapter achieve this to varying degrees. The more important and less well documented goal is to prevent cases in which an initial superficial cancer progresses to invasive disease, which is the primary goal of any novel therapy for superficial bladder cancer. The important work of pooling the extensive European Organization for Research and Treatment of Cancer (EORTC) and MRC [3] prospective randomized studies in superficial bladder cancer, has clearly defined patients that can be apportioned to low-, intermediate-and high-risk categories. In the high-risk category patients, up to 40% may subsequently demonstrate an invasive bladder cancer. The EORTC has also pioneered the utility of the marker lesion [43] and this enables novel therapies to be assessed for therapeutic utility against a marker lesion, but their ability to affect the most-at-risk patients can be decided by looking at them in high-risk category tumours in carefully constructed prospected phase II/III trials.

Although there still remains a place for a synthetic intravesical agent that can clear bladders and prevent recurrence, it is more likely, with our greater understanding, that the new era of biological therapy will actually produce the next generation of intravesical drugs. Intravesical treatment is useful because the bladder is accessible; has a large surface area, which enables prolonged contact with any novel therapy; and can rapidly and frequently be monitored for side-effect. Vectors such as a virus can be used to carry either replacement or genetically neutralizing proteins into the tumour to prevent progression of disease, because undoubtedly the bladder mucosa will be unstable. The possibility of modifying or reversing that instability should have a very fruitful opening and the benefits previously described for retinoids may, by utilizing new biological methods of transfection, enable these plastic and neoplastic changes to be reversed as they have been demonstrated to be reversed in the laboratory with retinoids more than 30 years ago. [44–48]

Conclusions

Thiotepa in the early 1960s and subsequently BCG in the mid-1970s have provided useful tools for the consistent reduction of superficial bladder cancer recurrence. No drug, however, has consistently prevented recurrence nor have they consistently prevented progression. Large trials carried out in the 1980s by the MRC and EORTC, which remain the bedrock of our understanding of the therapy of superficial bladder cancer, have identified three coherent and consistent groups of patients at low, intermediate and high risk of recurrence and subsequent progression. This means that with novel therapies, which may more effectively interfere and indeed reverse the processes leading to potential invasion, the right group of patients can be identified and in prospective randomized trials, hopefully, fruitful answers will come quickly rather than in the serendipitous way that drugs in superficial bladder cancer have evolved in the last 30 years.

References

1 Jones HC, Swinney J. Thiotepa in the treatment of tumours in the bladder. *Lancet* 1961; 2: 615.
2 Kurth KH, Schroder FH, De Bruyne F *et al.* Long-term follow-up in superficial transitional cell carcinoma of the bladder: prognostic factors for time to first recurrence rate and survival. *Prog Clin Biol Res* 1989; 303: 481.
3 Pawinski A, Stylvester R, Kurth KH *et al.* A combined analysis of EORTC and MRC randomised clinical trials for the prophylactic treatment of Ta T1 bladder cancer. *J Urol* 1997; 156: 1934.

4   Walker MC, Masters JRW, Paris CN. Intravesical chemotherapy: in vitro studies ion the relationship between dose and toxicity. *Urol Res* 1997; **14**: 137.

5   Groos E, Masters RJW. Intravesical chemotherapy studies on the relationship between osmolarity and cytoxicity. *J Urol* 1986; **136**: 399.

6   Klans JE, Wientjes MG, Badalament RA *et al*. Pharmacokinetic intervention to improve intravesical therapy of superficial bladder cancer. *J Urol* 1995; **153**: 232A.

7   Ritchie JP. Intravesical chemotherapy treatment selection, techniques, results. *Urol Clin North Am* 1992; **19**(3): 521.

8   Huland H, Kloppel G, Feddersen I *et al*. Comparison of different schedules of systematic intravesical installations in patients with superficial bladder carcinoma final evaluation of a prospective multi centre study with 419 patients. *J Urol* 1990; **144**: 68.

9   Bassi P, Piassa N, Pagano F. Retinoids and principles of intravesical therapy. In: Pagano F, Fair WR, eds. *Superficial Bladder Cancer*. Oxford: Isis Medical Media, 1997: 74.

10 Koontz WW, Prout GR, Smith W *et al*. The use of intravesical thiotepa in the management of non-invasive carcinoma of the bladder. *J Urol* 1981; **125**: 307.

11 Zincke H, Utz DC, Taylor WF *et al*. Influence of thiotepa and doxorubicin installation at time of transurethral surgical treatment of bladder cancer on tumour recurrence: a prospective, randomised, double blind controlled trial. *J Urol* 1983; **129**: 505.

12 Carter SK. Adriamycin – a review. *J Natl Cancer Inst* 1975; **55**: 1265.

13 Lamm DL, Crawford ED, Blumevstein B *et al*. SWOG 8795: a randomised comparison of bacillus Calmette–Guérin and mitomycin C prophylaxis in stage Ta and T1 transitional cell carcinoma of the bladder. *J Urol* 1993; **149**(2): 275A.

14 Matinez-Pineiro JA, Leon JJ, Martinez-Pineiro L *et al*. Bacillus Calmette–Guérin versus doxorubicin versus thiotepa: a randomised prospective trial in 202 patients with superficial bladder cancer. *J Urol* 1990; **143**: 502.

15 Lamm DL, Blumenstein BA, Crawford ED et al. A randomised trial of intravesical doxorubicin and immunotherapy with bacillus Calmette–Guérin for transitional cell carcinoma of the bladder. *N Engl J Med* 1991; **325**: 1705.

16 Cersosimo RJ, Hong WK. Epirubicin: a review of the pharmacology, clinical activity and adverse events of an Adriamycin analogue. *J Clin Oncol* 1986; **4**: 425.

17 Oosterlinck W, Kurth KH, Schroder FH *et al*. A prospective European Organisation for Research and Treatment of Cancer – Genito Urinary Group randomised trial comparing transurethral resection followed by a single intravesical installation of epirubicin or water in single stage Ta T1 papillary carcinoma of the bladder. *J Urol* 1993; **149**: 749.

18 Mishina T, Oda K, Murtata S *et al*. Mitomycin C bladder installation therapy for bladder tumour. *J Urol* 1975; **114**: 217.

19 Harrison GSM, Green DF, Newling DWW *et al*. A phase II study of intravesical mitomycin C in the treatment of superficial bladder cancer. *Br J Urol* 1983; **55**: 676.

20 Van der Meijden AMR. Overview on mitomycin C side effects profile. In: Pagano F, Fair WR, eds. *Superficial Bladder Cancer*. Oxford: Isis Medical Media, 1997: 117.

21 Navasivayam S, Whelan P. Intravesical Mitozantrone in recurrent superficial bladder cancer a phase II study. *Brit J Urol* 1995; **75**(6): 740–43.

22 Newling DWW, Hetherington JW, Sundara SK *et al*. The use of valrubicin for chemoresection of superficial bladder cancer. A marker lesion study. *Eur Urol* 2001; **39**: 643.

23 Morales A, Eidinger D, Bruce AW. Intracavitary Bacillus Calmette–Guérin on the treatment of superficial bladder tumours *J Urol* 1976; **116**: 180.

24 Lamm DL, Blumenstein BA, Crissman JD *et al*. Maintenance Bacillus Calmette-Guérin immunotherapy for recurrent Ta T1 and carcinoma in situ transitional cell carcinoma of the bladder, a randomised Southwest Oncology Group Study. *J Urol* 2000; **163**: 1124.

25 Brusman SA. Experience with bacillus Calmette–Guérin in patients with superficial bladder cancer. *J Urol* 1982; **128**: 27.

26 Di Marco A, Zunio F, Silvestrini R *et al*. Interaction of some davnomycin derivatives with deoxyribonucleic acid and their biological activity. *Biochem Pharmacol* 1971; **20**: 1323.

27 Lamm DL. Long term results of intravesical therapy for superficial bladder cancer. *Urol Clin North Am* 1992; **19**: 573.

28 Lamm DL. Carcinoma in situ. In: Lamm DL, ed. *The Urologic Clinic of North America*. Philadelphia: W.B Saunders, 1992; **19**: 499.

29 Lamm DL, Van der Meidden APM, Akaza LT *et al*. Intravesical chemotherapy and immunotherapy: how do we assess their effectiveness and what are their and uses? *Int J Urol* 1975; **2**: 23.

30 Sarodsy M. High dose versus low dose intravesical interferon-alpha 2b in the treatment of carcinoma in situ, a randomised controlled study. *Anticancer Drugs* 1992; 3(Suppl.): 13.

31 O'Donnell MA, Krohn J, De Wolf WC. Salvage intravesical therapy with interferon-alpha 2b plus low dose bacillus Calmette–Guérin is effective in patients with superficial bladder cancer in whom bacillus Calmette–Guérin alone previously failed. *J Urol* 2000; **166**: 1300.

32 Malmstrom PV. A randomised comparative dose-ranging study of interferon-alpha and mitomycin C as an initial control in primary or recurrent superficial transitional cell carcinoma of the bladder. *BJU Int* 2002; **89**: 681.

33 Olsson C, Chute R, Rao C. Immunologic reduction of bladder cancer recurrence rate. *J Urol* 1974; **111**: 173.

34 Jurinic CD, Engelmann V, Gasch J *et al*. Immunotherapy in bladder cancer with keyhole limpet haemocyanin: a randomised study. *J Urol* 1988; **139**: 723.

35 Olsson C, Rao C, Menzion J *et al*. Immunologic activity in bladder cancer patients. *J Urol* 1972; **107**: 607.

36 Kelly JF, Snell ME. Haemoporhyrin derivatives. A possible aid in the therapy of carcinoma of the bladder. *J Urol* 1976; **115**: 150.

37 Bonson RC. Treatment of bladder cancer with haemoporphyrins derivatives and laser light. *Urology* 1988; **31**: 13.

38 Harty J, Amin M, Wieman TJ *et al*. Complications of whole bladder dihaematoporphyrin ether photodynamic therapy. *J Urol* 1989; **141**: 1341.

39 Kriegmain M, Stepp H, Steinbach P *et al*. Fluorescence cystoscopy following intravesical instillation of 5 aminolevulinic and: a new procedure with high sensitivity if highly visible urothelial neoplasms. *Urol Int* 1995; **55**: 190.

40 Walther MM, Delaney TF, Smith PD *et al*. Phase I trial of photoluminescence therapy in the treatment of recurrent superficial transitional call carcinoma of the bladder. *Urology* 1997; **50**: 199.

41 Shackley DC, Briggs C, Gilholley A *et al*. Photodynamic therapy for superficial bladder cancer under local anaesthetic. *BJU Int* 2002; **89**: 665.

42 Vegt PDJ, Witjes WPJ *et al*. A randomised study of intravesical mitomycin C, Bacillus Calmette–Guérin TKC, and Bacillus Calmette–Guérin RIVM treatment in pTa T1 papillary carcinoma and carcinoma in situ of the bladder. *J Urol* 1995; **153**: 929.

43 Van der Meijden APM, Hall RR, Pavone-Macaluso M *et al*. Marker tumour response to the sequential combination of intravesical therapy with mitomycin C and BCG – RIV in multiple superficial bladder tumour reports from the European Organisation for Research and Treatment of Cancer – Genito-Urinary Group. (EORTC 30897). *Eur Urol* 1996; **29**: 199.

44 Morris BD, Drazan KE, Ceste ME et al. Adenoviral-mediated gene transfer to bladder in vivo. *J Urol* 1994; **152**: 506.

45 Messing EM. Clinical implication of the expression of epidermal growth factor receptors in human transitional cell carcinoma. *Cancer Res* 1990; **50**: 2530.

46 Camilleri-Broet S, Vanderwerff H, Caldwell C, Hockenbery D. Distinct alterations in mitochondrial mass and function characterise different models of apoptosis. *Exp Cell Res* 1998; **239**: 277–92.

47 Zhu P, Yu XD, Ling S *et al*. Mitochondrial Ca(2+) homeostasis in the regulation of apoptosis and reactive cell death. *Cell Calcium* 2000; **28**: 107.

48 Jones A, Fudiyama C, Turner K *et al*. Role of thymidine phosphatase in an in vitro model of human bladder cancer invasion. *J Urol* 2000; **167**: 1482.

12: Systemic Therapy for Bladder Cancer

J. D. Chester & M. G. Leahy

Introduction

Despite radical treatments with curative intent, the chance of long-term survival for patients with muscle-invasive bladder cancer remains disappointing. In a large series of more than 1000 patients with apparently organ-confined disease, 5-year overall survival was only 47% for all muscle-invasive tumours, ranging from 72% for T2 tumours to only 33% for T4 disease [1]. Death from bladder cancer following radical primary treatment is largely due to occult systemic disease, present at the time of surgery, which is below the limits of resolution of currently available cross-sectional imaging.

This chapter reviews systemic therapy for muscle-invasive cancer of the urothelium and describes the common drugs that are used, the various clinical scenarios when they may be indicated and the selection of patients for treatment.

Drugs in use

Orthodox cytotoxic agents

Transitional cell carcinoma (TCC) is sensitive to a variety of drugs as shown by complete or partial response in patients with measurable metastatic or locally advanced disease. Of the older cytotoxic drugs, cisplatin and methotrexate are the most active agents, with significant activity also seen with carboplatin, doxorubicin, vinblastine, cyclophosphamide, ifosfamide and 5-fluorouracil (Table 12.1). Newer agents with significant activity against bladder cancers include gemcitabine [2] and paclitaxel [3].

CISPLATIN

Cisplatin is a derivative of the heavy metal platinum. As a single agent, cisplatin produces objective response rates between 12% and 35% in bladder tumours [4,5]. Its activity as a DNA-modifying cytotoxic drug is as a bifunctional alkylating agent, which results in intra-strand cross-linking of DNA, thereby interfering with synthesis of new DNA during replication. It has a broad range of anti-tumour activity, being particularly effective in tumours that are defective in DNA repair.

188

Table 12.1 Efficacy of cytotoxic agents in TCC

Agent	Response rate (CR + PR) %
Cisplatin	24
Carboplatin	13
Methotrexate	29
Doxorubicin	17
Vinblastine	16
Cyclophosphamide	31
5-Fluorouracil	17
Mitomycin C	13
Ifosfamide	28
Paclitaxel	46
Docetaxel	31
Gemcitabine	22

Cisplatin is administered intravenously. Typical doses range from $40 \, mg/m^2$ to $100 \, mg/m^2$, either in a single dose, or divided over several days. Intravenous (IV) administration is almost invariably as a slow infusion over 2–4 h. When given as an IV bolus, nephrotoxicity is dose-limiting. Pre- and post-hydration with IV crystalloids is routinely employed to minimize nephrotoxicity. This usually means that the patient is admitted overnight, although recently, in selected patients, outpatient schedules have been explored. Cisplatin is not usually administered to patients with glomerular filtration rate (GFR) less than 40 ml/min [6].

Cisplatin is highly emetogenic; however, the introduction of effective anti-emetic regimens, based around combinations of corticosteroids such as dex-amethasone and 5-hydroxytryptamine-3 antagonists such as ondansetron or granisetron, have dramatically reduced acute nausea and vomiting, although 'delayed' effects 4–6 days after administration can still be troublesome.

Haematological toxicity (leukopenia, more than thrombocytopenia or anaemia) is not usually dose-limiting, and recovery from myelosuppression is usually sufficiently rapid to permit 3-week dosing. Alopecia, a side-effect often associated with chemotherapy, is rarely encountered with cisplatin.

Significant neurotoxicity is a common feature of treatment with cisplatin, being dose-limiting for a significant proportion of patients. Peripheral neur-opathy producing numbness and tingling in a glove-and-stocking distribu-tion is seen in up to 40% of long-term survivors, although it rarely severely compromises performance status. Autonomic neuropathy may result in postural hypotension. Central nervous system toxicity is also seen, with tinnitus and high-frequency hearing loss reported in up to 50% of patients, particularly in older age groups. Neurotoxicities may be permanent, and even when they are not, only resolve very slowly, over a period of many months.

Most patients treated with cisplatin have at least temporary reduction in fertility, but sperm counts back to pretreatment levels occur in 40% of younger patients treated with cisplatin, within 2 years. There is no convincing evidence of an increased incidence of second malignancies in long-term survivors following cisplatin-based chemotherapy. A frequently overlooked long-term side-effect of cisplatin is an increase in risk of thromboembolic events. These can often be attributed to comorbidity but careful series have shown a significant increase in myocardial infarction, pulmonary embolism and stroke after cisplatin chemotherapy.

METHOTREXATE

Until relatively recently, methotrexate was the only cytotoxic with single-agent activity comparable with cisplatin, with objective response rates in small studies ranging from 26% to 56% [7–10].

It is an antimetabolite cytotoxic that acts as specifically during the S phase (DNA synthesis) of the cell cycle as a folate antagonist via reversible inhibition of the enzyme dihydrofolate reductase (DHFR), the enzyme that is required to regenerate tetrahydrofolate for thymidine synthesis. By producing a metabolic block, methotrexate produces an accumulation of dihydrofolate, depletion of intracellular pools of reduced folate and reduced synthesis of both the pyrimidine nucleoside thymidine and the purine nucleotides. Methotrexate also inhibits another key nucleic acid–metabolizing enzyme, thymidine synthase, via the formation of polyglutamate derivatives.

Methotrexate can be administered either orally, as an IV solution, via intrathecal injection or, rarely, as an intramuscular injection. When used in chemotherapy for advanced bladder cancer it is usually given as an IV infusion, usually at 30 mg/m² bolus weekly for 2 out of a 3-week or 3 out of a 4-week cycle.

Clearance of methotrexate is predominantly renal, and elimination is inhibited by renal dysfunction but increased toxicity may also be seen in patients with liver dysfunction. Particularly at higher doses, adequate renal function is required for administration of the drug. Renal dysfunction results in slower clearance and prolonged exposure of normal tissues, resulting in increased toxicity. Free distribution into 'third-space' fluid compartments such as pleural fluid or ascites also prolongs drug exposure and increases toxicity. Methotrexate is readily absorbed by the gut. In bladder cancer patients who have had urinary diversion procedures involving the formation of reservoirs from segments of the gastrointestinal (GI) tract, such as an ileal conduit, reabsorption of the drug from the urine may also result in increased toxicity.

At high doses, good renal function and adequate hydration are required, with alkalinization of the urine. Unless this occurs, crystallization of the drug in the urine can cause nephrotoxicity. In contrast to many cytotoxic agents, methotrexate is not particularly myelotoxic and as a result can be successfully combined with other agents without a requirement for a reduction in dose.

Inhibition of DHFR in normal tissues as well as in tumours also accounts for much of the toxicity of methotrexate. GI tract toxicity is common, particularly stomatitis, oral mucositis, nausea and diarrhoea. Acute, reversible hepatitis and pneumonitis are also seen, although more rarely.

The metabolic block produced by methotrexate can be reversed by providing exogenous reduced folates. Folinic acid (leucovorin) 'rescue' can be administered to minimize stomatitis and GI tract toxicity. For lower doses of methotrexate, a 'flat' dose of folinic acid at 15–30 mg QDS for 4–6 doses is usually sufficient, but at higher doses, dose and duration of folinic acid rescue are based on plasma methotrexate levels. Despite some concern, there is no evidence that folinic acid rescue abrogates the therapeutic effect of methotrexate.

VINBLASTINE

Single-agent response rates for vinblastine range from 4% to 28% [3,11]. Vinblastine is a polycyclic organic base that belongs to the vinca alkaloid class of cytotoxic drugs, derived from the periwinkle plant, *Vinca rosea*. Like its formylated analogue vincristine, its mechanism of action is via inhibition of the polymerization of tubulin, thereby inhibiting the formation of microtubules, including the mitotic spindle required for cell division, although effects on microtubules may also produce other toxic effects in non-proliferating cells. However, its spectra of activity and of toxicity are significantly different from those of vincristine. It is usually administered intravenously as a bolus injection into a fast-running drip at a dose of 3–6 mg/m^2, with doses being given weekly in some regimens.

Vinblastine is extensively bound to serum proteins, and to platelets and red blood cells. Metabolism is predominantly hepatic, and it is excreted in the stools via the biliary tract, and, to a lesser extent, is also eliminated in the urine. Care must therefore be taken in administering the drug to patients with an obstructive pattern of liver function tests, and consideration given to dose reduction. Dose modification to take account of renal dysfunction is not usually required.

Extreme caution must be exercised to avoid extravasation, as vinblastine is a vesicant, capable of causing severe tissue necrosis if not promptly and appropriately treated. Principal toxicities of vinblastine are myelosuppression and GI disturbances. Mucositis and stomatitis are more frequently seen with vinblastine than with vincristine, whilst neuropathic effects such as sensory peripheral neuropathy and autonomic neuropathy, resulting in urinary retention or ileus, are seen less often than with vincristine. Like vincristine, vinblastine may cause hyponatraemia, secondary to a syndrome of inappropriate ADH secretion. Hypertension and Raynaud's phenomenon may also be induced, but alopecia is rare and usually only mild.

DOXORUBICIN

Doxorubicin belongs to the anthracycline class of microbially derived antitumour antibiotic compounds. It is composed of a tetracyclic chromophore, adriamycinone (which gives it its characteristic ruby colour), covalently linked to an aminosugar, daunosamine. It has multiple effects on cancer cells, via both the formation of free radicals and intercalation between the stacked base pairs of DNA. In addition to its effects on DNA, and subsequent DNA replication and transcription, it causes damage to mitochondria (where interaction of doxorubicin with the electron transport chain is important in the formation of free radicals), to cytoplasmic structures and to the cell membrane.

Administration of doxorubicin is usually via the IV route, most commonly as a bolus injection into a fast-running IV drip. IV dosing is usually on a 3-week basis, most commonly at doses in the range 45–90 mg/m². It has also been given intravesically as a treatment for superficial bladder cancer (see Chapter 11).

The major route of elimination is via the biliary tract, with no more than 10% being excreted in the urine. Consequently, dose adjustments are required in the case of abnormal hepatic biochemistry, but not in the case of impaired renal function.

The dose-limiting acute toxicities for the administration of doxorubicin are myelosuppression and mucositis/stomatitis. Nausea and vomiting can usually be well controlled with modern anti-emetic regimens. Alopecia is usually seen, although scalp cooling can been used to limit this. However, there is also a chronic dose-limiting toxicity of cardiomyopathy. This is dose-related and clinically significant in about 10% of cases above a cumulative dose of 550 mg/m² [12]. Transient acute dysrhythmias may also occur during the administration of the drug, which are not usually clinically significant. Like vinblastine, doxorubicin is vesicant. Another notable skin toxicity seen with doxorubicin is the so-called 'radiation recall phenomenon', observed 4–7 days after administration of doxorubicin in patients who have had previous external-beam radiotherapy. Patients experience an erythematous dermatitis, similar in appearance to radiation dermatitis, in the anatomical distribution of previous radiation exposure. The severity of the dermatitis is variable, from mild warmth and erythema to severe burning pain, occasionally accompanied by vesicle formation, ulceration or desquamation.

CARBOPLATIN

Carboplatin is an analogue of cisplatin that has shown higher efficacy when compared with cisplatin in some tumour types. Although carboplatin acts via a cell cycle–independent mechanism similar to cisplatin, it has a very different toxicity profile. Carboplatin is generally considered easier for frail or elderly patients to tolerate and can also be given to patients with impaired renal function. Like cisplatin it is predominantly cleared via the renal route, although with slower clearance than cisplatin and rarer nephro- or neurotoxicity. Myelosuppression, particularly thrombocytopenia, is the dose-limiting toxicity. The nadir is late compared with most other cytotoxics, with thrombocytopenia being maximal at around 21 days after administration. Carboplatin-based chemotherapy may therefore be given on a 4-week schedule. Most non-haematological toxicities of carboplatin are mild in comparison with cisplatin, for example, it is less emetogenic. Nevertheless, significant hypersensitivity reactions are seen in a proportion of patients, requiring cover with corticosteroids and antihistamines for subsequent chemotherapy cycles, and occasionally discontinuation of the use of carboplatin entirely.

Like cisplatin it is almost invariably administered via the IV route. Its reduced nephrotoxicity means that it can be administered as a short infusion, without pre- or post-hydration, and can thereby almost always be administered on a day-case basis, rather than requiring admission. Unlike most cytotoxic drugs, dosing of carboplatin is not based on body surface area, but upon renal function, which reliably predicts tissue exposure to a given dose of drug.

GEMCITABINE

Gemcitabine is a nucleoside analogue of deoxycytidine that belongs to the anti-metabolite class of cytotoxic drugs. The active metabolite acts as a chain terminator when DNA strands elongate during replication. Its action is, therefore, cell cycle phase–specific, acting predominantly in the S phase, but also blocking progression through the G1/S phase 'check-point'. It also competitively inhibits the DNA synthesis enzymes DNA polymerase and ribonucleotide reductase.

Like other cytotoxics used in the treatment of metastatic bladder cancer, gemcitabine is administered intravenously, as a short infusion. Typically, dosing is at 1000–1250 mg/m^2 on a weekly or 2 weeks in 3 schedule. Metabolism involves inactivation via deamination, forming difluorodeoxyuridine, which, along with the parent compound is excreted, predominantly (up to 98%) in the urine.

The dose-limiting toxicity of gemcitabine is myelosuppression, particularly neutropenia and thrombocytopenia. Non-haematological toxicities are usually mild. Commonly observed non-haematological adverse effects including nausea and vomiting, rash and flu-like symptoms. Toxicity is greater when longer infusion times are employed; this may be because shorter infusions swamp the capacity for activation and there may be a ceiling effect at about 10 mg/m^2/min [13].

Gemcitabine has shown single-agent response rates of 23–29% in patients pretreated with cisplatin [14,15] and 28–36% in previously untreated patients [2,16]. Complete responses have been reported between 4% and 13%.

PACLITAXEL

The taxanes (paclitaxel and docetaxel) have shown impressive activity both as single agents [17,18] and in combination with other agents [19–21]. Indeed, paclitaxel is the most active drug yet investigated as single-agent first-line therapy [3].

Paclitaxel is a semi-synthetic derivative of a naturally occurring antitumour agent, which is extracted from the bark and needles of the yew tree, *Taxus baccata*. Like vinblastine, its effect is on microtubules, but its mechanism of action is entirely different, causing stabilization of microtubules by preventing depolymerization, with consequent disruption of the intracellular cytoskeleton and of the mitotic spindle.

Paclitaxel is administered intravenously, in a variety of infusional schedules, including 1-, 3-, 6- and 24-h infusions. One of the commonest schedules involves administering at a dose of 175 mg/m^2 as a 3-h infusion, once every 3 weeks, but weekly schedules are also under investigation.

Hypersensitivity or anaphylactic reactions to the IV administration of paclitaxel were seen in 2–4% of patients receiving paclitaxel in early clinical trials. They are unrelated to dose or schedule of the drug, consistent with the hypothesis that they are due to the presence of polyoxyethylated castor oil (Cremophor® EL) required to improve the solubility in aqueous solution of the highly lipophilic paclitaxel molecule. Consequently, all patients receiving paclitaxel now receive premedication, which includes oral or IV corticosteroids and antihistamines. Paclitaxel is metabolized by cytochrome P450 enzymes in the liver and eliminated predominantly in the faeces, via biliary excretion. Very little of the drug or its metabolites is found in the urine. Consequently, dose modification is required for patients with an obstructive pattern of hepatic dysfunction, but is not necessary for patients with renal impairment. Paclitaxel is therefore an attractive drug for the treatment of advanced bladder cancer, where impaired renal function is commonly seen.

In addition to the acute hypersensitivity reactions discussed above, the common toxicities of paclitaxel are myelosuppression, alopecia, transient arthralgia or myalgia, nausea/vomiting, diarrhoea, mucositis and peripheral neuropathy, with neutropenia being the major dose-limiting toxicity. Neurotoxicity is seen in approximately 50% of patients without previous symptoms. It is severe in 2% and results in discontinuation of the drug in 1%. This neurotoxicity is thought to result from effects on microtubules involved in axonal transport of neurotransmitters. Interestingly, when used in combination with carboplatin, paclitaxel seems to interact to produce a platelet-sparing effect, with reduced incidence and severity of thrombocytopenia compared with carboplatin alone.

Relevant clinical trial data

Combination versus single-agent therapy

Cytotoxic chemotherapy with a single drug usually fails to achieve complete cure due to the development of drug-resistant clones. Combining a number of different agents results in an attack on the cancer cell on multiple fronts in the hope that at least one of these attacks will inflict a lethal injury to the largest possible number of cells. With respect to bladder cancer, this rationale has been supported in clinical trials, showing that single-agent regimens are inferior to combination regimens [4,22–26]. Importantly, combination chemotherapy containing cisplatin is superior to the same combination without cisplatin [27], and cisplatin is the foundation of all of the most effective regimens in systemic treatment of urothelial tumours.

Comparison of well-known combination regimens

CMV and MVAC

The CMV regimen [28] is a combination of cisplatin, methotrexate and, vinblastine. In the context of a randomized controlled phase III clinical trial, treatment with CMV resulted in an objective response rate of 46%, with a median survival of 7 months [27].

MVAC [28] combines cisplatin with methotrexate, vinblastine and doxorubicin (Adriamycin™). In randomized controlled trials, this regimen has been found superior to single-agent cisplatin [4,22], combination chemotherapy with cisplatin, cyclophosphamide and doxorubicin (CISCA) [30] and also methotrexate, carboplatin and vinblastine (MCAVI) [31]. For these phase III studies, overall response rates have varied between 39% and 65%, with median survivals up to 16 months [4,31,32]. Dose escalation of MVAC has been attempted using recombinant haematopoietic growth factors [33–35]. Better objective response rates have been reported with the more dose-intense regimen; this did not translate into improved time to disease progression or overall survival in a large randomized controlled trial. However, toxicity was significantly less in the accelerated arm, suggesting that the accelerated regimen may be a reasonable alternative to the classical MVAC [36].

Until recently, CMV has been regarded as a standard combination chemotherapy for advanced bladder cancer in the UK while MVAC has been more widely used in the USA. Unfortunately, these two regimens have never been compared head-to-head in a randomized controlled trial. MVAC is probably associated with more toxicity than CMV. The most significant side-effects (grade 3 and 4) include bone marrow suppression (causing anaemia, neutropoenia and thrombocytopenia), mucositis, alopecia, nausea, vomiting, infection and diarrhoea. As a result of these toxicities, only 37% of cycles of MVAC were given without a dose adjustment in a recent phase III study [37]. Furthermore, treatment-related mortality is 3–4% in most studies.

GEMCITABINE AND CISPLATIN

The therapeutic index of MVAC is therefore suboptimal. There has therefore been a search for novel cytotoxic agents with superior cost benefit ratio to MVAC. Several new cytotoxics, including gemcitabine and paclitaxel, are of particular interest, as they have single-agent response rates as high as, or higher, than those of cisplatin itself.

The combination of gemcitabine and cisplatin (GC) has been shown to be safe and effective in 119 patients between three phase II trials [38–40]. In a direct randomized comparison with MVAC, the combination was shown to have a superior toxicity profile and efficacy appeared equivalent although the trial was not powered to confirm equivalence. As a result of this, GC has now been adopted as a standard of care in many institutions [37].

New doublet and triplet combinations

The introduction of several new agents into the portfolio of drugs with activity in bladder cancer has given rise to a confusing plethora of small phase II trials testing new doublet and triplet (and even quadruplet) combinations. In many cases these have been tested in the second line and the results can only be interpreted as screening tests for activity. Not surprisingly, given the inherent chemosensitivity of TCC, most of these series confirm activity of the new combinations. Unfortunately, few large phase III trials have been performed to test whether any of these newer combinations are superior to those already described above. However, randomized comparison of taxane platinum doublets has shown inferiority in comparison to MVAC [41,42] although these trials were small. In a rare assessment of cisplatin versus carboplatin, a randomization of Gem Cis versus Gem Carbo [43] suggested inferior results for the carboplatin-containing regimen. Table 12.2 gives an overview of the important published doublets and triplets to date.

Sequential therapy

The disadvantage of combination treatment is that it may be necessary to reduce the dose of each component of the regimen, because of overlapping toxicity (usually myelosuppression) with other components. The more the components in a chemotherapy regimen, the more this is likely to be the case. An alternative to combination regimens with many agents is to treat sequentially with single-agent or doublet combinations using the highest possible dose to ensure the highest possible fractional cell kill of the clones that are sensitive to each agent. This approach is being explored at Memorial Sloan–Kettering (MSK), with encouraging results [44]. In this treatment patients receive six cycles of a combination of doxorubicin and gemcitabine every 2 weeks followed by six cycles of a combination of ifosfamide,

Table 12.2 New doublet and triplet cytotoxic combination chemotherapies for TCC

Combination regimen	RR
CisCA	51
CMV	36
MVAC	39–65
GemCis	57–66
Doublets	RR
Cisplatin and paclitaxel	62–72
Cisplatin and docetaxel	60
Carboplatin and paclitaxel	71.9
Carboplatin and gemcitabine	44
Gemcitabine and doctaxel	50
Triplets	RR
Cisplatin, gemcitabine and paclitaxel	60–79
Cisplatin, gemcitabine and docetaxel	65
Cisplatin, paclitaxel and ifosfamide	68
Carboplatin, gemcitabine and paclitaxel	49–58
Carboplatin, paclitaxel and methotrexate	56

paclitaxel and cisplatin every 3 weeks. All cycles of this treatment required support with granulocyte colony-stimulating factor.

Clinical scenarios when systemic chemotherapy is indicated

FIRST-LINE TREATMENT FOR PATIENTS WITH METASTATIC DISEASE

It is generally assumed that the confirmation of metastatic disease implies the patient is incurable and survival is short. Chemotherapy used in this setting may improve quality of life and survival by causing tumour deposits to shrink and thereby reducing both the local symptoms of cancer (e.g. pain) and the systemic symptoms (e.g. fatigue). Chemotherapy in this setting needs careful management as the burden of chemotherapy in terms of toxicity and hospital visits can easily outweigh the benefits. For some patients however, the rewards are definitely worthwhile.

However, in a large retrospective review of the patients treated at the memorial with the MVAC regimen, a small number of patients were alive and disease-free at 5 years [45]. It should be remembered therefore that selected patients, treated aggressively, often with a combination of chemotherapy and local therapy, can be cured.

SECOND-LINE TREATMENT FOR METASTATIC BLADDER CANCER

Given that even when chemotherapy produces a response in a metastatic tumour, it is usually partial and temporary, selection of patients for a second-line treatment at disease progression is difficult. This is an area with a weak evidence base and wide variation of practice around the world. Generally speaking, responses to second-line chemotherapy are less common than to first-line treatment and for that reason patients who have had a good response to previous treatment are usually selected, lasting a significant period of time (6 months). Re-challenge with cisplatin is an option for patients having a treatment-free interval of more than 6 months or a year. Another approach is to use drugs the patient has not previously received in the hope that mechanisms of drug resistance that developed during the previous course of chemotherapy will not apply to a different agent. Finally, a patient in this situation should be offered entry to clinical trials of new agents.

PATIENTS WITH CLINICALLY ORGAN-CONFINED DISEASE

Systemic treatment given after radical local therapy in an attempt to eradicate occult micro-metastatic disease and prevent treatment failure is called adjuvant therapy, while the same treatment given before local therapy is called neoadjuvant therapy. These two approaches have a number of similarities and differences, as shown in Table 12.3. These differences mean that each approach must be evaluated separately in clinical trials and results from adjuvant chemotherapy should not be extrapolated to neoadjuvant and vice versa.

ADJUVANT THERAPY

There is a good reason for thinking that adjuvant chemotherapy should improve the outcome for patients with bladder cancer since the risk of metastatic relapse is high, the disease is chemosensitive, but cures are rare in the setting of overt metastatic disease. Unfortunately, there is an absence

Table 12.3 Neoadjuvant versus adjuvant chemotherapy for locally advanced bladder cancer

Neoadjuvant		Adjuvant	
For	Against	For	Against
Eliminate micrometastases > improved survival		Eliminate micrometastases > improved survival	
Potential for 'downstaging' inoperable tumours to resectable disease or to allow bladder preserving surgery		Tumour burden is minimized before chemotherapy	
	Delays surgery with risk of tumour progression if failing to respond to chemotherapy	No delay to surgery	
	Modifies postsurgical pathological assessment of tumour with loss of prognostic information	No loss of prognostic information	
Brings forward treatment modality for most serious (systemic) aspect of disease			
Patient is generally fit and able to tolerate chemotherapy			Patient is recovering from major surgery and may not wish to undergo toxic therapy

of good clinical trial data to demonstrate benefits because of a lack of well-powered, well-designed trials.

To date, four randomized studies have assessed the role of adjuvant chemotherapy following cystectomy and two following radical radiotherapy, against an observation control arm [46–50] (Table 12.4). None of the trials individually had sufficient statistical power to conclusively demonstrate a significant survival advantage. Indeed, the combined accrual to all the published trials includes only a few hundred patients. Just considering the patients with high-risk disease whose 5-year survival is 35% would require more than 1300 patients to generate sufficient events to observe a 7% improvement in overall survival at a power of 80% with 95% confidence. Of the four published trials randomizing patients between surgery alone and surgery plus postoperative chemotherapy, three [46,47,50] employed cisplatin-based chemotherapy and reported improved disease-free survival. Significant improvements in overall survival were reported in only one [46]. However, the design and/or analysis of each of these trials has been questioned [51,52].

There is thus, to date, insufficient evidence to advocate the routine use of adjuvant chemotherapy for muscle-invasive bladder cancer outside of the context of a clinical trial. Nevertheless, the existing data can be interpreted as giving an encouraging suggestion towards improved survival with

Table 12.4 Previous randomized studies of adjuvant chemotherapy after cystectomy for bladder cancer

First author	Regimen	Number of patients	TTP	p	Survival	p
			Median (years)		Median (years)	
Skinner [45]	CisCA	44	4	0.001	4.3	0.006
	No chemo	47	2		2.4	
			Median (months)		Median EFS (months)	
Stockle [46]	MVA(E)C	23	66	0.001	40	0.004
	No chemo	26	18		18	
					At 5 years (%)	
Studer [48]	Cisplatin	37	NA		57	NS
	No chemo	40			54	
			Median (months)		Median (months)	
Freiha [49]	CMV	25	37	0.1	63	0.3
	No chemo	25	12		36	

CisCA: cisplatin, cyclophosphamide, and doxorubicin; MVA(E)C: methotrexate, vinblastine, doxorubicin or epirubicin, cisplatin; CMV: cisplatin, methotrexate, vinblastine; TTP: time to progression; EFS: event free survival.

chemotherapy, and a definitive trial with appropriate statistical power to answer the question of adjuvant chemotherapy for bladder cancer is therefore now vital. The European Organization for Research and Treatment of Cancer (EORTC) is currently coordinating an international intergroup trial and we look forward to the results of this in due course [53].

NEOADJUVANT THERAPY

In view of the difficulties of delivering chemotherapy after radical local therapy to the bladder, there are advantages to neoadjuvant therapy. Furthermore, this approach minimizes the delay before the introduction of a therapy that may have an effect on systemic disease and may initiate a response in the primary tumour, both reducing the chance of metastatic spread at surgery and maximizing the possibility of organ-sparing surgery. Clearly, there is a risk that if the chemotherapy is ineffective for a particular patient, the tumour may continue to progress and/or delay definitive treatment and allow an organ-confined cancer to progress. For this reason, more intense monitoring of the tumour is required when giving neoadjuvant chemotherapy so that, if there is evidence of continued progression, immediate salvage local therapy can be given.

As for adjuvant therapy, none of the individual trials of neoadjuvant chemotherapy for muscle-invasive bladder cancer published in the peer-reviewed literature, including the largest single trial of neoadjuvant chemotherapy for bladder cancer, the MRC BA06 trial, has achieved conventional statistical significance. The BA06 trial randomized 976 patients with locally advanced TCC (at least T2 G3, but node-negative and free of distant metastases) either to radical treatment alone (surgery or radiotherapy) or to local therapy plus three cycles of neoadjuvant CMV combination chemotherapy [54], demonstrated trends towards the neoadjuvant chemotherapy arm both for median survival (increased from 35.5 months to 44 months) and for 3-year survival from 50.5% to 55.5%. However, the trial did not reach statistical significance at a median follow-up of 4 years. It has been suggested that this failure to reach statistical significance may be due to the use of CMV, rather than MVAC chemotherapy and/or the fact that 34% of patients were in the relatively good prognosis T2 G3 group, for whom it would be more difficult to demonstrate a convincing treatment benefit. The SWOG 8710 trial [55] provided similar support for neoadjuvant chemotherapy, with an improvement in median survival from 3.8 years to 6.2 years and a 26% reduction in mortality in 624 node-negative T2-T4a patients treated with three cycles of preoperative MVAC, compared with patients who had surgery only. However, these data were obtained only over a recruitment period of 11 years, and randomized only a small proportion of the patients eligible for entry. Furthermore, they only reached statistical significance when analysed using a one-sided *t* test, whilst re-analysis of the SWOG data using two-sided tests, to permit comparison with the MRC BA06 trial data, showed that the SWOG 8710 data no longer achieved statistical analysis in their own right [56].

Recently, an updated meta-analysis of individual patient data on 2688 patients treated in ten published randomized controlled trials of neo-adjuvant chemotherapy for muscle-invasive bladder cancer has been published [57]. This showed that in patients treated with cisplatin-based combination chemotherapy (already demonstrated to be superior to single-agent cisplatin chemotherapy and to chemotherapy lacking cisplatin, as above) there was an absolute benefit in overall survival at 5 years of 5% in favour of neoadjuvant chemotherapy, compared with treatment with surgery alone. This has led to the suggestion that neoadjuvant chemotherapy be considered a new standard of care for muscle-invasive bladder cancer [58].

Principles of therapy

Selection of patients suitable to receive systemic chemotherapy

Bladder cancer is a condition associated with smoking, the incidence of which rises with age with no demonstrable peak. The average age of unselected patients in large institutions is over 75 years. It is not surprising then that up to half of all patients with locally advanced/metastatic TCC of the bladder are not fit to receive cisplatin-based chemotherapy [61]. Commonly encountered reasons for this include poor renal function due to renovascular disease or obstructive uropathy due to bladder cancer, poor cardiac status, inadequate bone marrow reserve, poor performance status and a variety of comorbid conditions. Various strategies have been considered to account for this problem. These include modulation of cisplatin's nephrotoxicity by using nephro-protective agents such as *N*-acetyl cysteine and amifostine, modifying the scheduling of cisplatin or use of less cisplatin-intense regimens. Other strategies avoid the use of cisplatin completely (e.g. the use of the MV regimen rather than CMV), but these are associated with inferior results [27]. Another strategy to attempt to improve the toxicity profile of combination chemotherapy regimens for bladder cancer is substituting carboplatin for cisplatin. In a small trial of methotrexate, vinblastine, epirubicin and cisplatin (MVEC) compared with (methotrexate, vinblastine, epirubicin and carboplatin (MVECA) [62], the overall response rate was 71% versus 41% ($p = 0.024$) in favour of the cisplatin-based MVEC regimen, but there was less toxicity in the MVECA arm.

The extent of disease may help predict response to treatment, with durable responses being generally confined to patients with nodal relapses. In a retrospective analysis of the MSK patients treated with the MVAC regimen, a scoring system has been proposed to help predict the long-term outcome from treatment in which good performance status and absence of visceral metastases were independently associated with a good outcome [45].

Other clinical issues

VARIANT HISTOLOGIES

While the vast majority of patients with invasive bladder cancer have TCC, a minority may present with pure adenocarcinoma, small cell carcinoma or squamous cell carcinoma and in many cases the histology shows a mixed picture. A frequently asked question is whether patients with these variant histologies should be treated any differently to those with the usual TCC morphology. This approach is certainly followed in other cancers, such as lung cancer, where small cell histology is treated quite differently from the other histological types. It is certainly reasonable to suppose that the different spectrum of activity seen in different cancers is at least partly due to the different response to chemotherapies attributable to differing histologies. Should small cell bladder cancer be treated with regimens designed for small cell cancers at other sites, such as lung, where drugs such as etoposide and ifosfamide are frequently used with good responses seen? Should adenocarcinoma of the bladder be treated with 5-fluorouracil, which is the most important drug used in the treatment of colorectal adenocarcinomas? Unfortunately, there are very little clinical trial data to guide us in answering these questions. Furthermore, while pure variant histologies are very rare (no more than 5% of all bladder cancers) mixed histology is much more common and in this situation it would perhaps make less sense to change the management plan. In the absence of a good evidence base, however, some oncologists would recommend treating patients with pure small cell cancer of the bladder differently to those with TCC, perhaps favouring an earlier use of chemotherapy and using the drugs mentioned above in regimens more usually applied to small cell lung cancer [63–65].

MANAGEMENT OF RENAL TRACT OBSTRUCTION IN PATIENTS WITH BLADDER CANCER HAVING CHEMOTHERAPY

Renal tract obstruction is such a common feature of patients with bladder cancer that it deserves special mention. As has been discussed, optimal chemotherapy is generally thought to include cisplatin and this may be

difficult if the GFR is much below 60 ml/min. Where impaired renal function is found in association with obstructed renal tracts, a commonly held
view is that it is generally preferable to intervene promptly and aggressively
to maximize the renal function, if optimal chemotherapy is to be given.
Options for optimizing renal function include percutaneous nephrostomies,
often followed by antegrade or retrograde ureteric stenting, extraanatomic
stents and direct surgical repair. Selection of the appropriate management
depends on a number of patient-specific factors including the cause of the
obstruction (due to the cancer or other causes such as postsurgical stricture)
and whether the patient has had cystectomy and ileal conduit formation or
has a native bladder. Appropriate diagnostic imaging and intervention
should be as speedy as possible, as the pace of the disease is often sufficiently
rapid for even small delays to be associated with further tumour progression. Even when renal function is optimized, extra complications can arise
during chemotherapy for patients who have stents or nephrostomies in
place as they are a potential source of infection.

Because of these difficulties, alternative approaches have been attempted.
Substitution of drugs not dependent on renal function is an obvious option
(see 'Carboplatin'). Unfortunately, direct comparisons of such drugs with
cisplatin suggest that carboplatin is an inferior drug in this disease and so
many oncologists are reluctant to make modifications that may abrogate the
effectiveness of therapy. Fractionation of the cisplatin dose reduces the
nephrotoxicity, although no comparison with unfractionated regimens has
been made to confirm that there is no loss of efficacy.

Future developments

Even with the latest developments in cytotoxic chemotherapy for bladder
cancer, many patients die from muscle-invasive disease, despite aggressive
therapy with curative intent. Durable long-term remissions due to chemotherapy in metastatic disease are the exception rather than the rule, and
median survival is approximately 14 months after commencement of
chemotherapy [37]. There remains a need for novel treatments that will
either improve survival or increase the therapeutic ratio of systemic therapy.
Potential new treatments include new cytotoxic drugs, new rationally
designed 'targeted' therapies with small molecules and new 'biological'
treatment modalities, including gene therapy.

Oxaliplatin

Given the established efficacy of cisplatin and carboplatin for patients with
advanced/metastatic bladder cancer, other platinum-based cytotoxic drugs

may have a role in the treatment of bladder cancer. The most promising of these is oxaliplatin, which is not associated with the nephrotoxicity of cisplatin, and is less myelosuppressive than carboplatin. However, in a small series of previously treated patients only 1 of 18 patients had a response to this agent [66]. Better results have been seen in combination with gemcitabine [67].

Vinflunine

Vinflunine is a third-generation vinca alkaloid with demonstrated single-agent activity (ORR 17%) in phase II trials in bladder cancer [68] and is now undergoing phase III evaluation in second line against best supportive care.

Chemoradiotherapy

The concurrent use of chemotherapy and radiotherapy may be of use in organ-confined or locally advanced bladder cancer. There is synergism between certain drugs and radiotherapy and this can be exploited either by allowing a reduction in the dose of the radiotherapy or by enhancing its therapeutic effect. A number of agents have this property including cisplatin and gemcitabine – both of which are known to have specific therapeutic activity in bladder cancer as discussed above – and also 5-fluorouracil which, although not highly active in bladder cancer on its own, has a well-established place in chemoradiotherapy in other diseases [59,60].

New treatment modalities

TARGETED THERAPIES

Our increasing understanding of the molecular pathogenesis of bladder cancer suggests that forthcoming developments in systemic therapy may employ molecularly targeted therapies, directed against specific molecular phenotypes. Of particular interest are therapies directed against bladder tumours, which overexpress members of the epidermal growth factor receptor (EGFR) family [69], and/or tumours with mutations in the p53 and pRB tumour suppressor genes and their associated cellular stimulus-response pathways [70].

It has long been appreciated that bladder tumours overexpress EGFR and EGFR-2 (her2/neu), and that this overexpression is associated with worse prognosis [69,71]. These cell surface receptors therefore represent attractive targets for rational drug design. Indeed, 'biological' therapies directed against the EGFR family, such as the use of the monoclonal antibody

C225 (Cetuximab) [72] and Trastuzumab(Herceptin) [73] and receptor tyrosine kinase inhibitors such as Iressa and Tarceva [74], are already in either early clinical trials or advanced preclinical development. However, in previously treated patients, only 1 partial response was seen in 29 patients and progression-free survival was only 4% at 6 months [75] despite demonstration of > 40% expression in the primary tumours of these patients.

Other agents of interest include farnesyl transferase inhibitors that in combination with gemcitabine led to ORR in 39% of 33 patients in a phase II trial [76].

GENE THERAPY

Another developing strategy for the treatment of metastatic cancers is gene therapy, and the first trial of gene therapy for bladder cancer was published recently [77]. Mutations in the p53 and pRB tumour suppressor genes are seen in up to 70% and 37% of bladder tumours, respectively [78], making them attractive targets for bladder cancer gene therapy. Indeed, the first trial of locally delivered gene therapy for bladder cancer, involving intravesical installation of an adenoviral vector encoding exogenous p53, has recently been reported [79,80]. Selectively replicating adenoviruses containing deletions in the E1A and E1B regions of the viral genome have been designed to preferentially kill tumour cells with mutations in the pRB and p53 tumour suppressor genes, respectively, rather than non-cancerous cells [81,82]. Although controversy surrounds the molecular mechanism of its action, the p53-selective oncolytic adenovirus dl1520 (ONYX-015) has been demonstrated to be safe in clinical trials when administered via a variety of routes, and has been demonstrated to be efficacious in combination with systemic cisplatin-based chemotherapy when injected directly into head and neck tumours [83]. It seems likely that cancer gene therapy will be an area of intense clinical research interest in a variety of tumours, including bladder cancer.

Conclusion

Combination chemotherapy is now well established as a useful treatment modality for advanced bladder cancer, which is moderately sensitive to cytotoxic drugs. For patients with good performance status and adequate renal function, such systemic chemotherapy should be cisplatin-based, with two alternative regimens as treatment of choice: MVAC and gemcitabine/cisplatin. Many patients are unable to tolerate such relatively aggressive chemotherapy, and particularly in patients with renal impairment, combinations such as carboplatin, methotrexate and vinblastine can be valuable.

Newer cytotoxic drugs such as gemcitabine and paclitaxel may improve the therapeutic index of chemotherapies for metastatic TCCs, and are currently the subject of much clinical research activity.

The success of such chemotherapy regimens in bladder cancer raises the question of whether, in an analogous situation to the treatment of breast and bladder cancers, perioperative chemotherapy might improve the disappointing survival figures seen in muscle-invasive bladder cancer, treated with curative intent. Although a recent meta-analysis of randomized controlled trial data suggests that preoperative 'neoadjuvant' chemotherapy may become a new standard of care, adjuvant chemotherapy cannot currently be recommended outside the context of a clinical trial.

Despite these advances in treatment, survival rates for both advanced and muscle-invasive bladder tumours remain disappointing, and novel therapies are required. Potential future areas of promise include molecularly targeted therapies, targeting tumour phenotypes such as overexpression of EGFR at the cell surface or tumour suppressor gene mutations intracellularly. Therapies with orally bioavailable tyrosine kinase inhibitors and/or targeted cancer gene therapies are promising areas of development.

References

1 Stein JP *et al*. Radical cystectomy in the treatment of invasive bladder cancer: long-term results in 1,054 patients. *J Clin Oncol* 2001; **19**(3): 666–75.

2 Moore MJ *et al*. Gemcitabine: a promising new agent in the treatment of advanced urothelial cancer. *J Clin Oncol* 1997; **15**(12): 3441–5.

3 Bokemeyer C *et al* The role of paclitaxel in chemosensive urological malignancies: current strategies in bladder cancer and testicular germ-cell tumors. *World J Urol* 1996; **14**(6): 354–9.

4 Loehrer PJ Sr *et al*. A randomized comparison of cisplatin alone or in combination with methotrexate, vinblastine, and doxorubicin in patients with metastatic urothelial carcinoma: a cooperative group study. *J Clin Oncol* 1992; **10**(7): 1066–73.

5 Yagoda A *et al*. Cis-dichlorodiammineplatinum(II) in advanced bladder cancer. *Cancer Treat Rep* 1976; **60**(7): 917–23.

6 Royal College of Radiologists' COIN Chemotherapy Working Group. Guidelines for cytotoxic chemotherapy in adults. *Clin Oncol* 2001; **13**(1): S211–48.

7 Oliver RT *et al*. Methotrexate in the treatment of metastatic and recurrent primary transitional cell carcinoma. *J Urol* 1984; **131**(3): 483–5.

8 Natale RB *et al*. Methotrexate: an active drug in bladder cancer. *Cancer* 1981; **47**(6): 1246–50.

9 Hall RR *et al*. Methotrexate treatment for advanced bladder cancer. *Br J Urol* 1974; **46**(4): 431–8.

10 Turner AG *et al*. The treatment of advanced bladder cancer with methotrexate. *Br J Urol* 1977; **49**(7): 673–8.

11 Blumenreich MS *et al*. Phase II trial of vinblastine sulfate for metastatic urothelial tract tumors. *Cancer* 1982; **50**(3): 435–8.

12 Riggs C Jr. Antitumor antibiotics and related compounds, In: Perry MC, Editor *The Chemotherapy Source Book*, 1992, Williams and Wilkins: Baltimore. p. 318–358.

13 Tempero M *et al*. Randomized phase 11 comparison of dose-intense gemcitabine: thirty-minute infusion and fixed dose rate infusion in patients with pancreatic adenocarcinoma. *J Clin Oncol* 2003; **21**(18): 3402–8.

14 Lorusso V *et al*. A phase II study of gemcitabine in patients with transitional cell carcinoma of the urinary tract previously treated with platinum. Italian Co-operative Group on Bladder Cancer. *Eur J Cancer* 1998; **34**(8): 1208–12.

15 Gebbia V *et al*. Single agent 2′,2′-difluorodeoxycytidine in the treatment of metastatic urothelial carcinoma: a phase II study. *Clin Ter* 1999; **150**(1): 11–15.

16 Stadler WM *et al*. Phase II study of single-agent gemcitabine in previously untreated patients with metastatic urothelial cancer. *J Clin Oncol* 1997; **15**(11): 3394–8.

17 Roth BJ *et al*. Significant activity of paclitaxel in advanced transitional-cell carcinoma of the urothelium: a phase II trial of the Eastern Cooperative Oncology Group. *J Clin Oncol* 1994; **12**(11): 2264–70.

18 Dreicer R *et al*. Paclitaxel in advanced urothelial carcinoma: its role in patients with renal insufficiency and as salvage therapy. *J Urol* 1996; **156**(5): 1606–608.

19 Redman BG *et al*. Phase II trial of paclitaxel and carboplatin in the treatment of advanced urothelial carcinoma. *J Clin Oncol* 1998; **16**(5): 1844–8.

20 Pycha A *et al*. Paclitaxel and carboplatin in patients with metastatic transitional cell cancer of the urinary tract. *Urology* 1999; **53**(3): 510–15.

21 Zielinski CC *et al*. Paclitaxel and carboplatin in patients with metastatic urothelial cancer: results of a phase II trial. *Br J Cancer*, 1998; **78**(3): 370–74.

22 Saxman SB *et al*. Long-term follow-up of a phase III intergroup study of cisplatin alone or in combination with methotrexate, vinblastine, and doxorubicin in patients with metastatic urothelial carcinoma: a cooperative group study. *J Clin Oncol* 1997; **15**(7): 2564–9.

23 Hillcoat BL *et al*. A randomized trial of cisplatin versus cisplatin plus methotrexate in advanced cancer of the urothelial tract. *J Clin Oncol* 1989; 7(6): 706–709.

24 Troner M *et al*. Phase III comparison of cisplatin alone versus cisplatin, doxorubicin and cyclophosphamide in the treatment of bladder (urothelial) cancer: a Southeastern Cancer Study Group trial. *J Urol* 1987; **137**(4): 660–62.

25 Khandekar JD *et al*. Comparative activity and toxicity of cis-diamminedichloroplatinum (DDP) and a combination of doxorubicin, cyclophosphamide, and DDP in disseminated transitional cell carcinomas of the urinary tract. *J Clin Oncol* 1985; 3(4): 539–45.

26 Soloway MS *et al*. A comparison of cisplatin and the combination of cisplatin and cyclophosphamide in advanced urothelial cancer. A National Bladder Cancer Collaborative Group A Study. *Cancer* 1983; **52**(5): 767–72.

27 Mead GM *et al*. A randomized trial comparing methotrexate and vinblastine (MV) with cisplatin, methotrexate and vinblastine (CMV) in advanced transitional cell carcinoma: results and a report on prognostic factors in a Medical Research Council study. MRC Advanced Bladder Cancer Working Party. *Br J Cancer* 1998; **78**(8): 1067–75.

28 Harker WG *et al*. Cisplatin, methotrexate, and vinblastine (CMV): an effective chemotherapy regimen for metastatic transitional cell carcinoma of the urinary tract. A Northern California Oncology Group study. *J Clin Oncol* 1985; 3(11): 1463–70.

29 Sternberg CN *et al*. Methotrexate, vinblastine, doxorubicin, and cisplatin for advanced transitional cell carcinoma of the urothelium. Efficacy and patterns of response and relapse. *Cancer* 1989; **64**(12): 2448–58.

30 Logothetis CJ *et al*. The impact of chemotherapy on the survival of patients with metastatic urothelial tumors. *Prog Clin Biol Res* 1990; **350**: 107–14.

31 Bellmunt J *et al*. Carboplatin-based versus cisplatin-based chemotherapy in the treatment of surgically incurable advanced bladder carcinoma. *Cancer* 1997; **80**(10): 1966–72.

32   Logothetis CJ *et al*. A prospective randomized trial comparing MVAC and CISCA chemotherapy for patients with metastatic urothelial tumors. *J Clin Oncol* 1990; 8(6): 1050–55.

33   Logothetis CJ *et al*. Escalated MVAC with or without recombinant human granulocyte-macrophage colony-stimulating factor for the initial treatment of advanced malignant urothelial tumors: results of a randomized trial. *J Clin Oncol* 1995; 13(9): 2272–7.

34   Seidman AD *et al*. Dose-intensification of MVAC with recombinant granulocyte colony-stimulating factor as initial therapy in advanced urothelial cancer. *J Clin Oncol* 1993; 11(3): 408–14.

35   Loehrer PJ Sr *et al*. Escalated dosages of methotrexate, vinblastine, doxorubicin, and cisplatin plus recombinant human granulocyte colony-stimulating factor in advanced urothelial carcinoma: an Eastern Cooperative Oncology Group trial. *J Clin Oncol* 1994;. 12(3): 483–8.

36   Sternberg CN *et al*. Randomized phase III trial of high-dose-intensity methotrexate, vinblastine, doxorubicin, and cisplatin (MVAC) chemotherapy and recombinant human granulocyte colony-stimulating factor versus classic MVAC in advanced urothelial tract tumors: European Organization for Research and Treatment of Cancer Protocol no. 30924. *J Clin Oncol* 2001; 19(10): 2638–46.

37   von der Maase H *et al*. Gemcitabine and cisplatin versus methotrexate, vinblastine, doxorubicin, and cisplatin in advanced or metastatic bladder cancer: results of a large, randomized, multinational, multicenter, phase III study. *J Clin Oncol* 2000. 18(17): 3068–77.

38   von der Maase H *et al*. Weekly gemcitabine and cisplatin combination therapy in patients with transitional cell carcinoma of the urothelium: a phase II clinical trial. *Ann Oncol* 1999; 10(12): 1461–5.

39   Moore MJ *et al*. Gemcitabine plus cisplatin, an active regimen in advanced urothelial cancer: a phase II trial of the National Cancer Institute of Canada Clinical Trials Group. *J Clin Oncol* 1999; 17(9): 2876–81.

40   Kaufman D *et al*. Phase II trial of gemcitabine plus cisplatin in patients with metastatic urothelial cancer. *J Clin Oncol* 2000; 18(9): 1921–7.

41   Bamias A *et al*. Docetaxel and cisplatin with granulocyte colony-stimulating factor (G-CSF) versus MVAC with G-CSF in advanced urothelial carcinoma: a multicenter, randomized, phase III study from the Hellenic Cooperative Oncology Group. *J Clin Oncol* 2004; 22(2): 220–28.

42   Dreicer R *et al*. Phase III trial of methotrexate, vinblastine, doxorubicin, and cisplatin versus carboplatin and paclitaxel in patients with advanced carcinoma of the urothelium. *Cancer* 2004; 100(8): 1639–45.

43   Carteni G *et al*. Phase II randomised trial of gemcitabine plus cisplatin (GP) and gemcitabine plus carboplatin(GC) in patients (pts) with advanced or metastatic transitional cell carcinoma of the urothelium (TCCU). *Proc Am Soc Clin Oncol* 2003; 22: 384 (Abstract 1543).

44   Dodd PM *et al*. Phase I evaluation of sequential doxorubicin gemcitabine then ifosfamide paclitaxel cisplatin for patients with unresectable or metastatic transitional-cell carcinoma of the urothelial tract. *J Clin Oncol* 2000; 18(4): 840–46.

45   Bajorin DF *et al*. Long-term survival in metastatic transitional-cell carcinoma and prognostic factors predicting outcome of therapy. *J Clin Oncol* 1999; 17(10): 3173–81.

46   Skinner DG *et al*. The role of adjuvant chemotherapy following cystectomy for invasive bladder cancer: a prospective comparative trial. *J Urol* 1991; 145(3): 459–464.

47   Stockle M *et al*. Advanced bladder cancer (stages pT3b, pT4a, pN1 and pN2): improved survival after radical cystectomy and 3 adjuvant cycles of chemotherapy. Results of a controlled prospective study. *J Urol* 1992; 148(2 Pt 1): 302–306.

48   Stockle M *et al.* Adjuvant polychemotherapy of nonorgan-confined bladder cancer after radical cystectomy revisited: long-term results of a controlled prospective study and further clinical experience. *J Urol* 1995; **153**(1): 47–52.

49   Studer UE *et al.* Adjuvant cisplatin chemotherapy following cystectomy for bladder cancer: results of a prospective randomized trial. *J Urol* 1994; **152**(1): 81–84.

50   Freiha F, Reese J, Torti FM. A randomized trial of radical cystectomy versus radical cystectomy plus cisplatin, vinblastine and methotrexate chemotherapy for muscle invasive bladder cancer. *J Urol* 1996; **155**(2): 495–9.

51   Sylvester R, Sternberg C. The role of adjuvant combination chemotherapy after cystectomy in locally advanced bladder cancer: what we do not know and why. *Ann Oncol* 2000; **11**(7): 851–6.

52   Dimopoulos MA, Moulopoulos LA. Role of adjuvant chemotherapy in the treatment of invasive carcinoma of the urinary bladder. *J Clin Oncol* 1998; **16**(4): 1601–12.

53   de Wit R. Overview of bladder cancer trials in the European Organization for Research and Treatment. *Cancer* 2003; **97**(8 Suppl.): 2120–26.

54   International Collaboration of Trialists. Neoadjuvant cisplatin, methotrexate, and vinblastine chemotherapy for muscle-invasive bladder cancer: a randomised controlled trial. *Lancet* 1999; **354**(9178): 533–40.

55   Grossman HB *et al.* Neoadjuvant chemotherapy plus cystectomy compared with cystectomy alone for locally advanced bladder cancer. *N Engl J Med* 2003; **349**(9): 859–66.

56   Sternberg CN, Parmar MK. Neoadjuvant chemotherapy is not (yet) standard treatment for muscle-invasive bladder cancer. *J Clin Oncol* 2001; **19**(18 Suppl.): 21S-6S.

57   Advanced Bladder Cancer Meta-analysis Collaboration. Neoadjuvant chemotherapy in invasive bladder cancer: a systematic review and meta-analysis. *Lancet* 2003; **361**(9373): 1927–34.

58   Stadler WM, Lerner SP. Perioperative chemotherapy in locally advanced bladder cancer. *Lancet* 2003; **361**(9373): 1922–3.

59   Cowan R *et al.* A phase I trial of chemo-radiation with gemcitabine for muscle invasive bladder carcinoma. *Proc Am Soc Clin Oncol* 2003; **22**: 427 (Abstract 1715).

60   Sangar VK *et al.* An evaluation of gemcitabines differential radiosensitising effect in related bladder cancer cell lines. *Br J Cancer* 2004; **90**(2): 542–8.

61   Bellmunt J *et al.* A feasibility study of carboplatin with fixed dose of gemcitabine in 'unfit' patients with advanced bladder cancer. *Eur J Cancer* 2001; **37**(17): 2212–15.

62   Petrioli R *et al.* Comparison between a cisplatin-containing regimen and a carboplatin-containing regimen for recurrent or metastatic bladder cancer patients. A randomized phase II study. *Cancer* 1996; **77**(2): 344–51.

63   Salo JO *et al.* Primary small cell cancer of the bladder. Report of a case and review of literature. *Ann Chir Gynaecol* 1988; **77**(2): 81–4.

64   Siefker-Radtke AO *et al.* Evidence supporting preoperative chemotherapy for small cell carcinoma of the bladder: a retrospective review of the M. D. Anderson cancer experience. *J Urol* 2004; **172**(2): 481–4.

65   Asmis TR *et al.* Genitourinary (GU) small cell carcinoma (SCC): A retrospective review of treatment and survival patterns at the Ottawa Regional Cancer Center (ORCC). *Proc Am Soc Clin Oncol* 2004; **23**: (Abstract 4545).

66   Moore MJ *et al.* Phase II study of oxaliplatin in patients with inoperable, locally advanced or metastatic transitional cell carcionoma of the urothelial tract (TCC) who have received chemotherapy. *Proc Am Soc Clin Oncol* 2003; **22**: 408 (Abstract 1638).

67   Font A *et al.* Gemcitabine and oxaliplatin combination: a multicenter phase II trial in unfit patients with locally advanced or metastatic urothelial cancer. *Proc Am Soc Clin Oncol* 2004; **23**: (Abstract 4544).

68   Bui B *et al*. Preliminary results of a phase II study testing intravenous (iv) vinflunine (VFL) as second line therapy in patients with advanced transitional cell cancer (TCC) of the bladder. *Proc Am Soc Clin Oncol* 2003; **22**: 391 (Abstract 1571).

69   Nicholson RI, Gee JM, Harper ME. EGFR and cancer prognosis. *Eur J Cancer* 2001; **37** (Suppl. 4):S9–15.

70   Knowles MA. The genetics of transitional cell carcinoma: progress and potential clinical application. *BJU Int* 1999; **84**(4): 412–27.

71   Neal DE *et al*. Epidermal-growth-factor receptors in human bladder cancer: comparison of invasive and superficial tumours. *Lancet* 1985; **1**(8425): 366–8.

72   Mendelsohn J. Targeting the epidermal growth factor receptor for cancer therapy. *J Clin Oncol* 2002; **20**(18 Suppl.): 1S–13S.

73   Hussain M *et al*. Trastuzumab (T), paclitaxel (P), carboplatin (C) and gemcitabine (G) in patients with advanced urothelial cancer and overexpression of HER-2 (NCI study #198). *Proc Am Soc Clin Oncol* 2003; **22**: 391 (Abstract 1569).

74   de Bono JS, Rowinsky EK. The ErbB receptor family: a therapeutic target for cancer. *Trends Mol Med* 2002; **8**(4 Suppl.): S19–26.

75   Petrylak D *et al*. Evaluation of ZA1839 for advanced transitional cll carcinoma (TCC) of the urothelium: a Southwest Oncology Group Trial. *Proc Am Soc Clin Oncol* 2003; **22**: 403 (Abstract 1619).

76   Theodore C *et al*. A phase II multicentre study of SCH66336 in combination with gemcitabine as second line treatment in patients with advanced/metastatic urothelial tract tumor. *Proc Am Soc Clin Oncol* 2003; **22**: 415 (Abstract 1667).

77   Gomella LG *et al*. Phase I study of intravesical vaccinia virus as a vector for gene therapy of bladder cancer. *J Urol* 2001; **166**(4): 1291–5.

78   Knowles MA. What we could do now: molecular pathology of bladder cancer. *Mol Pathol* 2001; **54**(4): 215–21.

79   Kuball J *et al*. Successful adenovirus-mediated wild-type p53 gene transfer in patients with bladder cancer by intravesical vector instillation. *J Clin Oncol* 2002; **20**(4): 957–65.

80   Pagliaro LC *et al*. Repeated intravesical instillations of an adenoviral vector in patients with locally advanced bladder cancer: a phase I study of p53 gene therapy. *J Clin Oncol* 2003; **21**(12): 2247–53.

81   Hernandez-Alcoceba R *et al*. A novel, conditionally replicative adenovirus for the treatment of breast cancer that allows controlled replication of E1a-deleted adenoviral vectors. *Hum Gene Ther* 2000; **11**(14): 2009–24.

82   Heise C *et al*. ONYX-015, an E1B gene-attenuated adenovirus, causes tumor-specific cytolysis and antitumoral efficacy that can be augmented by standard chemotherapeutic agents. *Nat Med* 1997; **3**(6): 639–45.

83   Khuri FR *et al*. A controlled trial of intratumoral ONYX-015, a selectively-replicating adenovirus, in combination with cisplatin and 5-fluorouracil in patients with recurrent head and neck cancer. *Nat Med* 2000; **6**(8): 879–85.

13: Testicular Cancer

Jourik A. Gietema & Dirk Th. Sleijfer

Introduction

A germ cell tumour of the testis is a rare disease although it is the most common tumour in men aged 20–35 years. The incidence of testicular cancer is about 4–5 per 100000 men per year, but there is a geographical and racial variation. Most patients present themselves with a painless lump in the testicle. Sometimes the first symptoms are related to retroperitoneal lymph node metastasis (back pain) or to lung metastasis (haemoptysis or breathlessness). A few patients present with gynaecomastia as a result of an elevated level of the tumour marker human chorionic gonadotrophin (HCG).

The diagnosis is established after an inguinal orchiectomy, and germ cell tumours are distinguished into seminomas and non-seminomas, each accounting for about 50% of the total. Staging includes, next to physical examination, computed tomographic (CT) scanning of the chest, the abdomen and the pelvis and determination of the serum levels of lacto-dehydrogenase (LDH), alpha-fetoprotein (AFP) and HCG. The Royal Marsden staging system is widely used [1]. In stage I there is no evidence of metastatic disease and the tumour is confined to the testicle. In stage II there is abdominal metastasis and in stage III supradiaphragmatic metastasis. In stage IV extralymphatic metastasis are present. Furthermore, this staging system also quantifies the volume of metastatic disease. In 1997, the International Germ Cell Cancer Collaborative Group published a prognostic classification system for patients with disseminated disease based on histology (seminoma vs non-seminoma), origin of the primary (gonadal vs extra-gonadal), place of metastases and the level of serum tumour markers. Patients can be divided into three prognostic groups: good, intermediate and poor [2] (Table 13.1).

Because the histopathology of testicular cancer is complex, as is the treatment, referral to a specialist centre is frequently advised [3], especially because survival of patients with testicular cancer appears to be related to the experience of the treating institution [4] and because of the need for long-term medical care of survivors [5].

Table 13.1 Staging and classification of testicular cancer [2,60,61]

Royal Marsden Hospital staging (seminoma and non-seminoma)	International Germ Cell Consensus classification	
	Non-seminoma	Seminoma
I Testicular involvement alone, no evidence of metastases	Good prognosis: all of the following	Good prognosis: all of the following
	αFP < 1000 ng/ml and βHCG < 5000 IU/L LDH < 1.5 × upper limit of normal (ULN)	Normal αFP, any βHCG and any LDH Any primary site
	Non-mediastinal primary and no non-pulmonary visceral metastases present	No non-pulmonary visceral metastases present
Im+ Stage I on CT scan but marker-positive	Intermediate prognosis: all of the following	Intermediate-prognosis:
II Infradiaphragmatic lymph node involvement	αFP 1000–10 000 ng/ml or βHCG 5000–50 000 IU/ L or LDH 1.5–10 × ULN	Non-pulmonary visceral metastases present
Stage IIA/B/C: maximum diameter < 2 cm/2– 5 cm/> 5 cm	Non-mediastinal primary site and no non-pulmonary visceral metastases present	
III Supradiaphragmatic lymph node involvement Stages IIIA/B/C as for stage II		
IV Extranodal metastases	Poor prognosis: any of the following αFP > 10 000 ng/ml or βHCG > 50 000 IU/L or LDH > 10× ULN Mediastinal primary site Non-pulmonary visceral metastases present	

Seminoma stage I

Radiation to the para-aortic and ipsilateral lymph nodes is the standard treatment for stage I seminoma, the so-called 'dogleg' field. Doses of 25–30 Gy are given and provide excellent local control. In order to reduce haematologic, gastrointestinal and gonadal toxicity and to maintain efficacy, a recent randomized prospective trial compared the conventional 'dogleg' field with a field limited to the para-aortic region alone. It was found that the limited field produced statistically less significant morbidity while the 3-year relapse-free survival was identical (96%), as was the overall survival (99–100%). The more limited field radiation, however, had a nonsignificant increased risk of pelvic recurrences (1.8% vs 0%) [6].

Concerns regarding acute and chronic toxicity of radiation have resulted in interest in surveillance for stage I seminoma. Several large surveillance series showed a recurrence rate in the range of 15–20% with a median follow-up of 4–6 years, but nearly all patients with recurrent disease can be cured by radiation therapy or cisplatin-containing chemotherapy, leading to a survival rate of more than 99% [7]. The risk of recurrence in patients on surveillance seems to be related to several adverse prognostic factors, such as tumour size, tumour invasion of small vessels and age at presentation, but in a multivariate analysis tumour size (more than 4 cm) and invasion of the rete testis were the only important factors [7]. Nevertheless, surveillance is not yet an accepted alternative to radiation.

The effectiveness of one or two courses of adjuvant chemotherapy with the single-agent carboplatin in stage I seminoma has been studied in 160 patients [8]. Although only two patients developed a recurrence, the use of adjuvant carboplatin should be considered as investigational until the results of randomized trials are available.

Standard treatment options

For patients with stage I: Radical inguinal orchiectomy, followed by radiation to para-aortic and ipsilateral lymph nodes, 'dogleg' field, with a dose range from 25 to 30 Gy.

Seminoma stage IIA/B with lymph node metastasis < 5 cm

In stage II seminomatous testicular cancer, retroperitoneal or para-aortic lymph nodes are usually present in the region of the kidney. Retroperitoneal involvement should be further characterized by the size of the involved nodes. For treatment planning and estimation of prognosis, stage II seminoma is divided into bulky (IIC) and nonbulky (IIA/B) disease. Radiotherapy alone is standard in seminoma stage IIA/B. The risk of recurrence after radiotherapy is increased if more than five nodes are involved, or if the maximal size of the lymph node metastasis is greater than 5 cm in diameter [9]. Stage IIA/B disease has a cure rate of more than 90% with radiation alone and chemotherapy cures more than 90% of patients who have a relapse after radiation therapy [10].

Bulky stage II (IIC) disease describes patients with extensive retroperitoneal nodes (< 5 cm) who require primary chemotherapy and who have a less favourable prognosis.

Standard treatment options

For patients with stage IIA/B: Radical inguinal orchiectomy followed by radiation to the retroperitoneal and ipsilateral pelvic lymph nodes. (Radiation to inguinal nodes is not standard unless there has been some damage to the scrotum, putting inguinal lymph nodes at risk.)

Seminoma advanced disease: stage IIC with lymph node metastasis > 5 cm to stage IV

Patients with stage IIC seminomatous testicular cancer have metastatic tumours greater than 5 cm on a CT scan. Historically, radiotherapy was used for all stages of seminoma; however, the success of the radiation is inversely related to the bulk of the disease. These studies suggest that radiotherapy had a high failure rate if the abdominal mass was more than 5 cm in diameter. Higher risk of relapse can amount to 35% for abdominal masses larger than 10 cm in diameter [9]. Another problem with the use of radiotherapy in the initial management of patients with an abdominal mass of more than 5 cm in diameter is the extent of the kidney within the radiation field. These considerations lead most authors to recommend primary chemotherapy for patients with bulky disease (IIC) [9]. Combination chemotherapy with cisplatin is an effective therapy in patients with stage IIC seminomas, leading to a probability of progression-free survival of ± 90%. Patients with stage III and IV disease are also treated primarily with combination chemotherapy. Chemotherapy combinations include BEP (bleomycin + etoposide + cisplatin) for four courses [11,12] and EP (etoposide + cisplatin) for four courses in good-prognosis patients only [13]. Other regimens, such as VIP (etoposide + ifosfamide + cisplatin), appear to produce similar survival outcomes but are less commonly used. A randomized study comparing four courses of BEP with four courses of VIP showed equivalent overall survival and time-to-treatment failure for the two regimens in patients with advanced disseminated germ cell tumours who had not received prior chemotherapy [14]. Haematologic toxic effects, however, were substantially worse with the VIP regimen. A recent study in patients with good-risk germ cell cancer (including seminoma) showed equivalence of three versus four courses of BEP chemotherapy [15]. Four hundred and six patients were compared in both arms; 23% of the randomized patients had seminoma in both arms. The projected 2-year progression-free survival was 90.4% for three cycles and 89.4% for four cycles of BEP.

Because of the toxicity of these cisplatin regimens in relatively old patients with seminoma, there is a need for less toxic treatments. Although monotherapy with carboplatin has a relatively high failure rate of about

23% [16], combinations of carboplatin-based chemotherapy have been propagated as active [17].

Residual radiologic abnormalities are common at the completion of chemotherapy, but many gradually regress over a period of months. Some clinicians advocate empiric radiation of persistent residual abnormalities or attempt to resect residual masses if the diameter is 3 cm or more [18]. Either approach is controversial. In a combined retrospective series of 174 seminoma patients with postchemotherapy residual disease treated in ten centres, empiric radiation was not associated with any significant improvement in progression-free survival after completion of the chemotherapy [19]. In some other series, surgical resection of specific masses has yielded a significant number with residual seminoma that requires additional therapy [20]. Nevertheless, other reports indicate that size of the residual mass does not correlate well with active residual disease; most residual masses do not grow and frequent marker and CT scan evaluation is a viable option even when the residual mass is 3 cm or more in diameter.

Table 13.2 Common chemotherapy regimens for patients with disseminated non-seminomatous testicular cancer in different prognostic groups

Prognosis group	Regimen	Days of administration	Interval (weeks)	Number of courses
Good prognosis	**BEP***		3	3
	Bleomycin 30 mg	Days 2, 8 and 15		
	Etoposide 100 mg/m^2	Days 1–5		
	Cisplatin 20 mg/m^2	Days 1–5		
	Bleomycin 30 mg	Days 2, 8 and 15	3	3
	Etoposide 165 mg/m^2	Days 1–3		
	Cisplatin 50 mg/m^2	Days 1 and 2		
	EP		3	4
	Etoposide 100 mg/m^2	Days 1–5		
	Cisplatin 20 mg/m^2	Days 1–5		
Intermediate and poor prognosis	**BEP**		3	4
	Bleomycin 30 mg	Days 2, 8 and 15		
	Etoposide 100 mg/m^2	Days 1–5		
	Cisplatin 20 mg/m^2	Day 1–5		
	VIP**		3	4
	Etoposide 75 mg/m^2	Days 1–5		
	Ifosfamide 1.2 g/m^2	Days 1–5		
	Cisplatin 20 mg/m^2	Days 1–5		

*de Wit *et al.* [15].
**Nichols *et al.* [14]

Standard treatment options

For seminoma patients with stage IIC–IV: Radical inguinal orchiectomy followed by combination chemotherapy (with a cisplatin-based regimen). Chemotherapy combinations include BEP for three or four courses in good- or intermediate-prognosis patients (Table 13.2) or EP for four courses in good-prognosis patients. There is controversy whether any residual masses present at the completion of chemotherapy should be empirically irradiated, or whether masses greater than 3 cm should be resected.

Non-seminoma stage I

The cure rate for patients with non-seminomatous tumours in clinical stage I exceeds 95%. About 20% of patients with stage I disease without lymphatic or vascular invasion or without invasion into the tunica albuginea, spermatic cord or scrotum are discovered to have regional lymph node metastases at surgery. Nerve-sparing retroperitoneal lymph node dissection and surveillance are both standard treatment options [1].

Nerve-sparing retroperitoneal lymph node dissection

A primary retroperitoneal lymph node dissection after orchiectomy allows careful pathological staging, while at the same time offering a therapeutic benefit if the retroperitoneal lymph nodes are positive. A nerve-sparing retroperitoneal lymphadenectomy (RPL) that preserves ejaculation in virtually every clinical stage I patient appears to be as effective as the standard RPL. Despite the improved accuracy of clinical staging methods about 20% of patients with clinical stage I have pathological stage II disease at RPL. Many of these patients are cured surgically without subsequent chemotherapy. However, approximately 80% of clinical stage I patients who undergo primary RPL are found to have pathological stage I disease and do not benefit from the surgical procedure [21].

In case of a pathological stage I after RPL, patients can go into follow-up without additional treatment. In a large study, 15% of patients with a negative lymph node dissection experienced recurrence, usually pulmonary and usually within 18 months [22]. The overall survival rate of patients with pathological stage I is about 99% [23].

In case of tumour in the resected lymph nodes in patients with a clinical stage I, a pathological stage II is documented. The relapse rate of a pathological stage II not treated with adjuvant chemotherapy is related to the volume of retroperitoneal disease up to 30% [21]. These patients are therefore further treated with two courses of adjuvant cisplatin-combination chemotherapy [24].

Prognostic factors for patients with stage I disease that may predict the likelihood of occult metastases are the presence of lymphatic or venous invasion in the primary tumour, the presence of embryonal cell carcinoma and the absence of yolk sac elements in the primary tumour [23]. A more sophisticated way to stain proliferating tumour cells in testicular tumours with a monoclonal antibody MIB-1 against Ki-67 in combination with the volume of embryonal cell carcinoma and the transaxial diameter of retroperitoneal lymph nodes in the predicted landing zone allows a low-risk clinical stage I classification [25]. However, none of these strategies reliably predicts the presence of occult metastases in clinical stage I disease.

If performed, surgery should be followed by monthly determination of serum markers and chest X-rays for the first year and 1- to 2-month determinations for the second year, every 6 months in years 3 to 5, and follow-up is then indicated yearly thereafter [26].

Surveillance

Approximately 75–80% of patients with clinical stage I disease who undergo RPL have negative lymph nodes [26]. The rational for surveillance is to avoid surgical 'overtreatment' of patients with clinical stage I disease. In this strategy, radical inguinal orchiectomy without retroperitoneal node dissection is followed by regular follow-up (e.g. every 1–2 months) consisting of history, physical examination, determination of serum tumour markers, and during the first year, abdominal CT scans [27]. Intervals for abdominal CT scans have varied from every 2 months to scans only at 3 and 12 months post-orchiectomy, with apparently similar outcomes [27]. Disease recurrence is rarely detected by chest X-ray alone, so chest X-ray may play little or no role in routine surveillance [28]. In a Medical Research Council (MRC) surveillance study of non-seminomatous germ cell tumours (NSGCTs), 396 patients with a median follow-up of 4 years had a 25% recurrence rate and a mortality rate of less than 2% [29]. Long-term follow-up is important, since relapses have been reported more than 5 years after the orchiectomy in patients who did not undergo a retroperitoneal dissection.

Surveillance should be considered only if:

1 CT scan and serum markers are normal;

2 the patient and the physician accept the need for repeating CT scans as necessary to continue the periodic monitoring of the retroperitoneal lymph nodes up to 24 months;

3 the patient diligently follows a programme of regular check-ups, which includes history, physical examination, radiology and determination of serum markers;

4 the physician accepts responsibility for seeing that a follow-up schedule is maintained as noted for 2 years and then periodically beyond 2 years.

Data suggest that relapse rates are higher in patients with histological evidence of lymphatic or venous invasion and lower when the primary tumour contains mature teratoma [30]. Some investigators have reported higher relapse rates in patients with embryonal cell histology and recommend RPL for such patients [22,29]. Other investigators have not found a higher relapse rate for this subgroup [30]. Additionally, some investigators recommend RPL in patients with a normal pre-orchiectomy AFP, because they feel this marker cannot be used as an indicator of relapse during follow-up [22,29]. However, since marker-negative patients may be marker-positive at relapse and marker-positive patients may be marker-negative at relapse, other investigators do not view a normal pre-orchiecomy AFP as a contraindication to a surveillance policy.

Adjuvant therapy consisting of two courses of BEP has been administered to patients with clinical stage I disease who were considered at high risk of relapse (about 50% predicted relapse rate based on presence of vascular invasion and histologic type) [31]. In 114 such patients, the relapse-free survival at 2 years was 98%. Another study of high-risk clinical stage I patients treated with two adjuvant courses of BEP [32] reported a relapse rate of less than 5%, while in historical series of high-risk patients followed without adjuvant chemotherapy the relapse rate was 50%. However, in the historical series, cure rates have also been 95% and greater after chemotherapy is given for relapse. Given the present criteria, high-risk patients will relapse, at most, around 50% of the time, and thus approximately 50% of patients who would not have relapsed would receive chemotherapy 'unnecessarily'.

It is unclear which approach is superior in outcome. The adjuvant chemotherapy series are too small to draw definite conclusions about ultimate efficacy and about the risk of chemotherapy-induced long-term toxicity, secondary malignancies, impact on fertility or risk of late relapse.

Standard treatment options

For patients with non-seminoma stage I: Radical inguinal orchiectomy followed by either retroperiotoneal lymph node dissection (in case of pathological stage I: follow-up, in case of pathological stage II: two adjuvant courses of BEP) or surveillance.

Non-seminoma stage II–IV

Disseminated non-seminoma is highly curable. In most patients, an orchiectomy is performed before starting chemotherapy. However, if the diagnosis has been made by biopsy of a metastatic site and chemotherapy initiated, subsequent orchiectomy is generally performed due to the fact that chemotherapy may not eradicate the primary cancer. This is illustrated by case reports in which viable tumour was found on postchemotherapy orchiectomy despite complete response of metastatic lesions [33].

After the introduction of cisplatin, vinblastine and bleomycin (PVB) combination chemotherapy, consisting of a remission–induction part and a maintenance part, the strategy for treatment outcome improvement had focused on less toxicity with similar efficacy. It was shown that the dosage of vinblastine could be reduced (0.3 mg/kg vs 0.4 mg/kg) and that maintenance chemotherapy does not prevent relapses but adds significantly to the toxicity [34]. Later on vinblastine has been replaced by etoposide; based on the efficacy of etoposide in salvage therapy, and based on the results of a randomized study with BEP, this combination became the new standard [34].

Other centres have developed their own combinations such as the Memorial Sloan–Kettering Cancer Center, New York, using the so-called VAB schemes [35], or Charing Cross Hospital, London, using the POMB-ACE combination [36], but most often the BEP regimen is used.

The success of treatment of disseminated testicular cancer has led to refinements in treatment, with a greater importance on prognostic factors. Several groups have devised schema for stratifying patients into prognostic groups. Although each prognostic system has advantages and disadvantages, several characteristics are common. On the other hand, substantial differences occur between the various classifications in their use of prognostic variables and in their ability to separate patients into good-and poor-prognostic groups. This means that the description of a good prognosis differs, depending on the prognostic system used. To achieve more uniformity in classifying the prognosis of patients with metastatic disease, the International Germ Cell Cancer Collaborative Group (IGCCCG) recently developed a prognostic classification for germ cell tumours based on a large analysis of more than 5000 patients who were treated in prospective studies in North America, Europe, New Zealand and Australia. Primary tumour site, degree of elevation of serum tumour markers (AFP, HCG and LDH) and the presence or absence of non-pulmonary visceral metastases were identified as the most important independent prognostic variables. Integration of these prognostic factors produced three groupings of testicular cancer patients with good, intermediate and poor prognosis, with 5-year overall survival rates of 92%, 80% and 48%, respectively [2]. Since then this system is used by all collaborative groups.

Good-risk patients with metastatic non-seminomatous testicular cancer

The strategy for treatment outcome improvement in 'good-risk patients' has focused on less toxicity with the same efficacy compared with the standard treatment of BEP. Attempts to improve the toxicity profile have focused on the role of bleomycin (especially because of bleomycin-induced pulmonary fibrosis). The European Organization of Research and Treatment of Cancer (EORTC) compared four courses of BEP with four courses of EP in patients with a 'good prognosis'. The total dose of etoposide per course, however, was 360 mg/m^2 compared with 500 mg/m^2, as is the US standard. In total, 419 patients were randomized. In the EP arm 87% of the patients achieved a complete response, if necessary followed by surgical resection of residual disease; in the BEP arm this was the case in 95% of the patients. This difference is significant. Due to the low number of relapses (4%) no difference in progression-free survival was found [37]. An Eastern Cooperative Oncology Group (ECOG) study compared three cycles of BEP with three cycles of EP [38]. In the BEP arm 94% of the patients achieved a complete response versus 88% in the EP arm. The progression-free survival of the BEP group was significantly higher than that of the EP group (86% vs 68% after 5 years). So bleomycin is an essential part of the standard BEP regimen.

To address the question whether cisplatin can be replaced by the less-toxic analogue carboplatin, an MRC–EORTC study was performed. Almost 600 patients with a 'good prognosis' were randomized between four courses of BEP and four courses of carboplatin–etoposide–bleomycin (CEB) [39]. Significantly less patients in the CEB arm achieved a complete response (94% vs 88%). After 1 year, the progression-free survival was significantly lower in the CEB arm compared with the BEP arm. These data demonstrate that cisplatin cannot be substituted by carboplatin. To assess the optimal number of courses of BEP (Table 13.2) a study was performed in which three courses of BEP have been shown to be equivalent to four courses in patients with minimal or moderate extent of disseminated germ cell tumours [40]. To estimate equivalence of three and four courses of BEP, an EORTC–MRC study was performed randomizing three courses of BEP with three courses of BEP plus one course of EP [15]. The median 2-year progression-free survival was 90.4% versus 89.4%. Therefore it can be concluded that for good-risk patients based on the IGCCCG criteria these regimens are equivalent.

One question remaining is whether in good-risk patients three courses of BEP are equivalent to four courses of EP (Table 13.2). Probably this question will never be answered and the choice is based on personal preferences.

The standard treatment options for 'good-prognosis' patients

Radical inguinal orchiectomy followed by chemotherapy. Chemotherapy regimens include BEP for three courses or EP for four courses (Table 13.2). If these patients do not achieve a complete radiological response on chemotherapy, surgical removal of all residual masses should be performed.

'Intermediate- and poor-risk' patients with metastatic non-seminomatous testicular cancer

Compared with good-risk non-seminoma patients, patients with intermediate or poor risk have a worse prognosis. This is a strong argument for treating patients as soon as possible after being diagnosed as having metastatic disease. IGCCCG data show that intermediate prognosis accounts for ± 28% of the non-seminomatous testicular cancer patients and the 5-year survival of this group is 80%. The non-seminomatous testicular cancer patients with a poor prognosis (± 16% of the patients) have a 5-year survival of 48% [2]. The patients who are not cured with standard chemotherapy usually have widespread visceral metastases, high tumour marker levels or mediastinal primary tumours at presentation. Some retrospective data suggest that the experience of the treating institution may impact the outcome of non-seminoma. Data from 380 patients treated from 1990 to 1994 on the same study protocol at 49 institutions were analysed [4]. Overall, 2-year survival for the patients treated at institutions that entered less than five patients onto the protocol was 62% (95% CI = 48–75%) versus 77% (95% CI = 72–81%) in the institutions that entered at least five patients. As in any nonrandomized study design, patient selection factors and factors leading patients to choose treatment at one centre over another can make interpretation of results difficult.

Although the standard treatment for patients with an intermediate or poor prognosis has been four courses of BEP chemotherapy, the strategy for treatment outcome improvement has focused on non-cross-resistant chemotherapy combinations, and dose escalation or intensification. A study in which 244 patients were randomized between four courses of BEP and four alternating courses of PVB and BEP showed no significant differences in complete remission numbers: 72% versus 76%, respectively. The progression-free survival was 80% in both groups [41]. Because of its activity in second-line treatments, ifosfamide was incorporated into first-line treatments. A randomized study comparing four courses of BEP with four courses of VIP showed equivalent overall survival (83% vs 85%, respectively) and time-to-treatment failure for the two regimens in patients with advanced disseminated germ cell tumours who had not received prior chemotherapy. Haematologic toxic effects were substantially worse with the VIP regimen [14].

In patients with poor-risk germ cell tumours, the standard dose cisplatin regimen has been shown to be equivalent to high-dose cisplatin (40 mg/m^2 daily $\times$ 5 per course) in terms of complete response, cure rates and survival; moreover, patients in the high-dose cisplatin regimen experienced significantly more toxic effects [42]. A randomized comparison of an intensive induction-sequential chemotherapy schedule BOP/VIP-B (bleomycin, vincristine, cisplatin, etoposide, ifosfamide) with BEP in patients with poor-prognosis non-seminomatous testicular cancer showed more toxicity without evidence of an improved response rate or survival for the BOP/VIP-B regimen [43].

Based on its activity in patients with a relapsed or refractory germ cell tumour, paclitaxel is an interesting drug to add to the first-line regimen in patients with intermediate- or poor-prognosis disease [44]. The EORTC is currently performing a study in which intermediate-risk patients are treated with standard BEP versus BEP plus paclitaxel (T-BEP).

More intensive approaches are explored in several studies, including high-dose chemotherapy with peripheral stem cell transplantation. This approach has been fuelled by results from small studies in patients who failed second- or third-line cisplatin-containing regimens. Long disease-free periods were established in 10–20% of patients who were treated with high-dose chemotherapy and peripheral stem cell rescue [45,46]. This approach has also been used in a French study in which patients with poor prognostic factors were randomized between conventional dose chemotherapy and conventional dose combined with high-dose chemotherapy as first-line treatment [47]. The 2-year survival rate was not different in both treatment arms; however, the trial was inconclusive because the dose of cisplatin was lower in the experimental arm compared with the standard arm. A dose-intense regimen using the VIP combination has been exploited by a German study group [48]. The dose intensity of etoposide was three times higher and that of ifosfamide two times higher compared with standard VIP. The EORTC is currently performing a randomized study in poor-prognosis testicular cancer patients, comparing standard BEP with high-dose VIP and peripheral stem cell rescue. Patients who present with brain metastases as a poor prognostic factor should be treated with chemotherapy and simultaneous whole-brain irradiation (5000 cGy/25 fractions) [49].

The standard treatment options for 'intermediate- and poor-prognosis' patients

Radical inguinal orchiectomy followed by chemotherapy with postchemotherapy surgery for removal of residual masses (if present). Chemotherapy regimens include BEP for four courses and VIP for four courses (Table 13.2).

Surgery after chemotherapy

If patients do not achieve a complete radiological response after chemotherapy, surgical removal of residual masses should be performed. The timing of such surgery requires clinical judgement, but occurs most often after three or four cycles of combination chemotherapy and after normalization of serum marker levels. The probability of finding residual teratoma or carcinoma after chemotherapy may depend on the histology of the primary tumour [50]. However, others have reported that irrespective of initial histology there is a significant risk of teratoma or carcinoma in residual masses. Moreover, neither size of the initial metastasis nor degree of shrinkage while on therapy appears to accurately identify patients with residual teratoma or carcinoma. This has led some authors to recommend surgery with resection of all residual masses apparent on scans in patients who have normal or normalized markers after chemotherapy [51]. The presence of persistent viable tumour cells in the resected specimen seems to be an indication for additional chemotherapy [52], although this strategy may not improve overall survival [53]. Surgical removal of residual masses is also necessary to prevent regrowth of teratomas and growth of non-germ cell elements present in some of these masses [54]. Some patients may have discordant pathological findings (fibrosis/necrosis, teratoma or carcinoma) in residual masses in the abdomen versus the chest; some medical centres therefore perform simultaneous retroperitoneal and thoracic operations. However, most centres do not perform simultaneous retroperitoneal and thoracic resections. Although the agreement among the histologies of residual masses above, versus below, the diaphragm is only moderate, there is some evidence that if retroperitoneal resection is performed first, results can be used to guide decisions about whether to perform a thoracotomy [55]. In a multi-institutional case series of surgery to remove postchemotherapy residual masses in 159 patients, only necrosis was found at thoracotomy in about 90% of patients who had also only necrosis in their retroperitoneal masses. This figure was about 95% if the original testicular primary tumour did not contain teratomatous elements. Conversely, the histology of residual masses at thoracotomy was not nearly as good a predictor of the histology of retroperitoneal masses [55].

The standard treatment options

If patients with disseminated non-seminomatous testicular cancer do not achieve a complete radiological response on chemotherapy, surgical removal of residual masses should be performed. The timing of such surgery should be done after three or four cycles of combination chemotherapy and after normalization of serum tumour marker levels.

Treatment of recurrent disease

Deciding on further treatment in case of recurrent testicular cancer depends on many factors, including the histology, prior treatment, site of recurrence, as well as individual patient considerations. Salvage regimens consisting of ifosfamide, cisplatin and either etoposide or vinblastine can induce long-term complete responses in about one quarter of patients with disease that has persisted or recurred following first-line cisplatin-based regimens. Patients who have had an initial complete response to first-line chemotherapy and those without extensive disease have the most favourable outcome [56]. The VIP regimen is now the standard initial salvage regimen [56]. However, few, if any, patients with recurrent NSGCTs of an extragonadal origin achieve long-term disease-free survival using VIP if their disease recurs [56]. High-dose chemotherapy with autologous stem cell transplantation has also been used with some success in the setting of refractory disease [46]. Durable complete remissions may be achievable in 10–20% of patients. The durable complete remission rate may even exceed 50% in selected patients if high-dose chemotherapy is used as salvage chemotherapy at the first relapse of primary testicular cancer [57]. In general, patients with progressive tumours during frontline or after salvage treatment and those with refractory mediastinal germ cell tumours do not appear to benefit as much from high-dose chemotherapy with autologous stem cell transplantation as those who relapse after an initial response [58]. In some highly selected patients with chemorefractory disease confined to a single site, surgical resection may yield long-term disease-free survival [52]. The choice of salvage surgery versus high-dose chemotherapy with autologous stem cell transplantation for refractory disease is based on resectability, the number of sites of metastatic disease and the degree to which the tumour is refractory to cisplatin.

A special case of late relapse may be patients who relapse more than 2 years after achieving complete remission; this population represents less than 5% of patients who are in complete remission after 2 years. Results with chemotherapy are poor and surgical treatment appears to be superior, if technically feasible [59]. This may be because mature teratoma may be amenable to surgery at relapse and also has a better prognosis than carcinoma. Mature teratoma is a relatively resistant histologic subtype, so chemotherapy may not be appropriate.

Clinical trials are appropriate and should be considered whenever possible, including phase I and II studies for those patients not achieving a complete remission with induction therapy or not achieving a complete remission following salvage treatment for their first relapse or for patients who have a second relapse.

Patients who relapse with brain metastases after a complete initial response to chemotherapy require further chemotherapy, with simultaneous whole-brain irradiation and consideration of surgical excision of solitary lesions [49].

The standard treatment options

Patients with recurrent non-seminomatous testicular cancer can be treated with a salvage VIP regimen. However, since only few of these relapsed patients achieve a long-term disease-free survival, high-dose chemotherapy with autologous stem cell transplantation can also be used. Participation of these patients in clinical trials should be considered whenever possible.

Follow-up

The aim of follow-up care in patients treated for testicular cancer is to detect a relapse at a stage where salvage treatment has the best chance of being effective, to monitor and treat treatment-related toxicity, to detect cancers in the contralateral testicle and to offer support and counselling about issues such as fertility and employment. Recently minimal recommendations have been published by the European Society for Medical Oncology (ESMO) [60,61], but the optimal timing of clinical, biochemical and radiological follow-up is still under investigation.

Early detection of recurrence of testicular cancer after successful treatment with cisplatin combination chemotherapy is beneficial if there is a chance of achieving another durable remission with salvage treatment [58]. The possibility of early recognition of recurrence and subsequent treatment prolonging survival will increase with more effective salvage therapies [57]. However, the optimal regimen of physical examination, tumour marker estimations and chest X-rays for use in the follow-up of patients after initial treatment has not been determined. The widely used follow-up strategies come from large multi-institutional chemotherapy trials that defined the optimal chemotherapy combination for disseminated non-seminomatous testicular cancer during the last 2 decades. However, the primary focus of this particular follow-up was to define the efficacy of the first-line treatment regimen and not to evaluate the value of follow-up examinations. Furthermore, there are few data in the medical literature concerning the effectiveness of these follow-up regimens. In daily practice, the aim of follow-up after successful chemotherapy is to detect a tumour relapse in time without unnecessary procedures. Recent data suggest that routine chest X-rays (CXR) have limited or no additional value in the detection of a relapse during follow-up in patients who have a complete biochemical response and no residual masses [62]. The value of CXR in follow-up of clinical stage I patients with non-seminomatous testicular cancer also does not show additional value in detection of disease recurrence [28]. So tumour marker measurements, medical history and physical examination seem to be of key value.

From an oncologic point of view, recent data and recommendations suggest that it is reasonable to discharge patients with stage I non-seminomatous testicular tumours and all stages of seminoma from follow-up after 5 years [28,60,61]. Metastatic non-seminomatous testicular cancers seem to have a continuing annual relapse rate of 1–2% even after 10 years, suggesting that life-long follow-up might be needed [1,60]. However, an important part of the long-term follow-up is surveillance of long-term toxicity of administered treatment. Since most of the cured patients are men in their twenties or early thirties, long-term treatment-related toxicity is of growing importance.

Treatment toxicity and long-term side-effects

Chemotherapy with cisplatin causes significant side-effects both in the short and the long term. Acute side-effects include nausea and vomiting, alopecia, bone marrow suppression with risk for neutropenic fever, fatigue, renal toxicity and acute cardiovascular toxicity. A particular complication of the BEP combination chemotherapy is lung toxicity associated with bleomycin [63]; in most studies, 0.5–1% developed fatal bleomycin-induced pneumonitis. Bleomycin combined with cisplatin is also associated with the risk of developing Raynaud's phenomenon [64]. Cisplatin may also cause damage to both peripheral and auditory sensory nerves. This resolves in most patients over 6–12 months but long-term studies suggest persistent damage in a proportion of patients.

Infertility is one of the most distressing adverse effects of cancer therapy. Patients with germ cell tumour may have azoospermia related to the disease itself or to the sterilizing effects of chemotherapy [65]. Fertility is an important predictor of long-term health-related quality of life in testicular cancer survivors. Testicular patients undergoing chemotherapy are usually counselled about the risks of infertility and offered the opportunity for sperm banking before commencing therapy. For the azoospermic germ cell cancer survivor, donor insemination and adoption have historically been the main reproductive options. A recent report by Damani *et al.* explores the possibilities of testis sperm extraction in testicular cancer survivors. This assisted reproductive technology, initially developed for conditions such as congenital absence of the vas deferens, resulted in successful retrieval of sperm in approximately two-thirds of the patients [66]. Rather, it should be considered a reproductive option for the azoospermic cancer survivor without banked sperm. This technique represents the development of an effective intervention for an established treatment-related adverse effect, with the potential to improve the long-term well-being of the cancer survivor. For many other physiologic adverse effects of cancer treatment, the situation is not so clear.

The prevalence and time course for development of certain other late effects have not been well defined. The main concerns relate to the increased risk of second malignancies that can occur after treatment with chemotherapy or radiotherapy or of cardiovascular events in long-term survivors [67,68].

Cisplatin-containing chemotherapy for germ cell cancer has been associated with Raynaud's phenomenon, and serious vascular complications, including myocardial infarction, stroke and thromboembolic disease, have been reported [64]. Some, but not all, studies have suggested that after cisplatin-containing chemotherapy, patients may be at increased risk for the premature development of hypertension and lipid abnormalities, well-known major cardiovascular risk factors [68,69,70]. Testicular cancer survivors develop a metabolic syndrome or syndrome X-like state after chemotherapy, which makes them more prone to cardiovascular events [71,72]. However, does cisplatin combination chemotherapy result in an increased risk for early cardiovascular events? In one study of testicular cancer patients treated with surgery or surgery plus chemotherapy, no increase in cardiovascular events was noted in the chemotherapy group at a median follow-up of 5 years [73]. A more recent study reported an increased risk of cardiovascular events for testicular cancer survivors younger than 50 years of age who had received chemotherapy and were in remission for 10 or more years [68]. Further studies are needed to better define the actual risk, if any, of early cardiovascular events in these patients. What do these data tell us regarding the education and counselling of testicular cancer survivors concerning cardiovascular risk? Are there rational early intervention possibilities?

Who will be following the cancer survivor when these adverse effects become manifest? While the oncologist might be the most knowledgeable about the potential late adverse effects of cancer treatment, many survivors may not regularly see an oncologist once the risk of tumour recurrence is unlikely. Probably many of these patients are followed by primary care physicians, who may not be fully aware of the details of the patient's oncologic history and may not be familiar with the long-term sequelae of cancer and its treatment. Other patients may exit the health care system altogether. For uncommon cancers such as germ cell tumours, few centres have enough patients to define a large enough long-term cohort for studies. Our preference is to undertake the long-term follow-up at a cancer centre to allow the build-up of well-documented databases on the well-being and actual health status of testicular cancer survivors facilitating cancer survivor research.

For future well-defined health care problems of testicular cancer survivors, either primary care physicians with knowledge of testicular cancer and treatment sequelae or a cancer specialist with knowledge of general internal medicine should take care of treatment sequelae or risk factors for disease.

References

1 Dearnaley DP, Huddart RA, Horwich A. Managing testicular cancer. *BMJ* 2001; **322**: 1583–8.
2 International Germ Cell Cancer Collaborative Group. International germ cell consensus classification: a prognostic factor-based staging system for metastatic germ cell cancers. *J Clin Oncol* 1997; **15**: 594–603.
3 Mead GM. Who should manage germ cell tumours of the testis? *BJU Int* 1999; **89**: 61–7.
4 Collette L, Sylvester RJ, Stenning SP *et al*. Impact of the treating institution on survival of patients with 'poor-prognosis' metastatic nonseminoma. European Organization for Research and Treatment of Cancer Genito-Urinary Tract Cancer Collaborative Group and the Medical Research Council Testicular Cancer Working Party. *J Natl Cancer Inst* 1999; **91**: 839–46.
5 Vaughn DJ, Gignac GA, Meadows AT. Long-term medical care or testicular cancer survivors. *Ann Int Med* 2002; **136**: 463–70.
6 Fossa SD, Horwich A, Russell JM *et al*. Optimal planning target volume for stage I testicalar seminoma: a medical research council randomized trial. Medical Research Council Testicular Tumor Working Group. *J Clin Oncol* 1999; **17**: 1146.
7 Milosevic MF, Gospodarowicz M, Warde P. Management of testicular seminoma. *Semin Surg Oncol* 1999; **17**: 240–49.
8 Oliver RT, Edmonds PM, Ong JY *et al*. Pilot studies of 2 and 1 course carboplatin as adjuvant for stage I seminoma: should it be tested in a randomized trial against radiotherapy? *Int J Radiat Oncol Biol Phys* 1994; **29**: 3–8.
9 Horwich A, Dearnaley DP. Treatment of seminoma. *Semin Oncol* 1992; **19**: 171–80.
10 Mencel PJ, Motzer RJ, Mazumdar M *et al*. Advanced seminoma: treatment results, survival, and prognostic factors in 142 patients. *J Clin Oncol* 1994; **12**: 120–26.
11 Williams SD, Birch R, Einhorn LH, Irwin L, Greco FA, Loehrer PJ. Treatment of disseminated germ-cell tumors with cisplatin, bleomycin, and either vinblastine or etoposide. *N Engl J Med* 1987; **316**: 1435–40.
12 Einhorn LH, Williams SD, Loehrer PJ *et al*. Evaluation of optimal duration of chemotherapy in favorable-prognosis disseminated germ cell tumours: a Southeastern Cancer Study Group protocol. *J Clin Oncol* 1989; **7**: 387–91.
13 Bajorin DF, Geller NL, Weisen SF, Bosl GJ. Two-drug therapy in patients with metastatic germ cell tumors. *Cancer* 1991; **67**: 28–32.
14 Nichols CR, Catalano PJ, Crawford ED, Vogelzang NJ, Einhorn LH, Loehrer PJ. Randomized comparison of cisplatin and etoposide and either bleomycin of ifosfamide in treatment of advanced disseminated germ cell tumors: an Eastern Cooperative Oncology Group, Southwest Oncology Group, and Cancer and Leukemia Group B study. *J Clin Oncol* 1998; **16**: 1287–93.

15 de Wit R, Roberts JR, Wilkinson PM *et al.* Equivalence of three or four cycles of bleomycin, etoposide, and cisplatin chemotherapy and of a 3- or 5-day schedule in good-prognosis germ cell cancer: a randomized study of the European Organisation for Research and Treatment of Cancer Genitourinary Tract Cancer Cooperative Group and the Medical Research Council. *J Clin Oncol* 2001; **19**: 1629–40.

16 Horwich A, Dearnaley DP, A'Hern R *et al.* The activity of single-agent carboplatin in advanced seminoma. *Eur J Cancer* 1992; **28A**: 1307–10.

17 Sleijfer S, Willemse PH, de Vries EG, van der Graaf WT, Schraffordt KH, Mulder NH. Treatment of advanced seminoma with cyclophosphamide, vincristine and carboplatin on an outpatient basis. *Br J Cancer* 1996; **74**: 947–50.

18 Ravi R, Ong J, Oliver RT, Badenoch DF, Fowler CG, Hendry WF. The management of residual masses after chemotherapy in metastatic seminoma. *BJU Int* 1999; **83**: 649–53.

19 Duchesne GM, Stenning SP, Aass N *et al.* Radiotherapy after chemotherapy for metastatic seminoma – a diminishing role. MRC Testicular Tumour Working Party. *Eur J Cancer* 1997; **33**: 829–35.

20 Herr HW, Sheinfeld J, Puc HS *et al.* Surgery for a post-chemotherapy residual mass in seminoma. *J Urol* 1997; **157**: 860–62.

21 Foster RS, Roth BJ. Clinical stage I non-seminoma: surgery versus surveillance. *Semin Oncol* 1998; **25**: 145–53.

22 Klepp O, Olsson AM, Henrikson H *et al.* Prognostic factors in clinical stage I nonseminomatous germ cell tumors of the testis: multivariate analysis of a prospective multicenter study. Swedish–Norwegian Testicular Cancer Group. *J Clin Oncol* 1990; **8**: 509–18.

23 Sonneveld DJ, Koops HS, Sleijfer DT, Hoekstra HJ. Surgery versus surveillance in stage I non-seminoma testicular cancer. *Semin Surg Oncol* 1999; **17**: 230–39.

24 Williams SD, Stablein DM, Einhorn LH *et al.* Immediate adjuvant chemotherapy versus observation with treatment at relapse in pathological stage II testicular cancer. *N Engl J Med* 1987; **317**: 1433–8.

25 Leibovitch I, Foster RS, Kopecky KK, Albers P, Ulbright TM, Donohue JP. Identification of clinical stage A nonseminomatous testis cancer patients at extremely low risk for metastatic disease: a combined approach using quantitive immunohistochemical, histopathologic, and radiologic assessment. *J Clin Oncol* 1998; **16**: 261–8.

26 Chang SS, Roth B. Treatment of clinical stage I germ cell tumors. *Urology* 2002; **59**: 173–9.

27 Francis R, Bower M, Brunstrom G *et al.* Surveillance for stage I testicular germ cell tumours: results and cost benefit analysis of management options. *Eur J Cancer* 2000; **36**: 1925–32.

28 Gels ME, Hoekstra HJ, Sleijfer DT *et al.* Detection of recurrence in patients with clinical stage I nonseminomatous testicular germ cell tumors and consequences for further follow-up: a single-center 10-year experience. *J Clin Oncol* 1995; **13**: 1188–94.

29 Read G, Stenning SP, Cullen MH *et al.* Medical Research Council prospective study of surveillance for stage I testicular teratoma. Medical Research Council Testicular Tumors Working Party. *J Clin Oncol* 1992; **10**: 1762–8.

30 Alexandre J, Fizazi K, Mahe C *et al.* Stage I non-seminomatous germ-cell tumours of the testis: identification of a subgroup of patients with a very low risk of relapse. *Eur J Cancer* 2001; **37**: 576–82.

31 Cullen MH, Stenning SP, Parkinson MC *et al.* Short-course adjuvant chemotherapy in high-risk stage I nonseminomatous germ cell tumors of the testis; a Medical Research Council report. *J Clin Oncol* 1996; **14**: 1106–13.

32 Pont J, Albrecht W, Postner G, Sellner F, Angel K, Hotl W. Adjuvant chemotherapy for high-risk clinical stage I nonseminomatous testicular germ cell cancer: long-term results of a prospective trial. *J Clin Oncol* 1996; **14**: 441–8.

33 Oliver RT, Ong J, Blandy JP, Altman DG. Testis conservation studies in germ cell cancer justified by improved primary chemotherapy response and reduced delay, 1978–1994. *Br J Urol* 1996; **78**: 119–24.

34 Einhorn LH. Treatment of testicular cancer: a new and improved model. *J Clin Oncol* 1990; **8**: 1777–81.

35 Bosl GJ, Geller NL, Bajorin D *et al*. A randomized trial of etoposide + cisplatin versus vinblastine + bleomycin + cisplatin + cyclophosphamide + dactinomycin in patients with good-prognosis germ cell tumors. *J Clin Oncol* 1988; **6**: 1231–8.

36 Hitchins RN, Newlands ES, Smith DB, Bengent RH, Rustin GJ, Bagshawe KD. Long-term outcome in patients with germ cell tumours treated with POMB/ACE chemotherapy: comparison of commonly used classification systems of good and poor prognosis. *Br J Cancer* 1989; **59**: 236–42.

37 de Wit R, Stoter G, Kaye SB *et al*. Importance of bleomycin in combination chemotherapy for good-prognosis testicular nonseminoma: a randomized study of the European Organization for Research and Treatment of Cancer Genitourinary Tract Cancer Cooperative Group. *J Clin Oncol* 1997; **15**: 1837–43.

38 Loehrer PJ Sr, Johnson D, Elson P, Einhorn LH, Trump D. Importance of bleomycin in favorable-prognosis disseminated germ cell tumors: an Eastern Cooperative Oncology Group trial. *J Clin Oncol* 1995; **13**: 470–76.

39 Horwich A, Sleijfer DT, Fossa SD *et al*. Randomized trial of bleomycin, etoposide, and cisplatin compared with bleomycin, etoposide, and carboplatin in good-prognosis metastatic nonseminomatous germ cell cancer: a multiinstitutional Medical Research Council/European Organization for Research and Treatment of Cancer Trial. *J Clin Oncol* 1997; **15**: 1844–52.

40 Einhorn LH, Williams SD, Loehrer PJ *et al*. Evaluation of optimal duration of chemotherapy in favorable-prognosis disseminated germ cell tumors: a Southeastern Cancer Study Group protocol. *J Clin Oncol* 1989; **7**: 387–91.

41 de Wit R, Stoter G, Sleijfer DT *et al*. Four cycles of BEP versus an alternating regime of PVB and BEP in patients with poor-prognosis metastatic testicular non-seminoma; a randomised study of the EORTC Genitourinary Tract Cancer Cooperative Group. *Br J Cancer* 1995; **71**: 1311–14.

42 Nichols CR, Williams SD, Loehrer PJ *et al*. Randomized study of cisplatin dose intensity in poor-risk germ cell tumors. A Southeastern Cancer Study Group and Southwest Oncology Group protocol. *J Clin Oncol* 1991; **9**: 1163–72.

43 Kaye SB, Mead GM, Fossa S *et al*. Intensive induction-sequential chemotherapy with BOP/VIP-B compared with treatment with BEP/EP for poor-prognosis metastatic nonseminomatous germ cell tumor: a randomized Medical Research Council/European Organization for Research and Treatment of Cancer study. *J Clin Oncol* 1998; **16**: 692–701.

44 Bokemeyer C, Beyer J. Metzner B *et al*. Phase II study of paclitaxel in patients with relapsed or cisplatin-refractory testicular cancer. *Ann Oncol* 1996; **7**: 31–4.

45 Nichols CR, Tricot G, Williams SD *et al*. Dose-intensive chemotherapy in refractory germ cell cancer – a phase I/II trial of high-dose carboplatin and etoposide with autologous bone marrow transplantation. *J Clin Oncol* 1989; **7**: 932–9.

46 Rodenhuis S, de Wit R, de Mulder PH *et al*. A multi-center prospective phase II study of high-dose chemotherapy in germ-cell cancer patients relapsing from complete remission. *Ann Oncol* 1999; **10**: 1467–73.

47 Chevreau C, Droz JP, Pico JL *et al*. Early intensified chemotherapy with autologous bone marrow transplantation in first line treatment of poor risk non-seminomatous germ cell tumours. Preliminary results of a French randomized trial. *Eur Urol* 1993; **23**: 213–17.

48   Bokemeyer C, Harstrick A, Beyer J *et al.* The use of dose-intensified chemotherapy in the treatment of metastatic nonseminomatous testicular germ cell tumors. German Testicular Cancer Study Group. *Semin Oncol* 1998; **23**(2 Suppl. 4): 24–32.

49   Spears WT, Morphis JG, Lester SG, Williams SD, Einhorn LH. Brain metastases and testicular tumors: long-term survival. *Int J Radiat Oncol Biol Phys* 1992; **22**: 12–22.

50   Steyerberg EW, Keizer HJ, Fossa SD *et al.* Prediction of residual retroperitoneal mass histology after chemotherapy for metastatic nonseminomatous germ cell tumor: multi-variate analysis of individual patient data from six study groups. *J Clin Oncol* 1995; **13**: 1177–87.

51   Toner GC, Panicek DM, Heelan RT *et al.* Adjunctive surgery after chemotherapy for nonseminomatous germ cell tumors: recommentations for patient selection. *J Clin Oncol* 1990; **8**: 1683–94.

52   Fox EP, Weathers TD, Williams SD *et al.* Outcome analysis for patients with persistent nonteratomatous germ cell tumor in postchemotherapy retroperitoneal lymph node dissections. *J Clin Oncol* 1993; **11**: 1294–9.

53   Fizazi K, Tjulandin S, Salvivioni R *et al.* Viable malignant cells after primary chemotherapy for disseminated nonseminomatous germ cell tumors: prognostic factors and role of postsurgery chemotherapy – results from an international study group. *J Clin Oncol* 2001; **19**: 2647–57.

54   Einhorn LH, Williams SD, Mandelbaum I, Donohue JP. Surgical resection in disseminated testicular cancer following chemotherapeutic cytoreduction. *Cancer* 1981; **48**: 904–908.

55   Steyerberg EW, Donohue JP, Gerl A *et al.* Residual masses after chemotherapy for metastatic testicular cancer: the clinical implications of the association between retroperitoneal and pulmonary histology. Re-analysis of histology in Testicular Cancer (ReHiT) Study Group. *J Urol* 1997; **158**: 474–8.

56   Loehrer PJ Sr, Gonin R, Nichols CR, Weathers T, Einhorn LH. Vinblastine plus ifosfamide plus cisplatin as initial salvage therapy in recurrent germ cell tumor. *J Clin Oncol* 1998; **16**: 2500–504.

57   Rick O, Bokemeyer C, Beyer J *et al.* Salvage treatment with paclitaxel, ifosfamide, and cisplatin plus high-dose carboplatin, etoposide, and thiotepa followed by autologous stem-cell rescue in patients with relapsed or refractory germ cell cancer. *J Clin Oncol* 2001; **19**: 81–8.

58   Beyer J, Kramer A, Mandanas R *et al.* High-dose chemotherapy as salvage treatment in germ cell tumors: a multivariate analysis of prognostic variables. *J Clin Oncol* 1996; **14**: 2638–45.

59   Baniel J, Foster RS, Gonin R, Messemeer JE, Donohue JP, Einhorn LH. Late relapse of testicular cancer. *J Clin Oncol* 1995; **13**: 1170–76.

60   ESMO minimum clinical recommendations for diagnosis, treatment and follow-up of mixed non-seminomatous germ cell tumours (NSGCT). *Ann Oncol* 2001; **12**: 1215–16.

61   ESMO minimum clinical recommendations for diagnosis, treatment and follow-up of testicular seminoma. *Ann Oncol* 2001; **12**: 1217–18.

62   Gietema JA, Meinardi MT, Sleijfer DT, Hoekstra HJ, van der Graaf WT. Routine chest X-rays have no additional value in detecting a relapse during the routine follow-up of patients treated with chemotherapy for disseminated non-seminomatous testicular cancer. *Ann Oncol* 2002; **13**: 1616–20.

63   Sleijfer S. Bleomycin-induced pneumonitis. *Chest* 2001; **120**: 617–24.

64   Meinardi MT, Gietema JA, van Veldhuisen DJ, van der Graaf WT, de Vries EG, Sleijfer DT. Long-term chemotherapy-related cardiovascular morbidity. *Cancer Treat Rev* 2000; **26**: 429–47.

65   Petersen PM, Skakkebaek NE, Vistisen K, Rorth M, Giwercman A. Semen quality and reproductive hormones before orchidectomy in men with testicular cancer. *J Clin Oncol* 1999; **17**: 941–7.

66 Damani MN, Masters V, Meng MV, Burgess C, Turek P, Oates RD. Postchemotherapy ejaculatory azoospermia: fatherhood with sperm from testis tissue with intracytoplasmic sperm injection. *J Clin Oncol* 2002; **20**: 930–36.

67 Travis LB, Curtis RE, Storm H *et al.* Risk of second malignant neoplasms among long-term survivors of testicular cancer. *J Natl Cancer Inst* 1997; **89**: 1429–39.

68 Meinardi MT, Gietema JA, van der Graaf WT *et al.* Cardiovascular morbidity in long-term survivors of metastatic testicular cancer. *J Clin Oncol* 2000; **18**: 1725–32.

69 Gietema JA, Sleijfer DT, Willemse PH *et al.* Long-term follow-up of cardiovascular risk factors in patients given chemotherapy for disseminated nonseminomatous testicular cancer. *Ann Int Med* 1992; **116**: 709–15.

70 Raghavan D, Cox K, Childs A, Grygiel J, Sullivan D. Hypercholesterolemia after chemotherapy for testis cancer. *J Clin Oncol* 1992; **10**: 1386–9.

71 Gietema JA, Meinardi MT, van der Graaf WT, Sleijfer DT. Syndrome X in testicular-cancer survivors. *The Lancet* 2001; **357**: 228–9.

72 Nuver J, Smit AJ, Postma A, Sleijfer DT, Gietema JA. The metabolic syndrome in long-term cancer survivors, a target for secondary preventive measures. *Cancer Treat Rev* 2002; **28**: 195–214.

73 Nichols CR, Roth BJ, Williams SD *et al.* No evidence of acute cardiovascular complications of chemotherapy for testicular cancer: an analysis of the Testicular Cancer Intergroup Study. *J Clin Oncol* 1992; **10**: 760–65.

14: Renal Cancer

Naveen S. Vasudev & Poulam M. Patel

Introduction

Renal cancer is a relatively rare cancer accounting for approximately 3% of all adult malignancies. There are more than 5000 new cases diagnosed per year in the UK and the incidence is increasing. It most commonly affects people in their fifth to seventh decades with a male-to-female ratio of approximately 2:1.

Renal cell carcinoma (RCC) (also known as clear cell carcinoma or hypernephroma) accounts for 80–85% of all kidney cancers. Papillary renal carcinoma constitutes approximately 10%, with the remainder including chromophobe and collecting duct carcinomas. Transitional cell carcinomas, squamous cell carcinomas and lymphomas can also arise in the kidney.

Risk factors for the development of RCC include smoking, obesity, adult polycystic kidney disease and long-term renal replacement therapy. Approximately 1% of RCCs are hereditary, the most commonly associated syndrome being the von Hippel–Lindau (VHL) syndrome. It has recently been demonstrated that most cases of sporadic RCC have mutations in the VHL gene, located on the short arm of chromosome three, which normally acts as a tumour suppressor gene.

The most commonly used method of staging renal cancer is the Robson staging system. Stage of disease and prognosis are closely linked. For tumours confined to the kidney (stage I) and with tumours that involve perinephric fat (stage II) the 5-year survival is 50–80% [1]. In patients with distant metastatic disease (stage IV) the median survival is just 8 months with a 5-year survival of less than 10% [2].

Approximately one quarter of patients present with metastatic disease. A further 30–40% of patients present with apparently localized disease but eventually develop distant metastases [3]. The lung is the most common site of metastasis (50–60%), followed by bone (30–40%), liver (30–40%) and brain (5%) [4].

Whilst radical nephrectomy can be curative in patients presenting with localized disease, the treatment options available to those with metastatic disease remain limited and far from ideal.

RCC is notoriously resistant to conventional chemotherapy agents and these drugs are not commonly used in disease management. Radiotherapy has a useful palliative role in a limited capacity, used mainly in the treatment of painful bony metastases, localized subcutaneous metastases and brain metastases. Hormonal agents, in particular medroxyprogesterone acetate and tamoxifen (more commonly used in mainland Europe) are often used to palliate the systemic effects of cancer. Their anticancer activity however is very limited, with objective response rates (RRs) of approximately 1%.

Attention has largely focused on the use of biological agents. Interferon-alpha (IFN-α) and interleukin-2 (IL-2) have both been used extensively in RCC over the past 2 decades, with encouraging results. It is well established that the use of such agents, termed immunotherapy, can induce complete and durable responses in a small number of patients. In the UK, IFN-α is now widely accepted as standard first-line therapy.

Whilst some progress has been made in recent years, the prognosis for patients with metastatic (m) RCC remains poor. Thus there remains an urgent need for the development of novel, more active agents. A greater understanding of the biology of this and other cancers has lead to the recent development of a number of new and promising strategies.

Principles of therapy

Chemotherapy

Cytotoxic chemotherapy remains the mainstay of systemic treatment for most solid cancers. RCC however is a characteristically unresponsive tumour and at present, these agents are not routinely used.

A comprehensive review of chemotherapy in RCC, performed by Yagoda *et al.*, included 4093 patients in 83 trials between 1983 and 1993. The trials included every class of anticancer agent. The overall RR was 6% (1.3% complete response (CR); 4.7% partial response (PR)) [5]. Similarly, a review of published literature between 1990 and 1998 showed no survival benefit for any single-agent chemotherapy drug [6].

Vinblastine (VLB) is a cytotoxic drug with some activity in RCC. For a time it was regarded as the best available agent. However, it is clear that RRs are low, typically between 2% and 7% [5], and VLB is no longer routinely used in the treatment of RCC.

5-Fluorouracil (5-FU) is a cytotoxic drug that has some single-agent activity (approximately 10% RR) in RCC. Introduced in the 1950s, it represents one of the first rationally designed anti-tumour agents. 5-FU is a fluorinated analogue of uracil, a pyrimidine base essential for nucleic acid metabolism. Through a number of mechanisms it interferes with DNA, RNA and protein synthesis. Myelosuppression and gastrointestinal (GI) toxicity are the predominant side-effects. The role of 5-FU, in combination with IFN-α and IL-2, is currently being investigated.

Renal cancer cells have an intrinsic resistance to chemotherapy. Classical multi-drug resistance (MDR) is associated with a membrane-bound protein, P-glycoprotein, that functions as a drug efflux pump. P-glycoprotein, and its encoding gene, MDR-1, have been shown to be overexpressed in many tumours, including RCC [7].

This is one of a number of mechanisms of drug resistance that has been described although several others have also been implicated. Until our understanding of these pathways improves, standard chemotherapy drugs are likely to remain largely obsolete in the treatment of renal cancer.

Immunotherapy

Scientists have long suspected that there is considerable interaction between tumour cells and the host's immune system. The small but significant number of spontaneous regressions of tumours, the increased incidence of malignancy in immunosuppressed patients and the presence of lymphoid infiltrates in solid tumours lent early support to this notion.

In recent years, greater understanding of basic immunology and of the host tumour relationship has lead to the development of immunotherapeutic approaches to cancer treatment. Biotherapy can be broadly defined as the use of natural substances that, by modifying the host's biological response to tumour cells, leads to therapeutic benefit. The term immunotherapy can be encompassed within this and relates specifically to approaches aimed at stimulating immune defence mechanisms.

The ability to differentiate tumour cells from normal cells is based on the ability of the immune system to detect tumour cells expressing abnormal proteins or abnormally expressed normal proteins (tumour antigens). Tumour antigens expressed on the cell surface can be detected by antibodies. Expression of intracellular tumour antigens is detected by T cells. Intracellular proteins are proteolytically degraded into small peptides, and a proportion of these are assembled into the groove of human leucocyte antigen (HLA) molecules. This HLA molecule/peptide complex is transported to the cell surface where it can be recognized by the T cell receptor (TCR) of cytotoxic T cells. The binding of the TCR to the major histocompatibility complex (MHC)/peptide complex triggers T cell activation and release of cytotoxic factors that induce death of the target cell. T cells however require other signals to give full activation, including cytokines and costimulatory signals from specialized antigen-presenting cells (APCs) such as dendritic cells (DCs). Indeed, effective T cell activation involves several steps.

Antigens shed by dying tumour cells are picked up by DCs and processed into HLA molecules. DCs migrate to the lymph nodes where the antigens are presented to T cells along with the appropriate costimulatory signals. These partially activated T cells can then circulate and when they encounter tumour cells expressing these antigens they are fully activated and kill the tumour cell. This whole process is controlled by a network of cytokines. Cytokines are a broad class of soluble proteins produced primarily by T cells, APCs, monocytes and macrophages and act as signals between cells of the immune system.

Tumour antigens have now been identified in many cancers and cytotoxic T cells specific for these can be isolated from patients with cancer. Unfortunately, in the majority of cancer patients there are defects in this immune response, and to date many different mechanisms of immune evasion have been identified. The aim of immunotherapy is to overcome these to allow effective immune stimulation.

Several approaches have been tried. These include specific and non-specific immunotherapies. Non-specific immunotherapies include cytokines such as IFN and IL-2 that enhance the immune response by a range of different mechanisms. Immunotherapies that enhance the immune response to specific antigens include vaccination with antigens in the form of whole cell vaccines, specific protein or specific peptides. Although many approaches have been tried in renal cancer the current mainstay of immunotherapy in renal cancer is the cytokines IFN-α and IL-2.

Surgery

The role of surgery in the management of localized RCC is well established. Radical nephrectomy is potentially curative for many patients with early stage disease. For patients with metastatic disease, decisions regarding surgery are more complicated.

At one time, nephrectomy was carried out in the hope of inducing a spontaneous regression of metastases. In fact, the frequency of this phenomenon is less than 1% [8] whilst the surgery itself carries a mortality of between 1% and 5%. There is therefore no justification for nephrectomy based solely on this assumption.

More recently however, data from two randomized trials have been published suggesting that nephrectomy in patients with metastatic disease can increase the likelihood of an objective response to immunotherapy at metastatic sites.

The European Organization for Research and Treatment of Cancer (EORTC) 30 947 trial randomized 83 patients with mRCC to either radical nephrectomy plus IFN-based immunotherapy versus IFN-α alone. Time to progression (5 vs 3 months) and median duration of survival (17 vs 7 months) were significantly better in the study patients than in the controls [9].

The results of a trial by the Southwest Oncology Group (SWOG) were similar. In that study of 245 patients, median survival was 12.5 months in the combined treatment arm compared with 8.1 months in patients who had interferon only and no nephrectomy [10].

It is important to note that only patients with a WHO performance status of 0–1 were eligible for these trials. In addition, both studies recruited relatively small numbers of patients over a very long time period.

Nevertheless, the current weight of evidence is in favour of nephrectomy before commencing immunotherapy for patients of good performance status. However, this approach is not appropriate or feasible in all cases and requires careful patient selection.

Adjuvant treatment

Adequate surgical excision is the only effective means of curing RCC. Approximately 70% of patients have nonmetastatic disease at the time of first presentation. However, of those who undergo tumour nephrectomy 2–14% relapse locally and 31–36% develop distant metastatic disease [3].

The concept of adjuvant therapy is well established in several tumours, such as of the breast and colon. In RCC however, chemotherapy, hormone therapy and radiotherapy have all failed to show a survival benefit when used in this setting. It remains unclear whether immunotherapy can make an impact in patients with RCC at high risk of relapse.

Pizzocaro *et al.* randomized 247 patients with Robson stage II and III RCC to 6 months of thrice-weekly IFN-α versus observation after radical nephrectomy. Overall, no advantage for adjuvant interferon was demonstrated in terms of overall and event-free survival [11]. Other similar studies using single-agent interferon in this setting have failed to demonstrate a survival advantage [12,13].

The EORTC 30955 trial is currently open and is using combination therapy in an adjuvant setting. Eligible patients should have a pT3b, pT3c or pT4 stage tumour; any pT stage and nodal status pN1or 2; or any pT stage and microscopic positive margins or evidence of microscopic vascular invasion. Patients are randomized either to an 8-week regimen of triple therapy with IFN-α, IL-2 and 5-FU or to observation.

There is currently no evidence to support the routine use of adjuvant therapies in RCC and observation remains the standard of care. Suitable patients should however be considered for participation in clinical trials.

Drugs available

Interferons

Interferons are a heterogeneous group of glycoproteins produced by mammalian cells in response to viral infections or other inducers. Three major types have been identified – interferon-α, interferon-β (class I) and interferon-δ (class II).

As well as helping to fight viruses, interferons have anti-tumour properties. These may be mediated through a direct cytotoxic effect on tumour cells or through augmentation of the immunogenicity of tumours by upregulation of histocompatibility and tumour-associated antigens (TAAs), and/or activation of macrophages, T lymphocytes and natural killer cells [14]. It is also thought that interferons possess anti-angiogenic properties.

The anti-neoplastic activity of IFN-α was first shown in hairy cell leukaemia and Kaposi's sarcoma. Subsequent studies have documented its activity in chronic mylogenous leukaemia, B and T cell lymphomas and melanoma. IFN-α is the most extensively tested IFN in clinical studies of patients with mRCC.

The use of IFN-α in RCC first began in the 1980s. It is now widely accepted in the UK as first-line treatment for metastatic renal cancer. A series of phase I and II studies have shown overall objective RRs for single-agent IFN-α in the region of 15%, with CRs in approximately 1%. The best responses have been achieved in patients with a good performance status and limited metastatic disease. Prognostic factors that help to predict response include prior nephrectomy, performance status, sites of metastatic disease and interval from presentation to the development of metastases. However, the modest increases in survival can be offset by treatment-related side-effects and the fact that responses are often not durable. Two large randomized phase III trials have been published demonstrating a clear survival advantage with the use of IFN-α.

Pyröhnen *et al.* prospectively randomized 160 patients with either locally advanced RCC or mRCC to receive either VLB alone or IFN-α plus VLB for 12 months or until disease progression. At the time, many considered VLB to be standard treatment. In both groups, intravenous VLB was given at 0.1 mg/kg every 3 weeks, and in the combination arm IFN-α was administered subcutaneously (s.c.) at 3 mega units (MU) three times a week for 1 week and 18 MU three times a week thereafter. The median survival was 67.6 weeks in the combination arm and 37.8 weeks in the VLB arm ($p < 0.0049$). Overall RRs were 16.5% in the combination arm and 2.5% in the VLB arm ($p < 0.0025$). Survival rates for patients treated with the combination or with VLB alone were 55.7% and 38.3%, respectively, after 1 year, and 11.7% and 5.1%, respectively, after 3 years. Survival was prolonged in the overall patient population, even in the subset of patients who did not have objective tumour responses, and was not decreased in patients who required a reduction of their IFN-α dose from 18 to 9 MU to improve tolerability [15].

A subsequent multicentre randomized trial by the Medical Research Council Renal Cancer Collaborators (MRC RE01) randomized 335 patients with mRCC to receive either s.c. IFN-α (three doses – 5, 5, 10 MU – for week 1, then 10 MU three times per week for a further 11 weeks) or MPA 300 mg once a day for 12 weeks. A survival advantage of IFN-α over MPA was demonstrated, with an absolute improvement in 1-year survival of 12% (43% vs 31%). The median survival time was 8.5 months for patients treated with IFN and 6 months for patients treated with MPA. The time to relapse, however, was short, and progression-free survival at 2 years was 5% or less for both groups. Side-effects were also more marked in the IFN-α group, notably tiredness, anorexia, loss of energy and nausea. The difference was most significant at 4 weeks, persistent at 12 weeks but had resolved by 6 months [16].

Treatment-related toxicity can be marked and, whilst rarely life-threatening, does affect quality of life. Acutely, patients suffer from flu-like symptoms, namely fevers, rigors and myalgia that can be largely alleviated by coadministration of paracetamol. These symptoms usually resolve within approximately 2 weeks of treatment. Lethargy is common and tends to accumulate with repeated injections. In addition, anorexia, weight loss, depression and loss of libido can occur. At higher doses, hepatotoxicity and myelosuppression may be seen.

Several dose schedules have been investigated. Overall, the differences in terms of RRs have been modest. The most commonly used regimen in the UK is 9–10 MU s.c., three times per week. Patients typically self-administer their interferon on an outpatient basis. Injecting at night means that patients can sleep through the worst of the acute side-effects.

Single-agent IFN-α produces a small but consistent response in renal cancer. Efforts to increase the proportion of patients who respond and to make responses more durable have largely focused around using interferon in combination with other active agents.

Interleukin-2

IL-2 is a 15 000-Da glycoprotein secreted predominantly by T helper-1 (Th1) lymphocytes. It is a potent growth factor that causes activation and proliferation of cytotoxic T lymphocytes, natural killer cells and macrophages. The first clinical trials with IL-2 were carried out in 1984. Promising early results were reported by Rosenberg *et al.*, who used high-dose, intravenous bolus IL-2. A 22% overall RR was reported in 54 patients with mRCC treated with IL-2 [17].

A subsequent multicentre study by Fyfe *et al.* reported an overall RR of 14%. Two hundred fifty-five patients were treated with high-dose bolus IL-2, 600 000–720 000 IU/kg, administered intravenously for 14 consecutive doses over 5 days, and repeated after a 5- to 9-day rest period. A long-term follow-up showed that 15% of patients achieved a CR or a PR. Of those patients achieving a CR, the median duration of response exceeded 80 months and 60% remained in CR at 10-year follow-up. The associated toxicity was severe and treatment-related death was 4%. This was despite the study population consisting of a relatively young group of patients (median age 52 years) with a good performance status [18].

The side-effects of IL-2 therapy are dose-dependent and at high dose can be formidable. Toxicity is manifest by a vascular leak syndrome as a result of increased capillary permeability. This leads to fluid retention, pulmonary oedema, decreased peripheral vascular resistance, hypotension, tachycardia and oliguria. These in turn can lead to respiratory failure, cardiovascular collapse and renal impairment. Patients often require inotropic support to maintain adequate blood pressure, and occasionally may need transfer to the intensive care unit. As experience with the use of high-dose IL-2 has increased, treatment-related mortality has reduced considerably and is now less than 1%. Careful patient selection is important and all patients should have an adequate assessment of their cardiac, respiratory, renal and hepatic function before commencing treatment.

Since many patients are unsuitable for high-dose treatment, alternative lower-dose regimens have been developed. Continuous infusional IL-2 has been shown to have efficacy comparable to bolus regimens and, by avoiding high peak levels, carries less toxicity.

The use of daily, self-administered subcutaneous IL-2 in patients with mRCC has been widely tested. The convenience and reduced toxicity of this regimen has made it an attractive alternative; it is the commonest route of administration in use in Europe today.

Many phase II studies have been published using subcutaneous IL-2 [19–21]. Essentially these studies show that subcutaneous IL-2 monotherapy produces RRs of 15–20%, similar to those achieved with high-dose therapy. In addition, it is well tolerated. Typical side-effects include fever, malaise, nausea, vomiting and diarrhoea. Rises in serum creatinine, especially in those with pre-existing renal impairment, and thyroid dysfunction may also occur. These toxicities are generally not severe and do not require hospitalization.

It remains uncertain whether high-dose IL-2 confers any benefit over lower-dose regimens in terms of clinical outcome. Whilst RRs appear to be similar, it is not known whether response duration and overall survival are increased using high-dose treatments. IL-2 has been approved by the US Food and Drug Administration for use in patients with mRCC on the strength of studies showing that, in small numbers of patients, IL-2 can induce complete, durable responses, sometimes lasting more than 10 years. The challenge of identifying which patients will respond and of defining the optimal dose and route of administration remains.

Combined immunotherapy

After establishing the individual activity of IFN-α and IL-2 in mRCC, investigators have looked at using them in combination. Studies in *in vitro* and *in vivo* animal models were encouraging and showed synergism between the two cytokines. Clinical trials have been disappointing however. A series of small randomized studies have suggested no advantage to combination therapy over IL-2 alone [22,23].

However, in a large phase III trial, Negrier *et al.* randomized 425 patients to receive high-dose intravenous IL-2 alone, subcutaneous IFN-α alone or a combination of both agents. The RR was better for the combination arm (IFN-α 7.5%; IL-2 6.5%; combination 18.6%; $p < 0.01$) and event-free survival at 1 year also improved (IFN-α 12%; IL-2 15%; combination 20%; $p = 0.01$). This did not however translate into a significant increase in overall survival [24].

Biochemotherapy

The concept of combining immunotherapy with standard chemotherapy agents is one that has generated much interest over recent years. The theoretical rationale behind such a combination is that chemotherapy may enhance immunogenicity by causing cellular damage and release of tumour cell antigens that are processed by IFN-α-stimulated APCs and, in turn, activate IL-2-stimulated cellular effectors. This theory, however, has yet to be proven.

One of the more promising regimens in mRCC was first used by Atzpodien. Patients with mRCC were treated with a combination of IFN-α, IL-2 and 5-FU. Treatment was given in an outpatient setting with 8 weeks of IFN-α (6–9 MU/m^2 s.c., 1–3 times/week), IL-2 for 4 weeks (5–20 MU/m^2 s.c., 3 times/week, weeks 1–4) and intravenous 5-FU 750 mg/m^2 weekly for weeks 5–8. The regimen was well tolerated. For the first 35 patients treated, an overall RR of 48.6% was reported [25].

Since 1993, there have been several phase II trials using this triple-therapy regime with RRs in the range of 15–45% (Fig. 14.1) [26–30].

In a randomized trial comparing the triple-agent regimen against single-agent tamoxifen, enrolling a total of 78 patients, those patients receiving triple therapy were shown to have an overall RR of 39% compared with 0% in the tamoxifen-only arm. The overall survival (24 vs 13 months) was significantly increased in the triple-therapy arm [26].

However, one phase III study has been published showing no advantage for triple therapy over interferon plus IL-2 alone [31]. The study used different drug schedules, which may explain the difference.

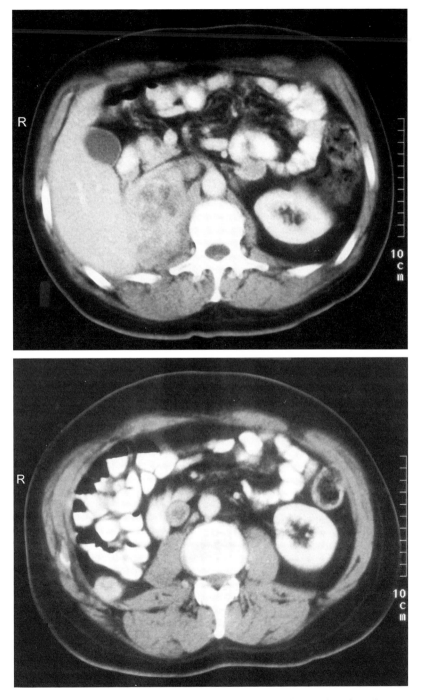

Figure 14.1 Computed tomographic (CT) scans of a 52-year-old man who relapsed 2 years after a right radical nephrectomy with renal bed, peritoneal and lung metastases. Scans show resolution of disease after three cycles of combination immunotherapy with interferon, interleukin-2 and 5-fluorouracil. Patient remains in remission 4 years after commencing treatment. (*Continued p. 244.*)

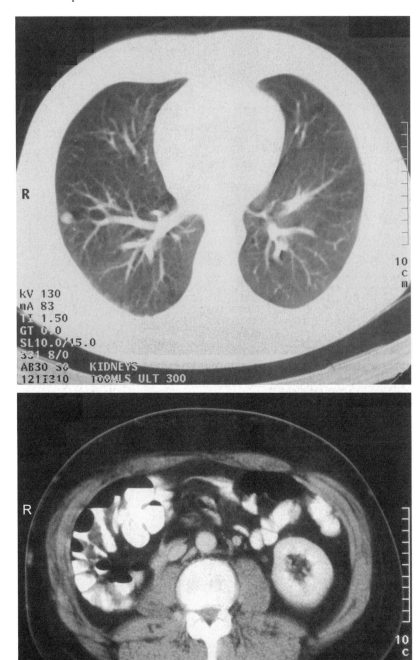

Figure 14.1   *Continued.*

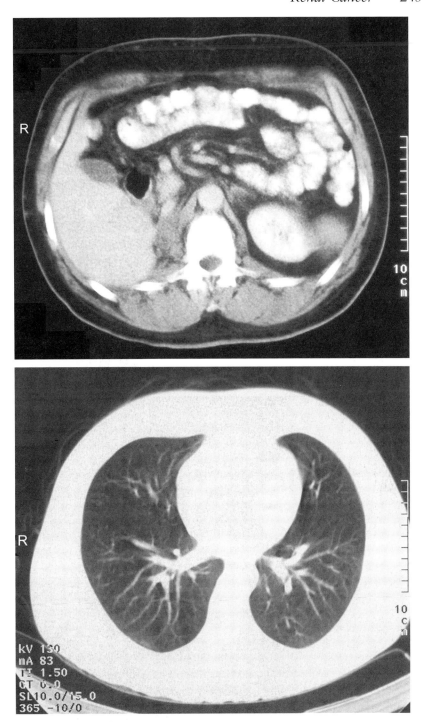

Figure 14.1 *Continued.*

RE04 is an MRC randomized controlled phase III clinical trial that is aimed at addressing these issues. The study, currently recruiting, will randomize 670 patients with mRCC to either triple therapy or standard single-agent IFN-α.

Medroxyprogesterone acetate

Medroxyprogesterone acetate (Provera) is a 17-OH progesterone derivative. The rationale for its use in mRCC is derived from the fact that a proportion of renal cancers express oestrogen and progesterone receptors. The exact mechanism of its anti-tumour effect is unclear.

At the time of its introduction there were few alternatives and hence Provera became widely used for patients with mRCC. The reality is that overall RRs with Provera are low (~2%) and short in duration [32].

At the standard dose of 300 mg daily, Provera is a well-tolerated drug. Its main side-effect is appetite stimulation, which may be beneficial in patients with tumour cachexia or anorexia. Nausea can be a problem early on but tends to improve with continued use. Fluid retention can occur but rarely requires intervention.

Today, Provera can be considered for use in those patients who have either progressed on, or are unsuitable for, first-line immunotherapy. For these patients it may provide a modest palliative benefit.

Future developments

Anti-angiogenesis agents

Angiogenesis refers to the formation of new blood vessels and is an important step in tumour growth. It is estimated that most tumours need to trigger angiogenesis in order to grow beyond 2 mm in diameter. The initiation and promotion of angiogenesis is under the control of a variety of cytokines and hormones, termed angiogenic factors, and include vascular endothelial growth factor (VEGF), basic fibroblast growth factor, IL-8 and a tumour necrosis factor (TNF-α). Renal tumours are highly vascular and this makes them an attractive target for inhibitors of angiogenesis.

The development of anti-angiogenesis agents is the focus of much research, both in RCC and in other solid malignancies. These novel approaches have burgeoned over recent years. Two such agents are discussed below.

Thalidomide is infamous as a drug that was prescribed to pregnant women in the late 1950s to combat morning sickness, which resulted in birth defects in thousands of children. We now know that thalidomide possesses anti-angiogenic properties and *in utero* this impaired limb development, with tragic consequences.

One mechanism through which thalidomide is thought to work is through the increased degradation of TNF-α mRNA. TNF-α plays a role in promoting new blood vessel formation and is also thought to account for many of the systemic effects of malignancy such as cachexia and fever.

There have been several small non-randomized phase II trials using thalidomide in patients with mRCC. Eisen *et al.* used thalidomide at 100 mg daily in 18 patients with advanced RCC. Three patients achieved a PR and three showed stable disease for up to 6 months [33].

In a study of 40 heavily pretreated patients with mRCC, 11 patients had at least stable disease at 6 months (2 out of 11 achieved PR). Thalidomide was given at 400 mg/day and increased to 800 mg/day or 1200 mg/day if patients progressed [34]. Motzer *et al.* recently published data on 26 patients (15 of whom had had prior systemic treatment) with mRCC treated with 200 mg/day of thalidomide, which was increased every 2 weeks to a maximum of 800 mg/day. No responses were seen but 32% of patients had stable disease at 6 months [35].

Thalidomide is a relatively well tolerated drug, particularly at a low dose. The most common side-effects include lethargy, sedation, constipation and skin rash. At higher doses peripheral neuropathy and venous thromboembolism are occasionally seen.

The monoclonal antibody (mAb) bevacizumab (Avastin) is an anti-VEGF antibody that is currently in phase II trials in RCC. In a randomized placebo-controlled trial, 110 patients with mRCC were treated with either high-(10 mg/kg) or low-(3 mg/kg) dose bevacizumab, or placebo. The time to progression was significantly increased in the high-dose group compared with the placebo group (hazards ratio = 2.3, p = 0.001). Only three PRs were observed, all in the high-dose arm. Toxicity at both doses of antibody was minimal [36].

It is too early to know whether such agents will become a recognized treatment option in RCC. The use of thalidomide in combination with other agents, such as IFN, is being investigated. It appears that inhibiting angiogenesis may result in stabilization of disease over long periods. If this is true then these drugs may represent a useful option in adjuvant therapy.

Dendritic cell vaccines

Harnessing the immune system to specifically target and destroy cancer cells has long been the goal of tumour immunologists. Approaches using systemic IFN-α and IL-2 lead to non-specific immune activation and, whilst useful responses are achieved, there remains scope for improvement.

Recently, with the identification of TAAs), and an improved understanding of the processes underlying antigen acquisition and presentation, the potential for a more rational application of immune-based therapies is becoming possible.

DCs are 'professional' APCs. They play a pivotal role in the host tumour response by presenting TAAs to cytotoxic T cells. Advances in laboratory techniques have enabled investigators to culture DCs *in vitro*, 'load' them with TAAs, and re-infuse these cells back into patients. Antigen binding is achieved by pulsing DCs with known antigen peptide epitopes, whole-antigen proteins or even whole tumour cells or cell lysates.

Höltl *et al.* performed a pilot study of antigen-loaded DCs in 12 patients with metastatic RCC. DCs were loaded with cell lysate from cultured autologous tumour cells, then activated with a combination of tumour necrosis factor and prostaglandin E2. The vaccine was administered by three intravenous infusions at monthly intervals. Potent immunological responses against cell lysate could be measured *in vitro* after the vaccinations, suggesting that a DC vaccine can induce antigen-specific immunity in patients with metastatic RCC [37].

DC vaccines seem to be well tolerated and, to date, there have been no significant adverse events [38]. This makes them attractive, particularly for use in less-well patients and combination therapies. More work is needed and clinical studies using DC vaccines are being published in increasing numbers.

Mini allogeneic stem cell transplants

Stem cell transplants (SCTs) have, for many years, been used to salvage the bone marrow of patients who have undergone high-dose, myeloablative chemotherapy. They are most commonly used in haematological malignancies, where they form part of potentially curative treatment. The term allogeneic transplant refers to the use of donor stem cells, usually from HLA-matched siblings.

For a long time investigators suspected that the donor cell population itself may be capable of exerting a direct anti-neoplastic effect. Much work has since been carried out in patients with leukaemia, which has helped to confirm this. It is now clear that immunocompetent donor T cells within the SCT can exert an anti-tumour response, called the graft-versus-tumour response.

Allogeneic SCTs are now an accepted treatment modality in many haematological malignancies that are refractory to standard chemotherapy. Infusions of donor lymphocytes alone are capable of inducing remissions in patients with relapsed leukaemias.

A similar approach has more recently been tested in patients with solid malignancies, with the most promising results achieved in patients with

RCC. Since high-dose chemotherapy is not beneficial in RCC, less toxic non myeloablative conditioning regimens (hence the term 'mini') have been developed. This significantly reduces the morbidity and mortality of the procedure.

In a phase II study of 19 patients with mRCC resistant to IL-2, treated with mini allogeneic SCT, a 53% RR (CR: three patients; PR: seven patients) was reported. Patients with a CR remained in remission over 2 years after transplant. There were two treatment-related deaths. The time to regression of metastases was delayed, occurring on average 5 months after transplant [39].

More recently Childs presented data on 47 patients treated to date. A 47% overall RR was achieved (CR: 4 patients; PR: 18 patients). The majority of the patients had failed standard immunotherapies. There were four treatment-related deaths (9%), two due to infection and two due to graft- versus-host disease. Again, the average time to response was delayed at a median of 6.5 months [40].

These RRs and their durability are impressive, especially in a study population that has failed conventional treatments. However, there are limitations. Firstly, patients usually require an HLA-matched or single-antigen mismatched sibling. The use of mismatched donors is possible but this increases the risks of an already hazardous procedure. Even in ideal circumstances the procedure carries a significant morbidity and mortality. Patients also need a life expectancy of at least 6 months to make the procedure worthwhile, due to the delayed time to response. Nevertheless, this is a promising new therapeutic option in the treatment of RCC.

Monoclonal antibodies

The concept of using mAbs in cancer treatment, the so-called 'magic bullet' approach, is in itself not new. For many years, investigators have been using monoclonals, alone or in combination with cytotoxic drugs, radioactive isotopes and toxins. To date, two mAbs have achieved broad market success, namely Rituximab in non-Hodgkin's lymphoma and Herceptin in Her-2-positive breast cancer.

mAbs remain under investigation in a number of tumour types, including renal cell cancer. Clinical experience with use of mAbs in RCC is most extensive with mAb G250. This antibody recognizes carbonic anhydrase IX, whose expression is suppressed in normal renal epithelium by pVHL. In RCC, loss of the VHL gene product leads to expression of the target antigen and, therefore reactivity with mAb G250. Phase I and II clinical trials with unlabelled or 131 I-labelled radioactive G250 antibody have shown some stable disease responses [41,42].

ABR-214936 is an mAb fused to a staphylococcal enterotoxin that is currently being tested in a phase II trial in patients with mRCC. The antibody is targeted to an oncofetal antigen, 5T4, which is expressed in non–small cell lung cancer, carcinomas of the kidney, pancreas and breast, but with limited normal tissue expression.

Another antibody in early development is ABX-EGF, which targets epidermal grown factor receptor (EGFR), a receptor tyrosine kinase. EGFR is overexpressed in many cancers, including RCC. In a phase II trial of 31 mRCC patients, treated with 8 weeks of ABX-EGF, 58% of patients showed minor response/stable disease whilst 36% progressed [43].

Conclusions

Renal cancer remains amongst the more difficult of cancers to treat. Effective therapies for the majority of patients with mRCC have not been found. Traditional chemotherapy drugs are ineffective and are not commonly used.

Currently, immunotherapy offers the best hope for patients. RRs may be increased by nephrectomy and should be considered before commencing systemic treatment. Standard first-line therapy in the UK is single-agent IFN-α, which has a modest overall RR of approximately 15%.

Atzpodien's triple therapy is a convenient, relatively well tolerated, outpatient-based regime that has shown high RRs in some studies. The MRC RE04 study will determine whether it confers a real advantage over single-agent interferon.

Beyond this, there are a wealth of new approaches being developed. A better understanding of the biology of cancer has lead to several novel therapies. Ultimately, success is likely to come from using a combination of agents that simultaneously target the multiple processes that drive the cancer cell.

References

1   Glaspy JA. Therapeutic options in the management of renal cell carcinoma. *Semin Oncol* 2002; **29**(3 Suppl. 7): 41–6.
2   Yagoda A. Chemotherapy of renal cell carcinoma: 1983–1989. *Semin Urol* 1989; **7**(4): 199–206.
3   Rabinovitch RA, Zelefsky MJ, Gaynor JJ, Fuks Z. Patterns of failure following surgical resection of renal cell carcinoma: implications for adjuvant local and systemic therapy. *J Clin Oncol* 1994; **12**(1): 206–12.
4   Ritchie AW, Chisholm GD. The natural history of renal carcinoma. *Semin Oncol* 1983; **10**(4): 390–400.
5   Yagoda A, Abi-Rached B, Petrylak D. Chemotherapy for advanced renal-cell carcinoma: 1983–1993. *Semin Oncol* 1995; **22**(1): 42–60.
6   Motzer RJ, Russo P. Systemic therapy for renal cell carcinoma. *J Urol* 2000; **163**(2): 408–417.

7 Mickisch G, Bier H, Bergler W, Bak M, Tschada R, Alken P. P-170 glycoprotein, glutathione and associated enzymes in relation to chemoresistance of primary human renal cell carcinomas. *Urol Int* 1990; **45**(3): 170–76.

8 Montie JE, Stewart BH, Straffon RA Banowsky LH, Hewitt CB, Montague DK. The role of adjunctive nephrectomy in patients with metastatic renal cell carcinoma. *J Urol* 1977; **117**(3): 272–5.

9 Mickisch GH, Garin A, van Poppel H, de Prijck L, Sylvester R; European Organisation for Research and Treatment of Cancer (EORTC) Genitourinary Group. Radical nephrectomy plus interferon-alpha-based immunotherapy compared with interferon-alpha alone in metastatic renal-cell carcinoma: a randomised trial. *Lancet* 2001; **358**(9286): 966–70.

10 Flanigan RC, Salmon SE, Blumenstein BA *et al.* Nephrectomy followed by interferon alfa-2b compared with interferon alfa-2b alone for metastatic renal-cell cancer. *N Engl J Med* 2001; **345**(23): 1655–9.

11 Pizzocaro G, Piva L, Colavita M *et al.* Interferon adjuvant to radical nephrectomy in Robson stages II and II renal cell carcinoma: a multicentric randomised study. *J Clin Oncol* 2001; **19**(2): 425–31.

12 Trump DL, Elson P, Propert R *et al.* Randomized controlled trial of adjuvant therapy with lymphoblastoid interferon (L-IFN) in resected high-risk renal cell carcinoma. *Proc Am Soc Clin Oncol* 1996 [Meeting Abstract]; **15**: 253 (Abstract 648).

13 Porzsolt F. Adjuvant therapy of renal cell cancer (RCC) with interferon alfa-2a. *Proc Am Soc Clin Oncol* 1992 [Meeting Abstract]; **11**: 202 (Abstract 622).

14 Haas GP, Hillman GG. Tumor biology for the clinician: update on the role of immunotherapy in the management of kidney cancer. *Cancer Control J* 1996; **3**(6): 536–41.

15 Pyrhönen S, Salminen E, Ruutu M *et al.* Prospective randomised trial of interferon alfa-2a plus vinblastine versus vinblastine alone in patients with advanced renal cell cancer. *J Clin Oncol* 1999; **17**(9): 2859–67.

16 Medical Research Council Renal Cancer Collaborators. Interferon-alpha and survival in metastatic renal carcinoma: early results of a randomised controlled trial. *Lancet* 1999; **353**(9146): 14–17.

17 Rosenberg SA, Yang YC, Topalian SL. Treatment of 283 consecutive patients with metastatic melanoma or renal cell cancer using high-dose bolus interleukin-2. *JAMA* 1994; **271**(12): 907–13.

18 Fyfe G, Fisher RI, Rosenberg SA, Sznol M, Parkinson DR, Louie AC. Results of treatment of 255 patients with metastatic RCC who received high-dose recombinant interleukin-2 therapy. *J Clin Oncol* 1995; **13**(3): 688–96.

19 Lissoni P, Bami S, Ardizzoia A *et al.* Second line therapy with low dose subcutaneous interleukin-2 alone in advanced renal cancer patients resistant to interferon-alpha. *Eur J Cancer* 1992; **28**(1): 92–6.

20 Buter J, Sleijfer DT, van der Graaf WT, de Vries EG, Willemse PH, Mulder NH. A progress report on the outpatient treatment of patients with advanced renal cell carcinoma using subcutaneous recombinant intereukin-2. *Semin Oncol* 1993; **20**(6 Suppl. 19): 16–21.

21 Sleijfer DT, Janssen RA, Buter J, de Vries EG, Willemse PH, Mulder NH. Phase II study of subcutaneous interleukin-2 in unselected patients with advanced renal cell cancer on an outpatient basis. *J Clin Oncol* 1992; **10**(2): 1119–23.

22 Atkins MB, Sparano J, Fisher RI *et al.* Randomised phase II trial of high-dose interleukin-2 either alone or in combination with interferon alfa-2b in advanced renal cell carcinoma. *J Clin Oncol* 1993; **11**(4); 661–70.

23 Jayson GC, Middleton M, Lee SM, Ashcroft L, Thatcher N. A randomized phase II trial of interleukin 2 and interleukin 2-interferon alpha in advanced renal cancer. *Br J Cancer* 1998; **78**(3): 366–9.

24 Negrier S, Escudier B, Lasset C *et al*. Recombinant human interleukin-2, recombinant human interferon alfa-2a, or both in metastatic renal-cell carcinoma. *N Engl J Med* 1998; **338**(18): 1272–1278.

25 Atzpodien J, Kirchner H, Hanninen EL, Deckert M, Fenner M, Poliwoda H. Interleukin-2 in combination with interferon-alpha and 5-fluorouracil for metastatic renal cell cancer. *Eur J Cancer* 1993; **29A**(Suppl. 5): S6–8.

26 Atzpodien J, Kirchner H, Illiger HJ *et al*. IL-2 in combination with IFN-alpha and 5-FU versus tamoxifen in metastatic renal cell carcinoma: long-term results of a controlled randomized clinical trial. *Br J Cancer* 2001; **85**(8): 1130–36.

27 Ellerhorst JA, Sella A, Amato RJ *et al*. Phase II trial of 5-fluorouracil, interferon-alpha, and continuous infusion interleukin-2 for patients with metastatic renal cell carcinoma. *Cancer* 1997; **80**(11): 2128–32.

28 Hofmockel G, Langer W, Theiss M *et al*. Immuno-chemotherapy for metastatic renal cell carcinoma using a regimen of interleukin-2, interferon-alpha and 5-fluorouracil. *J Urol* 1996; **156**(1): 18–21.

29 Sella A, Kilbourn RG, Gray I *et al*. Phase I study of interleukin-2 combined with interferon-alpha and 5-fluorouracil in patients with metastatic renal cell cancer. *Cancer Biother* 1994; **9**(2): 103–11.

30 Joffe JK, Banks RE, Forbes MA *et al*. A phase II study of interferon-alpha, interleukin-2 and 5-fluorouracil in advanced renal carcinoma: clinical data and laboratory evidence of protease activation. *Br J Urol* 1996; **77**(5): 638–49.

31 Negrier S, Caty A, Lesimple T *et al*. Treatment of patients with metastatic renal carcinoma with a combination of subcutaneous Interleukin-2 and Interferon-alpha with or without Fluorouracil. *J Clin Oncol* 2000; **18**(24): 4009–15.

32 Linehan WM, Zbar B, Bates SE, Zelefsky MJ, Yang JC. Cancer of the kidney and ureter. In: deVita VT Jr, Hellman S, Rosenberg SA, eds. *Cancer: Principles and Practice of Oncology*, 5th edn. Philadelphia: JB Lippincott, 1993: 1362–90.

33 Eisen T, Boshoff C, Mak L *et al*. Continuous low lose thalidomide: a phase II study in advanced melanoma, renal cell, ovarian and breast cancer. *Br J Cancer* 2000; **82**(4): 812–17.

34 Escudier B, Lassau N, Couanet D *et al*. Phase II trial of thalidomide in renal cell carcinoma. *Ann Oncol* 2002; **13**(7): 1029–35.

35 Motzer RJ, Berg W, Ginsberg M *et al*. Phase II trial of thalidomide for patients with advanced renal cell carcinoma *Clin Oncol* 2002; **20**(1): 302–6.

36 Yang JC, Haworth L, Steinberg SM *et al*. A randomized double-blind placebo-controlled trial of bevacizumab (anti-VEGF anti-body) demonstrating a prolongation in time to progression in patients with metastatic renal cancer. *Proc Annu Meet Am Soc Clin Oncol* 2002; 15.

37 Höltl L, Rieser C, Papesh C *et al*. Cellular and humoral immune responses in patients with metastatic renal cell carcinoma after vaccination with antigen pulsed dendritic cells. *J Urol* 1999; **161**(3): 777–82.

38 Melcher A, Bateman A, Harrington K, Ahmed A, Gough M, Vile R. Dendritic cells for the immunotherapy of cancer. *Clin Oncol* 2002; **14**(3): 185–192.

39 Childs R, Chernoff A, Contentin N. Regression of metastatic renal-cell carcinoma after nonmyeloablative allogeneic peripheral-blood stem-cell transplantation. *N Engl J Med* 2000; 14; **343**(11): 750–58.

40 Childs R. [oral presentation]. Kidney Cancer Association, Second International Kidney Cancer Symposium. 2001. Available at: http://player.eveo.com/presenter/kca/. Accessed 25 September 2002.

41 Steffens MG, Boerman OC, de Mulder PH *et al*. Phase I radioimmunotherapy of metastatic renal cell carcinoma with 131I-labeled chimeric monoclonal antibody G250. *Clin Cancer Res* 1999; **5**(Suppl. 10): 3268S–74S.

42 Wiseman GA, Scott AM, Lee F-T *et al.* Chimeric G250 (cG250) monoclonal antibody Phase 1 dose escalation trial in patients with advanced renal cell carcinoma (RCC). *Proc Annu Meet Am Soc Clin Oncol* 2001; **20**: 1027 (Abstract).

43 Schwartz G, Dutcher JP, Vogelzang NJ *et al.* Phase 2 clinical trial evaluating the safety and effectiveness of ABX-EGF in renal cell cancer (RCC). *Proc Annu Meet Am Soc Clin Oncol* 2002; 91 (Abstract).

Part 4
Analgesia

15: Postoperative Analgesia

Patrick McHugh

The definition of pain promulgated by the International Association for the Study of Pain is very appropriate in the context of postoperative pain management: 'Pain is an unpleasant sensory and emotional experience associated with actual or potential tissue damage, or described in terms of such damage' [1]. Pain may serve a number of functions including protection, defence and diagnosis, but it may also appear to be completely functionless and may in fact exacerbate other clinical problems for a patient. In dealing with the concepts of acute postoperative analgesia and pain management, it is important to remember that acute postoperative pain has a large component that is apparently 'useless', but definitely detrimental to the patient.

To understand the rationale for postoperative pain management, it is important to have a clear understanding of the neuroanatomy, neurophysiology and neuropharmacology of pain. This chapter deals with these aspects briefly before documenting the actual pharmacological management of postoperative pain.

Pain as a physiological entity

The sensation of pain involves the 'transduction' or conversion of external or internal energy by specific receptors into signals suitable for 'transmission' by the primary afferent neurones. These carry the signals to the central nervous system (CNS) where they are integrated and suitable responses propagated. In this system, there are a number of locations where signal modulation occurs and this is where the treatment of postoperative pain is targeted.

Neuroanatomy

SOMATIC PAIN

Physiological pain, often known as 'first' or 'fast' pain, is a protective response to tissue damage, facilitating withdrawal from the offending stimulus. It is mediated by thermo- and mechano-receptors, then transmitted by Aδ fast-conducting pain fibres. These fibres enter the dorsal horn of the spinal cord and synapse at Rexed's laminae I, V and X [2]. Local synaptic reflexes mediate withdrawal, while secondary afferent neurones travel up the spinal cord in the neo-spinothalamic tract to the posterior thalamic nuclei and the somatosensory postcentral gyrus at the cortical level. If the stimulus is short-lived and no tissue damage occurs, the sensation of pain disappears after the stimulus is withdrawn.

Pathophysiological, 'second' or 'slow' pain is caused by tissue injury and is a delayed, prolonged sensation. This is designed to protect tissue and encourage healing by immobilizing the affected area, but these actions also lead to some of the adverse effects of pain. This type of pain is mostly associated with surgery, inflammation and trauma.

Pain sensations, mediated by polymodal nocioceptors sensitive to mechanical, thermal and chemical stimuli, are then transmitted via slow-conducting C fibres to the dorsal horn of the spinal cord, synapsing in laminae II and III. The secondary fibres are polysynaptic and travel via the paleo-spinothalamic tract to medial thalamic nuclei with collaterals to many areas of the midbrain, pons and reticular formations and to the hypothalamus and limbic structures. This varied spread of the stimulus is accountable for the multitude of other effects found associated with this type of pain. There are respiratory, circulatory and endocrine responses and many emotional and behavioural patterns associated with pathophysiological pain.

VISCERAL PAIN

This type of pain is associated with poorly localized symptoms, diffuse spread and the referred pain phenomenon. Visceral nocioceptors are much fewer in number, and the stimulus is usually distension, chemical irritants, infection or ischaemia. Visceral pain is transmitted in nerves travelling along with the sympathetic, and in some cases parasympathetic (e.g. bladder neck, prostate, cervix and some colonic) nervous system, passing through, but not synapsing in, the sympathetic ganglia. These fibres are part of the sensory, not autonomic, nervous system. There is evidence that in the bladder the afferent fibres carry signals in a graded way from a mixed group of receptors that transmit throughout the biological and noxious range.

Neurophysiology and neuropharmacology

The physiology of pain transmission has been the subject of research and debate for many years and many theories have been postulated. With advances in scientific methods, new neurotransmitters, both excitatory and inhibitory, have been discovered. At a peripheral level, the existence of high-threshold nocioceptors, which are triggered by the inflammatory response mediators such as bradykinin, substance P, prostaglandins, IgE, 5-hydroxytryptamine (5HT), is well documented. Some agents directly trigger nociceptors (5HT, adenosine, protons, bradykinin, potassium) and some sensitize them (prostaglandins, leukotrienes, neuropeptides, cytokines, nerve growth factor), thus lowering the threshold and producing the sensation of primary hyperalgesia. There is no universal pain neurotransmitter [3].

It is known that the primary nociceptive neurones synapse with specific high-threshold nociceptive neurones in the superficial Rexed's laminae and with wide dynamic range (WDR) non-specific neurones that have a lower threshold. In 1965, Melzack and Wall postulated the gate theory of pain transmission, which is the best-fit theory to date [4]. They said that primary nociceptors synapse with specific (WDR) neurones in Rexed's laminae. These, in turn, also synapse with inhibitory interneurones. Activation of the Aβ neurones activate the inhibitory interneurones and thus reduce or 'gate' pain transmission. Transmission in the Aδ and C fibres directly inhibit the inhibitory interneurones. At the dorsal horn level, the known neurotransmitters include excitatory amino acids and neuropeptides. These include substance P, bombesin, vasoactive intestinal polypeptide (VIP), cholecystokinin, neurokinins A and B and calcitonin gene-related peptide (CGRP). These activate neurokinin1 and α-amino-3-hydroxy-5-methyl-4-isoxazoleproprionate (AMPA), which in turn activate N-methyl-D-aspartame (NMDA) receptors. Some neurotransmitters are anti-nociceptive, e.g. somatostatin, gamma-aminobutyric acid (GABA), glycine, β-endorphins, enkephalins, cannabinoids and galanin.

As one would expect, all the above substances are undergoing investigation, but to date there is no single clinically useful agent. Pharmacological manipulation at this level presently relies on global techniques such as local anaesthetics and opioids. Other drugs used at this level include α2-agonists clonidine and dexmedetomidine, the NMDA antagonists ketamine and memantine and benzodiazepines. Pain transmission is mainly via the spinothalamic, spinoreticular and spinomesencephalic pathways although other pathways have been implicated [5].

Supraspinal pain modulation and control seems to be mainly integrated in the thalamus, and cortex, through nuclei in the peri-aqueductal grey matter, locus ceruleus and medulla, which send inhibitory signals via the dorsolateral funuliculus to the dorsal horn. Neurotransmitters involved here include noradrenaline, 5HT and endogenous opioids.

Assessment of acute postoperative pain

Postoperative pain always occurs if there is a suitable surgical stimulus. Rawal [6] showed that 30–35% of patients undergoing day case or ambulatory surgery experienced moderate to severe pain at home; the incidence was even higher in children [7], at 50% plus. In fact, the most common reason for visits to the primary care physician after day surgery was post-operative pain [8]. It is also one of the most common reasons for decreased patient satisfaction with their surgical experience [9]. It is an accepted fact that the presence of pain in the postoperative period is harmful to patients, with the potential of inducing side-effects such as orthostatic pneumonia, immobility-related deep venous thrombosis (DVT) and pressure areas, and muscle weakness and contractures from prolonged underuse. It is also accepted that pain increases the neuro-humoral stress response with release of endogenous catecholamines, steroids and other neurotransmitters. This is associated with increased incidence of postoperative nausea and vomiting [10], agitation [11], delayed discharge [12] and unplanned admission after day case surgery [13]. These factors lead to increased postoperative mor-bidity and mortality, and for this reason there is much interest in the ablation of postoperative pain. For many years we have relied on phys-ician-prescribed drugs, with minimal monitoring and no allowance for interpersonal response variation. It has been shown that 'on demand' pre-scribing leads to underdosing, both in amount and time interval, and therefore to excess postoperative pain.

The assessment of pain is a very subjective experience and the best person to assess pain is the patient, if he or she has the ability to communicate effectively [14]. Health care professionals tend to underestimate pain, and parents or carers tend to overestimate suffering. Research into methods of scoring pain, and evaluating response to pain-relieving therapy, has led to the development of visual analogue scales, verbal rating scales, numerical rating scales and, for children, the 'smiley face' type of scale. It is also possible to measure complex scales of behaviour and physiological param-eters, but these can be biased by outside influences. The best approach is a combination approach, implemented by suitably trained staff. This ap-proach has led to the formation of the specialty of acute pain management. The first formal descriptions of multidisciplinary pain management teams came from Ready in Seattle [15] in 1988, and there are published national guidelines in many countries including Australia (Acute Pain Management – Scientific Evidence by the Australian National Health and Medical Research Council – ANHMRC) [16], and the Royal College of Anaesthetists [17]. The 'Report of the Working Party of Pain after Surgery' [18] from the Royal College of Surgeons and the College of Anaesthetists in 1990 documented very poor overall standards of postoperative pain management, including the presence of an acute pain team in only 57% of UK hospitals. Unfortu-nately, things have not changed dramatically in the intervening years. It is well known that pain is regularly underestimated by nursing [19] and medical staff, and in a small study from Italy it was reported that pain was underestimated and that the peak pain experience did not correlate with simple changes in cardiovascular parameters alone [20]. Effective assessment of pain is a skilled study including multidimensional tools such as the McGill pain questionnaire [21] or the Wisconsin brief pain inventory [22] along with scoring tools and history and patient examination. The multidimensional tools are too cumbersome for use as rapid tests in a clinical setting; therefore simplified unidimensional scales such as visual analogue scales have been designed [23]. It is essential that pain scoring be an ongoing process with adequate notice paid to response to therapeutic interventions.

Treatment of postoperative pain

The rationale behind treatment of postoperative pain is twofold. The humanitarian aspect is not supported by evidence-based medicine but is actually most relevant to patients. There is some anecdotal evidence of economic benefits with shorter hospital stays and more rapid return to independent status, and some evidence to support increased patient satisfaction [24]. The second facet is the reduction in postoperative neuro-humoral stress response. Postoperative pain is best addressed early in the patient's clinical course. The preoperative assessment of likely pain, patient characteristics and surgical procedures should be carried out at the preassessment clinic, if possible, by trained staff able to discuss treatment modalities and plans with the patient.

Treatment of pain starts with explanation and reassurance, and is assisted by a holistic approach to the care of the patient [25]. Infection, acidosis, cold and shivering, anxiety and any other cause should be looked for and treated. Only at this point does the pharmacological treatment of pain intervene. Route of administration is important and should take into account the following:

1 the condition of the patient, i.e. starvation, gut function, cold, peripheral perfusion;

2 the urgency of drug delivery, i.e. oral versus intramuscular (IM) versus intravenous (IV) administration;

3 the type of analgesic to be administered.

The use of a stepwise, planned approach should make the prescription of postoperative analgesia more efficient and therapeutic.

All patients should have simple analgesics such as paracetamol or paracetamol/weak opioid combinations prescribed on a regular basis as soon as they can be absorbed orally or rectally. A second line of therapy should be commenced using non-steroidal anti-inflammatory drugs (NSAIDs) prescribed on a regular basis, again orally or rectally.

In the past, the third line of analgesic prescription would have comprised an on-demand (p.r.n.) dosage of a narcotic analgesic such as morphine or pethidine. As previously described, there is evidence that p.r.n. prescribing results in underprescription by doctors, underadministration by nursing staff, and underrequesting by patients with a dislike for needles, injections and the side-effects of bolus narcotics. The advent of more technical methods of drug delivery, and an increased understanding of pharmacokinetics, has led to the use of IV boluses and infusions and the concept of patient-(or parent/nurse) controlled analgesia systems (PCASs) and other routes of drug delivery such as subcutaneous, paravertebral, epidural and intrathecal infusions.

Routes of administration

Buccal, sublingual or transmucosal routes can be very effective and avoid the delay in absorption associated with the oral route. There can also be an advantage in avoiding first-pass metabolism. The absorption depends on lipophilicity and amount of drug retained at the absorptive surface.

The rectal route is often overlooked for many reasons. It can be very useful as correct placement of the suppository in the distribution of the middle and inferior rectal veins allows absorption directly into the systemic circulation with avoidance of some first-pass metabolism. There are many rectal NSAID preparations with the advantage of less gastrointestinal tract (GIT) side-effects. There are also rectal preparations of opioids, with equivalent doses to oral preparations.

Topical or transdermal routes are sometimes used for narcotics, NSAIDs and local anaesthetics. The drug needs to be highly lipophilic, and the absorption depends on adequate blood flow to the area. This route has been well documented for NSAIDs [26] and fentanyl [27], although the pharmacokinetics of opioids makes this route more useful for chronic or malignant pain.

Intracavity use has been documented in orthopaedics for arthroscopic infiltration, for intrapleural use and for intranasal administration of many drugs. Intraperitoneal administration of local anaesthetics for laparoscopic surgery has had some success, but drug concentration and timing of the local anaesthetic instillation are critical [28].

Subcutaneous administration of analgesics, particularly opioids, is undergoing a revival at present. High concentrations of aqueous, non-irritating solutions are used, and absorption can sometimes be erratic.

IM routes of administration were for many years the gold standards of drug administration. With advances in pharmacology, drug delivery systems and monitoring, use of this route is reducing. The absorption can be erratic and pooling of drug can occur in poorly perfused sites, and occasionally neural damage has occurred. It necessitates repeated, often painful, injections, and is not well liked by patients.

Inhalational analgesia has been in use for many years in gaseous form, e.g. nitrous oxide, Entonox, Trilene. Recently it is being reapproached for opioids in particular, with some good evidence of adequate bioavailability [29]. It is characterized by rapid onset of action, but with variable effects and offset when the agents are discontinued.

Epidural and intrathecal analgesia is now provided postoperatively in many hospitals. This has been shown to provide better analgesia with less adverse effects than with PCA after general abdominal, thoracic and orthopaedic surgery [30]. The most commonly used agents are local anaesthetics, either alone or in combination with opiates. The drug is introduced into either the epidural space or the cerebrospinal fluid (CSF) in the intrathecal space. Intrathecal opioids work directly at the dorsal horn level, but epidural opioids have to cross the dura and some are lost to systemic absorption, and so on. For this reason, the doses required for intrathecal analgesia are much smaller. Other drugs are also found to provide good analgesia via the epidural and intrathecal route. These include the α2 agonist clonidine.

A systematic review by Rogers *et al.* found that neuraxial blockade reduced 30-day mortality, the risks of DVT and pulmonary embolism (PE), the need for transfusion and the morbidity associated with postoperative pneumonia [31]. However, a note of caution should be sounded in that up to 20% of postoperative patients get inadequate pain relief due to technical failures or system failures [32].

The IV route of administration is the gold standard for pain relief administration. Absorption is rapid and predictable. The plasma concentrations of drugs administered by bolus are short-lived, leading to the development of IV infusions. The recognition of minimum effective analgesic concentrations (MEAC) for most known analgesics has lead to more rational prescribing practice and better quality of pain relief.

A further development of IV infusions since the 1980s is the PCAS, where the patient is given some control of the rate of administration of the IV analgesic. This is an on-demand, intermittent self-administration of an analgesic used intravenously, subcutaneously (s.c.) and latterly epidurally. There is good quality analgesia, with allowances for interpatient variation. Most IV PCASs have standardized on the use of morphine, with 1-mg bolus doses, 5-min lockout periods, plus or minus a background infusion as the most common regime. This is believedto offer the best analgesic profile, with the minimum potential for side-effects for a majority of patients. The use of a regime like this relies for its success on the administration of adequate IV loading doses of morphine, either in the operating theatre or in the post-anaesthetic care unit.

Other narcotics such as pethidine (Demerol), fentanyl and tramadol are now being used in PCASs with no apparent differences to the patient [33,34]. The use of narcotic PCASs has an appreciable failure rate [35]; therefore the addition of adjuvant paracetamol or non-steroidal analgesia is beneficial. Other adjuvant drugs with evidence of benefit include clonidine, midazolam and ketamine.

It is important to remember that one of the most common side-effects, with incidences reported up to 30%, is nausea and vomiting, which is very distressing to the patient. In the past anti-emetics, particularly droperidol, were added to the PCAS mixture, but droperidol has recently been withdrawn from clinical use in a number of countries. It is helpful to prescribe regular and on-demand anti-emetics such as cyclizine, prochlorperazine or ondansetron.

Drugs and doses in postoperative pain relief

Oral analgesics

In 1997, McQuay *et al.* [36] reported a systematic examination of all published randomized controlled trials (RCTs) in the area of postoperative pain management. Using the concept of NNT (the number of patients with moderate or severe pain needing to receive a particular drug for 50% relief), they compared all the standard analgesic drugs prescribed postoperatively. An interesting point raised was that the use of regular oral non-steroidal analgesics or regular paracetamol in adequate doses was as effective as IM narcotics. The data suggest that paracetamol (NNT4) in adequate doses should be prescribed regularly for all surgical patients in view of its excellent therapeutic ratio.

NSAIDs (Ibuprofen NNT = 2) have a proven benefit in reducing pain and in reducing the use of opiate PCA by 15–60%. There is no evidence that they are better administered by injection or rectally over the oral route, but they have an appreciable incidence of side-effects especially GIT, renal and haematological problems.

A new class of oral and injectable analgesics are the recently introduced 'coxibs', a group of selective COX (cyclo-oxygenase)-2 inhibitors [37]. Cyclo-oxygenase is responsible for the generation of prostaglandin and is found in two forms, COX1 and COX2. COX1 is said to be responsible for effects on prostaglandin synthesis in gut, platelets and stomach. COX2 is the form found in response to inflammatory mediators, and is said to be responsible for the prostanoid mediators of pain, fever and inflammation. COX2 is also said to be involved in ovulation, implantation and CNS functions. Coxibs have been available orally for a number of years, but recently a new injectable form, Parecoxib, has been released.

Paracetamol (acetaminophen) is probably the most commonly prescribed analgesic and antipyretic worldwide. It has a very high therapeutic index and few adverse effects. It is a prostaglandin synthesis inhibitor, working in the CNS on cyclo-oxygenase pathways. It appears to have few peripheral effects. It is antipyretic and analgesic, but not anti-inflammatory. It acts synergistically with NSAIDs. It appears to have no GIT or haematological effects, and there are no absolute contraindications to its use except prior anaphylaxis. The major side-effect is very severe liver toxicity in acute overdose, a life-threatening emergency.

Dosage in adults is up to 1 g four times a day. In children, the maximum recommended dose for analgesia, in the short term, is 90 mg/kg/day in divided doses. This dose schedule is subject to change, as much research is under way on safe and effective dosages for children. Proparacetamol is available in an injectable formulation (propacetamol) in some countries, with known efficacy. The only risk is contact dermatitis amongst staff preparing the drug.

Acetyl salicylic acid (ASA) or **aspirin** is a very widely prescribed antipyretic and anti-inflammatory drug, also used in the treatment of thromboembolic disorders. ASA has the unique effect among non-steroidal analgesics of an irreversible inhibition of the COX1 enzyme. This means that even a single dose has effects on bleeding time for up to 1 week. On the balance of evidence, I would suggest that the incidence of side-effects with ASA outweighs the benefits in postoperative analgesia. In children there is good evidence that exposure to ASA during viraemia can lead to the development of Reye's syndrome, which has major morbidity and mortality.

Ibuprofen is the one of the most commonly prescribed oral anti-inflammatory agents. It is a prostaglandin synthetase inhibitor with antipyretic and analgesic properties. It is rapidly absorbed orally and is metabolized to propionic acid derivatives. It has been shown to be equivalent to aspirin as an analgesic, and has a much improved side-effects profile. Because of the low side-effects profile in wide exposure to the drug, it is available over the counter. GIT symptoms are the main side-effects limiting drug therapy. Dose is variable, varying from 1.2 g/day to 3.2 g/day in divided doses. As expected, side-effects increase with increasing daily dosage.

Naproxen is also a propionic acid derivative with a longer duration of action due to a half-life of 12–15 h, but with a slightly increased incidence of GIT and CNS side-effects. It is rapidly absorbed; so it has achieved popular status for analgesia and for migraines.

Ketoprofen is used primarily in oral and topical forms for the relief of inflammatory conditions and associated pain. An isomer, dexketoprofen, has been introduced and is gaining acceptance for postoperative pain management in some areas.

Indomethacin, an acetic acid derivative, was one of the earliest anti-inflammatory agents and one of the most potent. It has a very high incidence of toxic side-effects, particularly relating to the gut, liver and CNS. Although it is used in some countries, it is recommended in the UK for short-term use only and alternatives are preferred.

Diclofenac is an NSAID in use for many years. It has been the mainstay of second-line analgesics postoperatively. It has more activity against COX2 than against COX1, and so has a lower incidence of GIT side-effects. It has some effects on the lipo-oxygenase systems, and so has greater effects than other NSAIDs. Diclofenac can be administered orally, rectally or intramuscularly. Dosage is up to 1 mg/kg three times daily to a maximum of 150 mg/day.

Ketorolac is a very potent analgesic with some anti-inflammatory effects. It can be administered orally, intramuscularly or intravenously. It is licensed for the short-term treatment of pain, including postoperative pain. The dosage schedules vary from country to country, but usually comprise 10–30 mg every 4–6 h IV, with a maximum daily dose of 90–120 mg/day depending on the country. It is recommended that doses be changed to oral after 2–3 days with oral doses of 10 mg every 4–6 h, with a maximum of 40 mg/day. Ketorolac has been shown to have a marked opioid-sparing effect when used as combination therapy. In the UK, it is now recommended that ketorolac not be given preoperatively due to the risk of haemorrhage; and there are reports of acute reversible nephropathy, even with short-term use.

Piroxicam, tenoxicam and meloxicam are well-established NSAIDs for anti-inflammatory use. They are more suitable for chronic conditions, with long duration of action and slow time to maximal effect.

Over the past few years a new class of COX2-selective NSAIDs have been developed and marketed. A number have been licensed for the treatment of postoperative pain, including Celecoxib, Rofecoxib, Valdecoxib and particularly Parecoxib for intravenous use. Since 2004 serious concerns have been raised over a number of side effects including increased cardiovascular and cerebrovascular morbidity and mortality, acute skin reactions, and GIT bleeding in certain subgroups of patients. Some of these drugs have now been voluntarily withdrawn by the manufacturers and a question mark hangs over the long term future use of those remainig in clinical use. For these reasons I do not propose to identify dosing schedules or further information on this group of drugs.

Opioids

Many different types of opioids are available worldwide, but their actions are all very similar. Prescriptions of opioids for postoperative pain are very variable, with many non-clinical influences. Opioids, natural or synthetic, act on opioid receptors and are reversed to some degree by the effects of naloxone or other opioid antagonists. In 1976, Martin *et al.* described three groups of opioid receptors: μ, κ and σ. Shortly afterwards two other receptors, namely δ and ε were described [38]. Further research has limited the true receptors to three groups: μ, κ and δ. These groups have further subgroups but this is not particularly relevant to this discussion. Opioid receptors are widespread throughout the CNS, both central and spinal, and in some peripheral tissues [39]. Oral morphine in a short-acting, readily available form on demand can provide as good analgesia as IV PCAS. The longer duration of action gives a smoother pharmacokinetic profile for the patient. It is important to remember the conversion of IV dose:oral dose of 1:2 to 1:3. A newer atypical opioid, tramadol, first released in Germany in 1977, is a very useful alternative to morphine. It acts centrally, by opioid agonism and serotonin and noradrenaline re-uptake inhibition. It has a very high bioavailability of over 80%, so no dose conversions are necessary; and has a half-life of 6 h, so is appropriate for QDS dosing. It causes less sedation, constipation and respiratory depression and has less potential for abuse. It is approximately one-fifth as potent as morphine.

Codeine phosphate is a weak opiate, with some analgesic actions. It is used mainly as an anti-tussive and an anti-diarrhoeal as it has many side-effects but little analgesic effect.

Dextropropoxyphene is usually used orally as a constituent of compound analgesic preparations for mild to moderate pain. The dose is 65 mg every 6 h. Side-effects and precautions are as for all opiates.

Dihydrocodeine (DHC) is a weak opiate analgesic used on its own, but more commonly in combined preparations with paracetamol. It has analgesic actions, and in combination it is a very good background analgesic for moderate to severe pain postoperatively. It is given at a dose of 30–60 mg every 4–6 h. Higher doses give little additional analgesia but increased nausea, vomiting, constipation and other side-effects.

Morphine is still the gold standard for postoperative opioid use and is the drug all potencies are measured against. It can cause hypotension, and may precipitate coma in hepatic or renal impairment. The dose needs to be reduced for the elderly and debilitated. Severe withdrawal symptoms can occur if withdrawn abruptly. It may affect pupillary responses, vital for neurological assessment, and there is a risk of pressor response to histamine release in phaeochromatoma. Side-effects include nausea and vomiting (particularly in initial stages), constipation and drowsiness; larger doses produce respiratory depression and hypotension; other side-effects include difficulty with micturition, ureteric or biliary spasm, dry mouth, sweating, postural hypotension, hypothermia, hallucinations, dysphoria, mood changes, dependence, miosis, rashes, urticaria and pruritus. Dosage is 10–15 mg for adults, 2-to 4-hourly titrated to effect and may be administered orally, IM, IV, SC and now commonly by PCAS.

Buprenorphine is a mixed agonist/antagonist used in the management of postoperative and malignant pain. It has a slow onset of action and long half-life. As a partial agonist, the effects are not fully reversed by naloxone, and this can be a safety issue. It is often used sublingually and by transdermal patches for prolonged use. Dosage is up to 400 µg 6 hourly sublingually or by patches releasing up to 70 µg/h for up to 72 h. Due to the long half-life any patient having side-effects must be monitored for at least 30 h after withdrawal of the drug.

Meptazinol is used for moderate to severe pain and is often prescribed for renal or ureteric colic and for obstetric pain. It is a partial agonist, poorly reversed by naloxone. Dosage is up to 100 mg IV or IM and 200 mg PO, 2–4 hourly.

Nalbuphine has a profile similar to morphine. It causes less nausea and vomiting than other opioids, but respiratory depression is a similar problem.

Oxycodone is a very powerful oral opiate. It is used in the treatment of postoperative and terminal pain, and is available in slow-release formulations. Dosage is 5 mg 4 hourly up to 400 mg/day in terminal care. It is contraindicated in porphyrias.

Pentazocine is a mixed agonist/antagonist drug with a number of unique side-effects. It causes arterial and pulmonary hypertension, increases myocardial work load, and has a moderately high incidence of dysphoric and withdrawal type phenomena. Dosage is 30–60 mg 6 hourly by oral, rectal, IM or IV routes.

Pethidine is a powerful opiate, but with less potency than morphine even in high doses. It produces very rapid but short-lived analgesia, and was the drug of choice for many years in colic and in labour. It is metabolized to nor-pethidine, which can cumulate especially in renal dysfunction and which causes seizures and coma. Dosage is up to 100 mg IM, IV or s.c. 2–3 hourly, with a maximum of 400 mg/day, and up to 150 mg orally. Pethidine is sometimes packaged with an anti-emetic to minimize side-effects.

Tramadol is a newer atypical opioid, in use for the past 10 years. It has a high bioavailability and is useful for postoperative pain. Seizures have been reported with its use, usually after rapid IV bolus dosing. There have also been suspicions of enhanced intraoperative recall under light planes of general anaesthesia. Dosage is 50–100 mg 6 hourly up to 600 mg/day in short-term use. Respiratory depression and nausea are said to be less than with other opioids.

Local anaesthetics

Local anaesthetics provide good pain relief to allow early mobilization and so on. They have been shown to reduce the surgical stress response, myocardial ischaemic load and risk of thromboembolism [31]. They also increase the rate of recovery of bowel function postoperatively [40].

Local anaesthetic drugs can be divided into two classes depending on pharmacological structure. These are based on ester groups and amide groups. Esters include cocaine, procaine, tetracaine, amethocaine and chloroprocaine. Amides include lignocaine, bupivacaine and L-bupivacaine, prilocaine, ropivacaine and mepivacaine. Esters are unstable in solution and are hydrolysed in the body rapidly by plasma cholinesterases and other esterases. This gives a relatively short duration of action. One of the main breakdown products is para-amino benzoic acid (PABA), which is associated with an increased risk of hypersensitivity and allergic reactions. Amides are stable and slowly metabolized and so have a longer duration of action. They have a much lower incidence of untoward reactions. Amides are by far the most commonly used agents in modern clinical practice. Local anaesthetics work via blockade of sodium channels, thereby reversibly interrupting the transmission of impulses in peripheral nerves. The effect is mediated by the amount of free ionized form of the anaesthetic, which is related to alkalinity in the tissues. Local anaesthetics are prepared as hydrochloride salts as they are relatively insoluble in water. They are often mixed with vasoconstrictors as they have a vasodilatory effect (with the exception of ropivacaine and L-bupivacaine, which have intrinsic vasoconstriction effects), thus shortening their duration of action. Vasoconstrictors also reduce toxicity and increase safety margins. It should be remembered that solutions containing vasoconstrictors should never be injected into areas supplied by end arteries, such as digits, or the penis. Local anaesthetics are metabolized in blood (esters) and liver (amides), and are excreted via the kidney.

Local anaesthetics can be used topically, as infiltration, as wound irrigation or as nerve blocks on peripheral nerves and plexuses, and as more central regional blocks depending on the area to be anaesthetized and the type of operation. The time of onset, density of block and duration of action is determined by the specific agent used, the area blocked and the alkalinity of the tissues.

Toxicity of local anaesthetics is low if administered in appropriate doses in the appropriate route. Systemic reactions do occur, related to inadvertent intravascular or intrathecal injection, overdose or anaphylactoid type reactions. The reactions are predominantly cardiovascular or effect the CNS.

Lignocaine (lidocaine) is an aminoamide anaesthetic. It has a very rapid onset and short duration of action, although its effect can be prolonged by the use of vasoconstrictors such as epinephrine. It is administered for topical, infiltration and conduction blockade. The onset time is about 5–10 min, with a duration of action of 30–150 min without epinephrine. It is also used in eutectic mixtures such as EMLA cream for topical surface analgesia, particularly in children and needle phobics, or for skin-grafting sites and so on. It is also used as an anti-arrhythmic. Safe maximum dose for administration of lignocaine is 4 mg/kg without epinephrine and 7 mg/kg with epinephrine.

Prilocaine has a clinical profile similar to lignocaine. It causes less toxicity due to a larger volume of distribution, and so is considered safer for IV regional field blocks or field blocks. It causes little vasodilatation and so can be used without a vasoconstrictor. It is combined with lignocaine in EMLA cream for topical use. The unique feature of prilocaine is the ability to cause methaemoglobinaemia. At doses of greater than 8 mg/kg, cyanosis can be seen with prilocaine. This is usually reversible with methylene blue. The use of continuous spinal anaesthesia with prilocaine has recently been described for transurethral resection of the prostate with very successful results [41].

Bupivacaine is probably the most commonly used local anaesthetic for postoperative pain on a worldwide basis. It is a racemic mixture, with a long duration of action and a longer time of onset. In regional blockade, it has an onset time of 15–20 min and a duration of action of 4 h or more. Maximum safe dosage is approximately 2 mg/kg/4 h. Bupivacaine has the common side-effects of local analgesics, but additionally, it has a very slow rate of dissociation from myocardium and may act directly on the myocardium. Bupivacaine can be used for infiltration and conduction blockade in all age groups. The addition of epinephrine to bupivacaine is said to not affect duration of action or the safety profile. As little as 50 mg of bupivacaine injected intravenously has been shown to cause ventricular fibrillation [42].

L-bupivacaine is a newly released S-isomer of bupivacaine with a similar profile of action and reduced side-effects. It is said anecdotally to have less motor block and a more dense sensory block, but this remains to be proven. Dosage schedules are the same as for bupivacaine. Cardiac toxicity should be less in accidental intravascular injection and this is a major advantage.

Ropivacaine is an amide group local anaesthetic combining the long duration of action of bupivacaine with a side-effects profile somewhere between bupivacaine and lignocaine. It is produced as a pure S-enantiomer to reduce cardiovascular toxicity. It is said to produce a more differential block (sensory ≫ motor) than bupivacaine, and is not as potent as bupivacaine in spinal anaesthesia. A 0.75% solution of ropivacaine does not produce as much sensory or motor block as 0.5% bupivacaine in spinal anaesthesia, but there are no clinically apparent differences in epidural or plexus block uses. Ropivacaine causes some vasoconstriction, so the addition of epinephrine does not increase the duration of action.

Etidocaine is another amide group local anaesthetic. It has a very rapid onset of sensory and motor block at about 3–5 min, and a prolonged duration of action at about 6–9 h. Maximum recommended doses are 8 mg/kg with epinephrine and 6 mg/kg without epinephrine. Side-effects are as for other amide group anaesthetics.

Tetracaine is an ester group local anaesthetic used in some countries for long-acting intrathecal (spinal) anaesthesia.

The future of postoperative analgesia

Scientific evidence base for the drug treatment of postoperative pain

The National Health and Medical Research Council (NHMRC) in Australia has recently published a list of level 1 evidence-based postoperative analgesic interventions [16]. These include:

1 postoperative epidural analgesia, which can significantly reduce the incidence of pulmonary morbidity;
2 epidural opioids, which are more effective when used in conjunction with local anaesthetics in producing a synergistic analgesic action and in reducing the required dose and side-effects associated with either the local anaesthetic or the opioid alone;
3 PCA, which provides greater satisfaction and improved ventilation than conventional routes;
4 NSAIDs (although the currently used NSAIDs do not reduce severe pain when used alone, their efficacy as a component of multimodal analgesia is confirmed);
5 acetaminophen (paracetamol) as an effective postoperative analgesic and codeine; 60 mg produces additional analgesia.

Level II evidence statements were as follows:
1 multimodal analgesia improves the effectiveness of pain relief after surgery;
2 patients prefer the subcutaneous route of administration to IM injection;
3 the adverse effects of NSAIDs are serious and must be respected.

From these statements and a critical appraisal of the recent literature, it is obvious that we still have a long way to go before we adequately and reproducibly manage postoperative pain. To balance this however, the use of proper preoperative preparation, continual pain assessment and continual drug delivery devices have improved pain treatment immeasurably over the past 20 years.

In terms of pharmacological developments, there are new types of opioids, local anaesthetics and anti-inflammatory drugs under development. Otherwise, the fine-tuning of dosing schedules, drug delivery systems, adjuvant therapy and, above all, the increasing support for acute pain services should rapidly show further benefits for all our patients.

References

1   Merskey H. Pain terms: a list with definitions and notes on usage. Recommended by the IASP Subcommittee on Taxonomy. *Pain* 1979; **6**: 249–252.

2   Rexed B. The cytoachitectonic organisation of the spinal cord in the cat. *J Comp Neurol* 1952; **96**: 415–95.

3   Dickinson AH. Spinal cord pharmacology of pain. *Br J Anaesth* 1995; **75**: 193–200.

4   Melzack R, Wall PD. Pain mechanisms: a new theory. *Science* 1965; **150**(699): 971–9.

5   Hirshberg RM, Al-Chaer ED, Lawand NB *et al.* Is there a pathway in the posterior funiculus that signals visceral pain. *Pain* 1996; **67**: 291–305.

6   Rawal N, Hylander J, Nydahl PA *et al.* Survey of postoperative analgesia following ambulatory surgery. *Acta Anaesthesiol Scand* 1997; **41**: 1017–22.

7   Kotiniemi LH, Ryhanen PT, Valanne J. Postoperative symptoms at home following day case surgery in children: a multicenter survey of 551 children. *Anaesthesia* 1997; **52**: 963–9.

8   Ghosh S, Sallam S. Patient satisfaction and postoperative demands on hospital and community services after day surgery. *Br J Surg* 1994; **81**: 1635–8.

9   Tong D, Chung F, Wong D. Predictive factors in global and anaesthesia satisfaction in ambulatory surgical patients. *Ambul Surg* 1996; **3**: 127–30.

10 Anderson R, Krohg K. Pain as a major cause of postoperative nausea. *Can Anaesth Soc J* 1976; **23**: 366–9.

11 Lynch EP, Lazor MA, Gellis JE *et al.* The impact of postoperative pain on the development of postoperative delirium. *Anesth Analg* 1998; **86**: 781–5.

12 Chung F. Recovery pattern and home readiness after ambulatory surgery. *Anesth Analg* 1995; **80**: 896–902.

13 Chung F, Ritchie E, Su J. Postoperative pain in ambulatory surgery. *Anesth Analg* 1997; **85**: 808–16.

14 Farrar JT, Portenoy RK, Berlin JA *et al.* Defining the clinically important difference in pain outcome measures. *Pain* 2000; **88**: 287–94.

15 Ready LB, Oden R, Chadwick S *et al.* Development of an anaesthesiology based acute pain service. *Anaesthesiology* 1988; **68**: 100–106.

16 NHMRC Report Canberra. Acute pain management: the scientific evidence Australia. NHMRC 1999.

17 Provision of Pain Services. The Association of Anaesthetists of Great Britain and Ireland, and The Pain Society 1997.

18 The Royal College of Surgeons of England and The College of Anaesthetists. Report of the Working Party on Pain after Surgery. London: HMSO, 1990.

19 Field L. Are nurses still underestimating patients' pain postoperatively? *Br J Nurs* 1996; **5**: 778–84.

20 Dalpra A, Zampieron A. Post-operative pain in a urology department: evaluation by patients and nurses (Italian). *Prof Inferm* 1998; **51**(4): 3–6; Oct–Dec.

21 Melzack R. The McGill pain questionnaire: major properties and scoring scoring methods. *Pain* 1975; **1**(3): 277–99.

22 Daut RL, Cleeland CS, Flanery RC. Development of the Wisconsin brief pain question-naire to assess pain in cancer and other diseases. *Pain* 1983; **17**(2): 197–210.

23 DeLoach LJ, Higgins MS, Caplan AB, Stiff L. The Visual Analog Scale in the immediate postoperative period: intrasubject variability and correlation with a numeric scale. *Anesth Analg* 1998; **86**(1): 102–6.

24 Hug CC. Improving analgesic therapy. *Anesthesiology* 1980; **34**: 441–43.

25 Audit Commission. Anaesthesia under examination: The efficiency and effectiveness of anaesthesia and pain relief services in England and Wales. London: Audit Commission 1997.

26 Vaile JH, Davis P. Topical NSAIDs for musculoskeletal conditions. *Drugs* 1998; **56**: 783–99.

27 Jeal W, Benfield P. Transdermal fentanyl: a review of its pharmacological properties and therapeutic efficacy in pain control. *Drugs* 1997; **53**: 109–38.

28 Pasqualucci A, deAngelis V, Contardo R *et al*. Pre-emptive analgesia: intraperitoneal local anaesthetic in laparoscopic cholecystecyomy. A randomized, double-blind, placebo con-trolled study. *Anesthesiology* 1996; **85**: 11–20.

29 Chrubasik J, Wust H, Friedrich G, Geller E. Absorption and bioavailability of nebulised morphine. *Br J Anaesth* 1988; **61**: 230.

30 Liu S, Carpenter RL, Neal JM. Epidural anesthesia and analgesia: their role in post-operative outcome. *Anesthesiology* 1995; **82**: 1474–506.

31 Rodgers A, Walker N, Schug S *et al*. Reduction of postoperative mortality and morbidity with epidural or spinal anaesthesia: results from overview of randomized trials. *Br Med J* 2002; **321**: 1493–7.

32 Burstal R, Wegener F, Hayes C, Lantry G. Epidural analgesia: prospective audit of 1062 patients. *Anaesth Intensive care* 1998; **26**: 165–72.

33 Woodhouse A, Hobbes AF, Mather AE *et al*. A comparison of morphine, pethidine and fentanyl in the post surgical patient controlled analgesia environment. *Pain* 1996; **64**: 115–21.

34 Hopkins D, Shipton EA, Potgieter D *et al*. Comparison of tramadol and morphine via subcutaneous PCA following orthopaedic surgery. *Can J Anaesth* 1998; **45**: 435–42.

35 Sidebotham D, Dijkhuizen MR, Schug SA. The safety and utilisation of patient controlled analgesia. *J Pain Symptom Manage* 1997; **14**: 202–209.

36 McQuay HJ, Justins D, Moore RA. Treating acute pain in hospital. *Br Med J* 1997; **314**: 1531–5.

37 Langford RM, Evans N. Developments in specific cyclooxygenase therapy for acute pain. *Acute Pain* 2002; **4**: 1–4.

38 Martin WR, Eades CG, Huppler RE *et al*. The effects of morphine and nalorphine-like drugs in the nondependent and morphine-dependent chronic spinal dog. *J Pharm Exp Ther* 1976; **197**(3): 517–32.

39 Picard PR, Tramer MR, McQuay HJ, Moore RA. Analgesia efficacy of peripheral opioids (all except intra-articular): a qualitative systematic review of randomised controlled trials. *Pain* 1997; **72**: 308–18.

40 Jorgensen H, Wetterslev J, Moiniche S, Dahl JB. Epidural local anaesthetics versus opioid based analgesic regimens on post-operative gastrointestinal paralysis, PONV and pain after abdominal surgery. *Cochrane Database Syst Rev* 2000; **4**: CD001893.

41 Reisli R, Celik J, Tuncer S *et al*. Anaesthetic and haemodynamic effects of continuous spinal versus continuous epidural anaesthesia with prilocaine. *Eur J Anaesth* 2003; **20**: 26–30.

42 Whiteside JB, Wildsmith JAW. Developments in local anaesthetic drugs. *Br J Anaesth* 2001; **87**(1): 27–35.

16: Treatment of Pain in Urology

Adrian D. Joyce & William R. Cross

Introduction

As proposed by the International Association for the Study of Pain (ISAP) and the American Pain Society (APS), 'pain is an unpleasant sensory or emotional experience associated with actual or potential tissue damage, or described in terms of such damage' [1]. As this definition acknowledges, the perception of pain is a complex phenomenon involving biological, emotional, environmental and behavioural factors; therefore optimal pain management requires a holistic approach that is tailored to the individual. Increased understanding of the pathophysiology of pain, the development of more refined tools for the objective assessment of pain and the implementation of evidence-based therapies has recently led to dramatic improvements in clinical pain control [2]. The management of pain secondary to genitourinary pathology is no exception to this and is the focus of this chapter.

Classification and physiology of pain

Current classifications of pain are based on the temporal nature of the pain (acute and chronic) and on the underlying biological processes (nociceptive and neuropathic) [3]. From a temporal perspective, how and when acute pain becomes chronic is controversial and lacks clear definition. If pain persists beyond the usual course of an acute injury or disease, or recurs, it is often regarded as chronic. The distinction between acute and chronic pain has an impact on not only the choice of pharmaceutical agent but also the route of administration.

Nociceptive pain is elicited by the activation of highly specialized free endings of sensory nerve fibres (nociceptors), which are located in skin, muscle, connective tissue and bone (somatic nociceptors), and in viscera (visceral nociceptors) (Fig. 16.1). Noxious stimuli elicit the release of cell-bound mediators, including prostaglandins, bradykinin, serotonin, substance P and histamine, which facilitate the passage of primary nociceptive impulses along $A\delta$ and C fibres to the dorsal horn of the spinal cord [1]. Anti-inflammatory agents such as steroids and non-steroidal anti-inflammatory drugs (NSAIDs) exert analgesic affects at this peripheral site by decreasing

prostaglandin synthesis and by inhibiting phospholipase and cyclo-oxygenase (COX), respectively.

The Aδ fibres are sparsely myelinated, large-diameter, fast-conducting
fibres that transmit well-localized sharp pain. C fibres are unmyelinated,
small-diameter, slow-conducting fibres that transmit poorly localized dull
and aching pain. C fibres are sensitive to mechanical, thermal and chemical
stimuli, whereas Aδ fibres are sensitive principally to mechanical and thermal stimuli. In the dorsal horn of the spinal cord second-order neurons
originate and ascend to the brain stem and thalamus via the spinothalamic
tracts. From here information is relayed to the cortex where the sensation of
pain is perceived.

Ascending pain impulses are modulated at a number of sites in the
pathway, especially in the dorsal horn of the spinal cord. Here, descending
fibres from the brain stem release a variety of substances, including

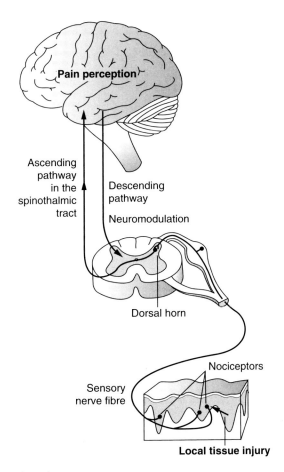

Figure 16.1 The pain pathway.

endogenous opioids, serotonin, norepinephrine, gamma-aminobutyric acid (GABA) and neurotensin, which have the capacity to inhibit neurotransmission of nociceptive impulses and thus produce analgesia [4]. Also at this site, as with endogenous opioids, exogenous opioids bind to opioid receptors and inhibit the release of neurotransmitters, principally substance P, resulting in a modulatory effect. C fibre neurotransmission of dull and diffuse pain is particularly sensitive to opioids, whereas well-localized sharp pain carried by Aδ fibres is less sensitive [1]. Tricyclic antidepressants, such as amitriptyline and imipramine, also inhibit noxious stimuli and produce analgesia by reducing the uptake of serotonin and norepinephrine in the dorsal root neuromodulatory complex.

The term neuropathic pain encompasses a diverse range of syndromes that are characterized by aberrant somatosensory processing in the peripheral or central nervous system (CNS). Neuropathic pain syndromes include the deafferentation pains (e.g. phantom pain and postherpetic neuralgia), peripheral mononeuropathies and polyneuropathies, and the complex regional pain syndromes (e.g. reflex sympathetic dystrophy). Although neuropathic pain is alleviated with conventional first-line analgesics, it often requires the coadministration of other pharmacotherapies, such as antidepressants and anticonvulsants, in order to achieve analgesic relief.

Overview of commonly used analgesics

Analgesics are commonly divided into three groups: nonopioids, opioids and adjuvants. Although this classification does not take into consideration the mechanism of action of the analgesics and hence its clinical value has been debated [5], it nevertheless forms the basis for most pain control programmes.

The nonopioid group includes paracetamol (acetaminophen) and NSAIDs. The opioid analgesic group is subdivided into mu agonists (mu is an opioid receptor in the CNS), which are also known as full agonists, pure agonists and morphine-like agonists, and a second group referred to as agonist antagonists. The adjuvant class includes a wide variety of medications whose primary indication is other than that of pain control, e.g. amitriptyline, which is principally used to treat depression but also has proven analgesic effects.

Examples from each of the different analgesic groups are listed below, with the indications, mechanism of action, dosage (adult), side-effects, contraindications and interactions [6].

Nonopioids

Paracetamol

Indications	Nociceptive and neuropathic pain
	Pyrexia
Mechanism	Little is known, but it primarily has a central action
Dosage	Oral and rectal routes: 0.5–1 g every 4–6 h to a maximum of 4 g daily
Side-effects	Rare, but include skin rashes and blood disorders; overdose is associated with liver and less frequently renal impairment
Contraindications	Paracetamol is to be used with
Interactions	caution in individuals with hepatic or renal impairment and those with alcohol dependence

Busulfan	Colestyramine
Coumarins	Domperidone
Metoclopramide	

NSAIDs

Indications	Nociceptive and neuropathic pain; particularly effective for inflammatory arthritides
	Pyrexia
Mechanisms	NSAIDs have both peripheral and central actions; in the periphery they inhibit prostaglandin synthesis and/or release in inflamed tissue, ultimately producing analgesia; centrally, they act by neuromodulation
Dosage	Aspirin: 0.3–1 g every 4 h with food. In acute conditions 8 g daily
	Ibuprofen: 1.2–1.8 g daily in 3–4 divided doses
	Voltarol: 75–150 mg daily in divided doses
Side-effects	About 60% of patients will respond to any NSAID; of the others, those that do not respond to one may well respond to another
	The main differences between NSAIDs are in the incidence and type of side-effects; side-effects include gastrointestinal discomfort, nausea, diarrhoea, and occasionally bleeding and ulceration occur; other side-effects include renal impairment, dizziness, drowsiness, hypersensitivity reactions and fluid retention

Contraindications	Should be used with caution in the elderly, in allergic disorders, during pregnancy and breast-feeding, in coagulation defects and those with renal impairment	
Interactions	ACE inhibitors	Adrenergic neurone blockers
	Alpha-blockers	Angiotensin-II receptor antagonists
	Antidepressants	Beta-blockers
	Cardiac glycosides	Calcium channel blockers
	Cyclosporin	Baclofen
	Clonidine	Corticosteroids
	Coumarins	Diuretics
	Heparin	Lithium
	Methotrexate	Methyldopa
	Nitrates	Nitroprusside
	Phenytoin	Quinolones
	Sulphonylurea	Venlafaxine

Cyclooxygenase-2 inhibitors

Indications	Primarily effective for inflammatory arthritides
Mechanism	Selectively inhibit COX-2, thus reducing the side-effect profile relative to NSAIDs that inhibit COX-1 and COX-2
Dosage	Celcoxib: 200–400 mg in 1–2 doses
	Etodolac: 600 mg in 1–2 divided doses
	Meloxicam: 7.5–15 mg a day
	Rofecoxib: 12.5–25 mg a day
	Parecoxib: IM/IV initially 40 mg then 20–40 mg every 6–12 h as required
Side-effects	Similar to NSAIDs; however improved gastrointestinal tolerance
Contraindications	The National Institute for Clinical Excellence (NICE; www.nice.org.uk) has recommended that the use of COX-2 inhibitors outside licensed indications should be discouraged
Interactions	Similar to NSAIDs

Opioids

Tramadol

Indications	Nociceptive and neuropathic pain
Mechanism	Weak mu receptor agonist; it is not as effective as other opioids in controlling severe pain
Dosage	Orally, 50–100 mg not more often than every 4 h. By intramuscular injection or

intravenous injection (over 2–3 min) or
intravenous infusion, 50–100 mg every 4–6 h

Side-effects,   See under morphine salts
contraindications
and interactions

Codeine

Indications   Mild to moderate pain
Mechanisms   Weak CNS opioid receptor agonist
Dosage   By mouth, 30–60 mg every 4 h, to a
maximum of 240 mg daily
By intramuscular injection 30–60 mg
every 4 h when necessary
Side-effects,   See under morphine salts
contraindications
and interactions

Morphine salts

Morphine is one of
the most
commonly used
opioids for severe
pain, particularly
chronic visceral
pain. It is also the
reference against
which other
opioid analgesics
are compared
Indications   Moderate to severe pain
Mechanism   CNS opioid receptor agonist
Dosage   Table 16.1 lists the approximate
equivalent single doses
In acute pain, by subcutaneous or intramuscular
injection, 10 mg every 4 h if necessary
In chronic pain, morphine is preferentially
administered by mouth either as an immediate
or as extended release preparation. The initial
dose largely depends on the patient's previous
analgesia therapy; 5–10 mg is often sufficient
to replace a weaker analgesic (e.g.
paracetamol), but 10–20 mg or more is
required to replace a stronger one. The
morphine dose should then be titrated to
achieve adequate analgesia
Breakthrough pain and pain associated
with activity (e.g. wound dressing) should be
managed with rescue doses of morphine
When the pain is controlled and the 24 h
morphine requirement is established, the
patient can be transferred to morphine given as
a modified-release preparation (12-h
administration)

If the patient becomes unable to swallow, the equivalent intramuscular dose of morphine is half the oral solution dose; in the case of the modified-release tablets it is half the total 24-h dose (which is then divided into six portions to be given every 4 h). Due to high solubility, diamorphine is often used in preference to morphine as it can be given in a smaller volume

Morphine can also be administered rectally as a suppository.

Another popular alternative to oral morphine is transdermal fentanyl. Conversion from oral morphine to fentanyl requires careful monitoring

The following 24-h doses of morphine are considered to be equivalent to the fentanyl patches shown:

Morphine salt 90 mg daily ≡ fentanyl '25' patch
Morphine salt 180 mg daily ≡ fentanyl '50' patch
Morphine salt 270 mg daily ≡ fentanyl '75' patch
Morphine salt 360 mg daily ≡ fentanyl '100' patch

Side-effects   The side-effect profile of the different opioid analgesics is very similar; however there is a degree of variability both qualitatively and quantitatively. The most common side-effects include nausea and vomiting (especially in the initial stages), constipation and drowsiness. Others include respiratory depression, hypotension, difficulty micturating, dry mouth, palpitations, rashes and pruritus

Contraindications   Avoid in respiratory depression, acute alcoholism, in raised intracranial pressure and head injury, and paralytic ileus

Interactions

Alcohol	Antipsychotics
Tricyclic antidepressants	Anxiolytics
Cimetidine	Ciprofloxacin
Domperidone	Monoamine oxidase inhibitors (MAOIs)
Metoclopramide	Mexiletine
Moclobemide	Ritonovir

Table 16.1 Approximate equivalent single doses of analgesics

Analgesic	Dose (mg)
Morphine salts (oral)	10
Oxycodone (oral)	5
Hydromorphone hydrochloride	1.3
Diamorphine hydrochloride	3

Adjuvants

Tricyclic antidepressants (e.g. amitriptyline)
Amitriptyline

Indications	Chronic pain syndromes (unlicensed indication in UK). Available evidence does not support its use as an analgesic for acute pain
Mechanism	The analgesic effect of amitriptyline, as with the other tertiary amine compounds, does not depend on the antidepressant activity. The most widely accepted hypothesis is that the tricyclic antidepressants enhance normal neuromodulation by interfering with the uptake of serotonin and norepinephrine in the CNS
Dosage	The starting dose should be low, 10 mg in the elderly and 25 mg in young patients. Doses can be increased gradually every few days, until pain relief is achieved or side-effects become troublesome. Often the dose needs to be titrated to antidepressant doses, which obviously should be considered in patients with coexisting depression
Side-effects	Serious adverse effects, especially cardiotoxicity, are very uncommon at the doses typically administered for pain. However, less serious side-effects are more frequent and include dry mouth, sedation, blurred vision, constipation, nausea, difficulty voiding, confusion, postural hypotension and sexual dysfunction
Contraindications	Recent myocardial infarction, arrhythmias (particularly heart block), and severe liver disease

Interactions

Amiodarone	General anaesthetics
Antidepressants, selective serotonin re-uptake inhibitors (SSRIs)	Antiepileptics
Antihistamines	Antimuscarinics
Antipsychotics	Anxiolytics and hypnotics
Barbiturates	Carbamazepine
Cimetidine	Clonidine
Diuretics	MAOIs
Thyroid hormones	Phenytoin
Flecainide	Sotalol

Anticonvulsant
   drugs (e.g.
   gabapentin)

Gabapentin

Indications	Neuropathic pain
Mechanism	Exact mechanism(s) of analgesic action remains to be established
Dosage	Usually start at 300 mg a day. Dose can be increased daily or more slowly depending on response. Daily doses required vary between 300 and 3600 mg/day (daily dose should be divided into three doses per day)
Side-effects	Usually well tolerated. Documented side-effects include drowsiness, dizziness, tremor, ataxia, dyspepsia and arthralgia
Contraindications	Caution in individuals with a history of psychotic illness, renal impairment and diabetes mellitus
Interactions	Antacids MAOIs
	Antidepressants, tricyclic and SSRIs

Pain assessment and measurement

Probably the most common cause of unrelieved pain and unnecessary suffering is the failure of health professionals to ask patients about their pain and to accept and act on individuals' reports of pain. As pain is so inherently subjective the patient's self-report should form the basis of any pain assessment. Although not required in all cases, two tools widely used for overall pain assessment are the Initial Pain Assessment tool and the Brief Pain Inventory [7]. These are often supplemented in research and clinical practice by the short-form McGill Pain Questionnaire [8].

The Initial Pain Assessment tool elicits from the patient information on location of the pain(s), pain intensity, quality of the pain, variations and rhythms, manner of expressing the pain, relieving and exacerbating factors, and the effects of the pain on sleep, appetite, physical activity, relationships, emotions and ability to concentrate. The tool acknowledges that it is not comprehensive and space is included for patients to document any other information or details that they wish. In contrast, the Brief Pain Inventory focuses on the nature and effects of the pain experienced by the patient during the previous 24 h.

Once an initial pain assessment has been made and a therapeutic management plan introduced, further evaluation is required to monitor the efficacy of the prescribed analgesics. This is most commonly performed by using one of many available validated pain rating scales (Fig. 16.2) [7]. These include:

- *The visual analogue scale*. This is a 10-cm line with phrases such as 'no pain' and 'pain as bad as it could be' at the line ends. The patient marks the line to represent pain intensity and a number is subsequently obtained by measuring up to the patient's point.
- *The graphic rating scale*. This scale builds on the visual analogue scale by adding to the measurement line either words (verbal graphic rating scale) or numbers (numerical graphic rating scale) between the ends of the scale.
- *The simple descriptor scale*. This is simply a list of adjectives describing different levels of pain intensity.
- Faces rating scales. These comprise a group of pictures or photographs of different facial expressions suggesting various pain intensities. Patients are asked to pick the face that best describes how they feel. The Wong–Baker faces rating scale may be used with children as young as 3 years [9].

As long as pain requires treatment, measuring pain intensity should be continued, especially in the hospital setting were it should be clearly documented on the patient's chart so that during ward rounds the results can be interpreted and, if required, analgesic therapy adjusted.

Pain management of common urological conditions

Renal colic

Acute ureteric obstruction induces intense activation of visceral nociceptors. The release of local and renal inflammatory mediators, especially prostaglandins, recruits additional nociceptors and produces an increase in renal blood flow with subsequent diuresis, further exacerbating the pain [10]. Traditionally, the standard treatment of renal colic was the administration of intravenous opioids. However, with greater appreciation of the pathophysiology of renal colic and the availability of nonopioid parental agents (e.g. ketorolac), NSAIDs have increasingly found application in the management of renal colic.

Holdgate and Pollock recently reported a meta-analysis of randomized controlled trials (RCTs) and quasi-RCTs that compared any NSAID with any opioid in the management of renal colic [11]. Twenty studies from nine countries, involving 1613 participants, met their selection criteria. Due to study heterogeneity the pooling of data was limited, which had a direct impact on statistical analysis. Nevertheless, it was found that in the 13 trials that reported patient-related pain scores, ten found lower pain scores in patients treated with NSAIDs, two demonstrated no difference and only one study found lower pain scores in patients treated with opioids. Patients treated with NSAIDs were significantly less likely to require rescue medication (analgesia administered to supplement the initial dose) and relative to those prescribed pethidine were less likely to experience adverse events,

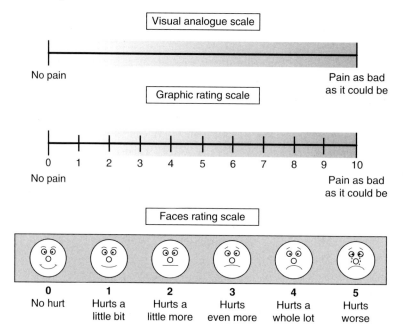

Figure 16.2 Pain rating scales.

especially nausea and vomiting. No study reported a case of gastrointestinal bleeding or drug-induced renal impairment. The reviewers concluded that both NSAIDs and opioids provide effective analgesia in acute renal colic. In addition, they emphasized that if opioids are used, pethidine should be avoided, as it is associated with a high incidence of nausea and vomiting. But before administering regular NSAIDs the patient's renal function should be assessed, as although healthy individuals may tolerate a temporary reduction in renal blood flow, those with pre-existing renal disease are at risk of developing acute renal failure [12].

It has been postulated that selective COX-2 inhibitors may have an application in renal colic; however this remains to be clinically established. Despite *in vitro* evidence that selective COX-2 inhibition reduces ureteric contractility [13,14] and therapeutically COX-2 inhibitors have a reduced gastrointestinal side-effect profile relative to nonselective COX inhibitors, cost-benefit analyses may restrict their routine use in renal colic.

The human ureter contains α-adrenergic receptors [15], the blockade of which decreases ureteral peristaltic frequency and amplitude, resulting in an increase in urine flow rate [16]. Based on these experimental findings Dellabella *et al.* evaluated the efficacy of the α1-adrenergic antagonist tamsulosin in the conservative management of ureteric stones [17]. In a prospective randomized trial, tamsulosin was compared with an anti-spasmotic agent (floroglucine–trimetossibenzene) in 60 patients with stones in the juxtavesical ureter. After 4 weeks, all patients in the tamsulosin group successfully passed their stones compared with only 70% in the anti-spasmotic group. Furthermore, patients in the tamsulosin group required significantly less pain medication than the anti-spasmotic group. The positive findings of this pilot study await validation in larger studies.

Kekeç *et al.* investigated the potential role of isosorbide dinitrite in the management of renal colic [18]. In a small double-blind trial, 50 patients were randomized to receive either 40 mg intravenous tenoxicam (NSAID) or tenoxicam and 5 mg sublingual isosorbide dinitrite. They found that the tenoxicam alone or in combination with isosorbide dinitrite was effective in relieving renal colic, but the pain relief obtained with the combination therapy was significantly greater than that with tenoxicam alone. The authors proposed that the therapeutic effect of isosorbide dinitrite was potentially due to ureteric smooth muscle relaxation and/or decreased urine output caused by reflex sympathetic vasoconstriction of the renal vasculature. Somewhat surprisingly none of the individuals who took isosorbide dinitrite experienced any side-effects, specifically orthostatic hypotension and headache. Considering the limited available data, it remains to be established whether isosorbide dinitrite has a role in routine clinical practice.

Two prospective double-blind RCTs have revealed that nifedipine, a calcium channel blocker, offers little in the management of renal colic [19,20]. Pain relief obtained with nifedipine did not significantly differ from that achieved with placebo [20].

The clinical efficacy of desmopressin, a synthetic analogue of ADH, in the management of renal colic has also been the focus of a number of studies [21–23]. In addition to decreasing the normal diuresis associated with renal colic, ADH may also reduce spontaneous contractions in the renal pelvis and increase secretion of β-endorphins by the hypothalamus. Lopes *et al.* randomly assigned 61 individuals with acute renal colic to receive intranasal desmopressin, intramuscular diclofenac or both [23]. Pain scores were assessed over a 30-min period and it was found that the analgesia obtained with combination therapy was not significantly different to that achieved with diclofenac monotherapy. Although desmopressin may not have a role in acute pain management, other studies are required to ascertain whether the drug facilitates stone passage.

Chronic nonbacterial prostatitis/chronic pelvic pain syndrome

Chronic nonbacterial prostatitis/chronic pelvic pain syndrome (CP/CPPS; National Institute of Health (NIH) category III prostatitis) is a common but poorly understood clinical entity characterized by pelvic pain and voiding symptoms [24,25]. Although progress has been made, the aetiology and pathophysiology of CP/CPPS still remain elusive and at present there are no evidence-based standardized medical or surgical therapies [26]. Empirical treatment often includes one or a combination of antibiotics, anti-inflammatory agents, α-blockers, finasteride, phytotherapy, behaviour modification, acupuncture and surgery [27].

Mehik *et al.* investigated the long-term efficacy of the α-blocker, alfuzosin, in patients with CP/CPPS [28]. The prospective placebo-controlled study revealed that at the end of 6 months of active treatment, the alfuzosin group had a statistically significant decrease in total NIH-Chronic Prostatitis Symptom Index (CPSI) score compared with the placebo group. The decrease in total NIH-CPSI score was predominantly due to a reduction in pain score; however, the improvement in pain did not translate into a significant quality of life improvement. The authors concluded that on the basis of their data, patients with CP/CPPS should not be managed with α-blocker monotherapy [28]. A more recent study has indicated that the selective $α_1$-adrenergic antagonist, tamsulosin, may have a role in providing symptomatic relief in certain men with CP/CPPS [29]. Tamsulosin was statistically and clinically superior to placebo in alleviating pain, but only in individuals with a 'severe' baseline NIH-CPPS score (mean score 31).

Finasteride has been investigated as a treatment option to reduce pain associated with CP/CPPS [30–32]. In a single-blind, randomized, prospective 1-year trial the efficacy of finasteride and of the phytotherapy agent, saw palmetto, was formally assessed [32]. Patients who received finasteride had a statistically significant improvement in pain score at 3 months that was maintained for the duration of the study, whereas individuals who took saw palmetto experienced an initial decrease in pain score, which returned to baseline before 12 months. Unfortunately, this study did not include a placebo arm, hence the potential therapeutic role of finasteride in the management of CP/CPPS remains to be clinically established in a large placebo-controlled trial.

The anti-inflammatory COX-2 inhibitor, rofecoxib, has been evaluated in the treatment of patients with chronic nonbacterial prostatitis [33]. In a multicentre study Nickel *et al.* randomized 161 patients to 6 weeks of rofecoxib (25 or 50 mg) or placebo [33]. The NIH-CPSI pain scores significantly decreased from baseline in all the groups and, although there was more improvement in the two rofecoxib arms, the difference was not statistically significant. In this relatively short study there was a marked placebo response that may have masked any treatment effect, indicating that more research is required to ascertain whether men with CP/CPPS may benefit from COX-2 inhibitors.

It has been proposed that CP/CPPS and interstitial cystitis share similar clinical characteristics and that they may be manifestations of the same disease process [34]. Based on the hypothesis that CP/CPPS may be secondary to dysfunctional epithelium, pentosan polysulphate sodium (PPS) has been investigated as a potential treatment [35]. A placebo-controlled trial revealed that although quality of life was significantly improved with PPS compared with placebo, there was no difference observed between the treatment groups in the pain domain of the NIH-CPSI. At present there is no evidence to support the routine use of PPS in CP/CPPS.

Pharmacotherapy for genitourinary cancer pain

Pain is one of the most prevalent symptoms experienced by patients with cancer, increasing in incidence from 50% to 75% as disease progresses from an intermediate to an advanced stage [36]. If inadequately controlled, pain can markedly impair physical and psychological functioning, which has a negative impact on the quality of life of the patient and his or her family. Optimal pain control is therefore an essential component in cancer care [37] and management of genitourinary malignancies is no exception to this.

In the early 1980s the WHO convened an expert committee to define the principles of cancer pain management. The report of that committee, entitled Cancer Pain Relief [38], recommended a methodology that has subsequently been validated and demonstrated to be effective for relieving cancer pain in 70–90% of patients [39]. The method can be summarized in five phrases:

• *By mouth.* Whenever possible oral or another non-invasive route of administration should be used.
• *By the clock.* Analgesia should be administered at fixed regular intervals of time. Less analgesia is required to prevent the recurrence of pain than to treat it after it recurs. Most patients who receive an 'around-the-clock' opioid regimen should also be provided with a so-called 'rescue dose', which is a supplemental dose offered on a as-needed basis for the treatment of breakthrough pain.
• *By the ladder.* Analgesia should be appropriate for the intensity of pain experienced by the individual (see 'WHO analgesic ladder').
• *For the individual.* With regard to the administration of opioid analgesia, there are no standard doses; the 'right' dose is the dose that relieves the individual's discomfort.
• *Attention to detail.* In addition to individualizing the doses of the analgesics, the administration times to the patient's normal routine should be tailored; the first and last doses of the day should be coordinated to the

waking time and bedtime. In addition, the patient and carers should be fully informed of the drug regimen, especially possible side-effects.

The WHO analgesic ladder

The analgesic ladder proposed by the WHO is based on the principle that the pain intensity experienced by an individual is the prime consideration in deciding the analgesic selection (Fig. 16.3). The approach advocates three basis steps.

Step 1   Patients with mild to moderate pain should be treated with a nonopioid analgesic. If indicated this can be combined with an adjuvant analgesic. The term adjuvant in this ladder refers to both the adjuvant analgesics and the adjuvant drugs that are used to reduce side-effects (e.g. laxatives for analgesia-induced constipation).

Step 2   Patients who present with moderate to severe pain, or fail to achieve adequate analgesia after a period of taking a nonopioid, should be treated with a weak opioid. Typically patients are managed with a combination product containing a nonopioid (e.g. aspirin or paracetamol) and an opioid (e.g. codeine or propoxyphene). As in step 1, these medications can be coadministered with an adjuvant medication.

Step 3   Individuals who present with severe pain, or fail to obtain adequate relief with medication on the second rung of the ladder, should be treated with a strong opioid, such as morphine. This can be combined with a nonopioid analgesic and/or an adjuvant agent.

Paracetamol and NSAIDs are widely used as monotherapy in the management of cancer pain, especially in the early stages of the disease. As pain increases, due to their maximum analgesic efficacy paracetamol and

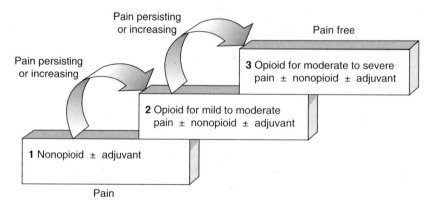

Figure 16.3 WHO analgesia ladder.

NSAIDs are supplemented with opioids, initially often as a combination drug (e.g. cocodamol). The dose of these combination products can only be increased until the maximum dose of the nonopioid coanalgesic is attained, thus limiting their application in individuals with severe pain. Although nonopioids are useful analgesics at all stages of cancer pain, ultimately their use is limited by the maximum efficacy and side-effects. With the advent of COX-2-selective inhibitors, which lack significant gastrointestinal and renal toxicity, the latest generation of NSAIDs may have increased application in cancer pain control [40]. This remains to be established in clinical trials.

It is now recognized that as individual patients vary considerably in their response to different opioids, sequential opioid trials (often referred to as opioid rotation) may be required to identify the drug that produces the most favourable balance between analgesia and side-effects. It is equally important not only to individualize the type of opioid administered but also to titrate the dose and deliver it via a route that is appropriate and acceptable to the patient. As there is no maximum or ceiling dose for the pure mu agonist opioids, the dose should be increased until the pain relief is satisfactory or intolerable side-effects occur. To maximize the opioid therapeutic window, by allowing increased and more effective doses, it is essential to appropriately manage side-effects [41].

Adjuvant analgesics are a diverse range of pharmaceuticals that can be coadministered with primary analgesics in any of the three steps of the analgesic ladder to optimize pain control [42]. The adjuvant analgesics can be classified into four broad groups:
1 multipurpose adjuvant analgesics;
2 adjuvant analgesics used for neuropathic pain;
3 adjuvant analgesics used for bone pain;
4 adjuvant analgesics used for visceral pain (Table 16.2).

For all the adjuvant analgesics, responses vary considerably from one individual to another in a rather unpredictable fashion. As a result, the administration of an optimal dosing regimen requires a comprehensive assessment of the patient both initially and during the course of therapy. And as with the opioid analgesics, sequential trials of different adjuvant analgesics are often needed to identify a useful drug.

The development of third-generation bisphosphonates, namely ibandronate and zoledronic acid, has recently generated increased interest in the application of bisphosphonates in the management of metastatic bone disease, a frequent cause of morbidity in patients with advanced genitourinary cancer [43]. Saad *et al.* conducted a study to define the role of zoledronic acid in patients with hormone-refractory prostate cancer with bone metastases [44]. The double-blind, placebo-controlled study reported

Group	Examples
Multipurpose drugs	Corticosteroids
	Dexamethasone
	Prednisolone
Neuropathic pain	Antidepressants
	Tricyclic antidepressants
	'Newer' antidepressants (e.g. SSRIs)
	NMDA receptor antagonists
	Ketamine
	Dextromethorphan
	Anticonvulsants
	Carbamazepine
	Phenytoin
	Gabapentin
	Valproate
	Clonazepam
	Neuroleptics
	Pimozide
	Fluphenazine
	Oral local anaesthetic agents
	Mexiletine
	Tocainide
	GABAergic
	Baclofen
	Topical agents
	Capsaicin
	Local anaesthetics
Drugs used for bone pain	Bisphosphonates
	Pamidronate
	Ibandronate
	Zoledronate
	Calcitonin
	Radiopharmaceuticals (e.g. strontium-89)
Drugs used for visceral pain	Scopolamine
	Octreotide
	Oxybutynin

Table 16.2 Adjuvant analgesics

a statistically significant reduction in the number of skeletal-related events in patients randomly assigned to the zoledronic acid arm compared with that in the placebo arm. Skeletal-related events were the primary end point and defined as pathologic fracture, spinal cord compression, surgery to bone, radiation therapy to bone, or a change in anti-neoplastic therapy to treat bone pain. Although assessed, the study did not focus on pain and analgesia use; hence, interpretation of the effect of zoledronic acid on these parameters was limited. Nevertheless, as noted, in other studies that used less potent bisphosphonates [45,46] Saad *et al.* found that the use of zoledronic acid did not reduce pain scores and analgesia use by a statistically significant amount [44]. In addition, bisphosphonates treatment did not significantly improve the quality of life [44].

Management of interstitial cystitis pain

Chronic bladder and pelvic pain in association with urinary frequency and urgency are the principal symptoms experienced by individuals with interstitial cystitis. The aetiology and pathogenesis of interstitial cystitis still remain elusive and present treatment strategies are far from evidence based [47]. Many of the proposed therapeutic regimes are empirical and result from anecdotal evidence, uncontrolled case series and small randomized clinical trials.

Peters *et al.* have explored the potential application of intravesical bacillus Calmette–Guérin (BCG) in the management of interstitial cystitis [48,49]. In contrast to a more recent study [50], the group from Michigan found that the majority of patients randomized to a 6-week course of intravesical BCG had a positive response (9/15 patients; 60% response rate relative to a 27% placebo response) [48]. At a mean follow-up of 27 months, the response was maintained in eight of the nine individuals [49]. Specifically, relative to baseline values, in the responders pelvic pain decreased 81%, vaginal pain decreased 71% and dysuria decreased 82% [49]. These improvements in pain scores were associated with an improvement in quality of life score. However, as indicated by the authors, although the data are encouraging the potential application of intravesical BCG therapy in interstitial cystitis remains to be confirmed in an appropriately powered, randomized, double-blind placebo-controlled trial [49].

A meta-analysis of four studies that individually investigated the efficacy of pentosan polysulphate in the treatment of interstitial cystitis found that, relative to placebo, PPS significantly improved pain, urgency and frequency [51]. With regard to pain, PPS improved the symptom in 37.3% of patients relative to 21.1% in the placebo group [51]. The authors calculated that seven individuals with interstitial cystitis would need to be treated with PPS for one person to achieve a 50% or greater improvement in pain score [51]. A more recent multicentre, randomized trial performed by the interstitial cystitis clinical trials group found no difference in pain scores in participants after receiving 24 weeks of placebo or PPS [52]. However, this study had strict eligibility requirements and despite an extension failed to recruit sufficient participants to demonstrate any significant treatment effects [52]. It is widely acknowledged that patients in interstitial cystitis trials are not representative of the 'typical' patient seen in clinical practice. Therefore in order to obtain statistical evidence for a clinically useful intervention, trials may have to relax their inclusion criteria beyond the National Institute for Diabetes and Digestive and Kidney Diseases diagnostic standard.

In conclusion, optimal pain management is that which is tailored to the individual patient and which takes into consideration biological, emotional, environmental and behavioural factors. With increased understanding of the pathophysiology of pain, the application of validated tools for the objective assessment of pain and the implementation of evidence-based therapies, the treatment of pain secondary to genitourinary pathology is achievable and an essential component of patient care.

References

1   Pasero C, Paice JA, McCaffery M. Basic mechanisms underlying the causes and effects of pain. In: McCaffery M, Pasero C, eds. *Pain: Clinical Manual,* 2nd edn. St Louis: Mosby; 1999, 15–34.

2   Holdcroft A, Power I. Recent developments: management of pain. *BMJ* 2003; **326**(7390): 635–9.

3   Shipton EA. *Pain: Acute and Chronic,* 2nd edn. London: Arnold; 1999.

4   Raj PP. Pain mechanisms. In: Raj PP, ed. *Pain Medicine: A Comphrensive Review.* St Louis: Mosby, 1996: 12–25.

5   McCaffery M, Portenoy RR. Overview of three groups of analgesics. In: McCaffery M, Pasero C, eds. *Pain: Clinical Manual,* 2nd edn. St Louis: Mosby, 1999: 103–28.

6   British National Formulary, 47th edn. London: British Medical Association, 2004.

7   McCaffery M, Pasero C. Assessment: underlying complexities, misconceptions, and practical tools. In: McCaffery M, Pasero C, eds. *Pain: Clinical Manual,* 2nd edn. St. Louis: Mosby, 1999: 35–102.

8   Melzack R. The short-form McGill Pain Questionnaire. *Pain* 1987; **30**(2): 191–7.

9   Wong DL, Baker CM. Pain in children: comparison of assessment scales. *Pediatr Nurs* 1988; **14**(1): 9–17.

10 Gulmi FA, Felsen D, Vaughan ED. Pathophysiology of urinary tract obstruction. In: Retik AB, Vaughan ED, Wein AJ, eds. *Campbell's Urology,* 8th edn. Philadelphia: Saunders, 2002: 411–62.

11 Holdgate A, Pollock T. *Nonsteroidal Anti-inflammatory Drugs (NSAIDs) versus Opioids for Acute Renal Colic (Cochrane Review).* Cichester: John Wiley & Sons, 2004.

12 Brater DC. Effects of nonsteroidal anti-inflammatory drugs on renal function: focus on cyclooxygenase-2-selective inhibition. *Am J Med* 1999; **107**(6A): 65S–70S; discussion 70S–1S.

13 Nakada SY, Jerde TJ, Bjorling DE, Saban R. Selective cyclooxygenase-2 inhibitors reduce ureteral contraction in vitro: a better alternative for renal colic? *J Urol* 2000; **163**(2): 607–12.

14 Mastrangelo D, Wisard M, Rohner S, Leisinger H, Iselin CE. Diclofenac and NS-398, a selective cyclooxygenase-2 inhibitor, decrease agonist-induced contractions of the pig isolated ureter. *Urol Res* 2000; **28**(6): 376–82.

15 Malin JM Jr, Deane RF, Boyarsky S. Characterisation of adrenergic receptors in human ureter. *Br J Urol* 1970; **42**(2): 171–4.

16 Morita T, Wada I, Saeki H, Tsuchida S, Weiss RM. Ureteral urine transport: changes in bolus volume, peristaltic frequency, intraluminal pressure and volume of flow resulting from autonomic drugs. *J Urol* 1987; **137**(1): 132–5.

17 Dellabella M, Milanese G, Muzzonigro G. Efficacy of tamsulosin in the medical management of juxtavesical ureteral stones. *J Urol* 2003; **170**(6 Pt 1): 2202–2205.

18 Kekec Z, Yilmaz U, Sozuer E. The effectiveness of tenoxicam vs isosorbide dinitrate plus tenoxicam in the treatment of acute renal colic. *BJU Int* 2000; **85**(7): 783–5.

19 Lloret J, Vila A, Puig X, Monmany J, Munoz J, More J. Nifedipine in the treatment of renal colic. *Methods Find Exp Clin Pharmacol* 1986; 8(9): 575–9.

20 Caravati EM, Runge JW, Bossart PJ, Martinez JC, Hartsell SC, Williamson SG. Nifedipine for the relief of renal colic: a double-blind, placebo-controlled clinical trial. *Ann Emerg Med* 1989; **18**(4): 352–4.

21 el-Sherif AE, Salem M, Yahia H, al-Sharkawy WA, al-Sayrafi M. Treatment of renal colic by desmopressin intranasal spray and diclofenac sodium. *J Urol* 1995; **153**(5): 1395–8.

22 Moro U, De Stefani S, Crisci A, De Antoni P, Scott CA, Selli C. Evaluation of the effects of desmopressin in acute ureteral obstruction. *Urol Int* 1999; **62**(1): 8–11.

23 Lopes T, Dias JS, Marcelino J, Varela J, Ribeiro S, Dias J. An assessment of the clinical efficacy of intranasal desmopressin spray in the treatment of renal colic. *BJU Int* 2001; 87(4): 322–5.

24 Batstone GR, Doble A, Batstone D. Chronic prostatitis. *Curr Opin Urol* 2003; **13**(1): 23–9.

25 Schaeffer AJ. Etiology and management of chronic pelvic pain syndrome in men. *Urology* 2004; **63**(3 Suppl. 1): 75–84.

26 McNaughton Collins M, MacDonald R, Wilt T. *Interventions for Chronic Abacterial Prostatitis (Cochrane Review)*. Chichester: John Wiley & Sons, 2004.

27 Hua VN, Schaeffer AJ. Acute and chronic prostatitis. *Med Clin North Am* 2004; **88**(2): 483–94.

28 Mehik A, Alas P, Nickel JC, Sarpola A, Helstrom PJ. Alfuzosin treatment for chronic prostatitis/chronic pelvic pain syndrome: a prospective, randomized, double-blind, placebo-controlled, pilot study. *Urology* 2003; **62**(3): 425–9.

29 Nickel JC, Narayan P, McKay J, Doyle C. Treatment of chronic prostatitis/chronic pelvic pain syndrome with tamsulosin: a randomized double blind trial. *J Urol* 2004; **171**(4): 1594–7.

30 Holm M, Meyhoff HH. Chronic prostatic pain. A new treatment option with finasteride? *Scand J Urol Nephrol* 1997; **31**(2): 213–15.

31 Leskinen M, Lukkarinen O, Marttila T. Effects of finasteride in patients with inflammatory chronic pelvic pain syndrome: a double-blind, placebo-controlled, pilot study. *Urology* 1999; **53**(3): 502–505.

32 Kaplan SA, Volpe MA, Te AE. A prospective, 1-year trial using saw palmetto versus finasteride in the treatment of category III prostatitis/chronic pelvic pain syndrome. *J Urol* 2004; **171**(1): 284–8.

33 Nickel JC, Pontari M, Moon T, Gittelman M, Malek G, Farrington J *et al.* A randomized, placebo controlled, multicenter study to evaluate the safety and efficacy of rofecoxib in the treatment of chronic nonbacterial prostatitis. *J Urol* 2003; **169**(4): 1401–405.

34 Parsons CL, Albo M. Intravesical potassium sensitivity in patients with prostatitis. *J Urol* 2002; **168**(3): 1054–7.

35 Nickel JC, Forrest J, Tomera KM. Effects of pentosan polysulfate sodium in men with chronic pelvic pain syndrome: a multicenter randomized, placebo-controlled study [abstract]. *J Urol* 2002; **167**: 63.

36 Daut RL, Cleeland CS. The prevalence and severity of pain in cancer. *Cancer* 1982; **50**(9): 1913–18.

37 Portenoy RK, Lesage P. Management of cancer pain. *Lancet* 1999; **353**(9165): 1695–700.

38 WHO. *Cancer Pain Relief*. Geneva: World Health Organization, 1986.

39 Grond S, Zech D, Schug SA, Lynch J, Lehmann KA. Validation of World Health Organization guidelines for cancer pain relief during the last days and hours of life. *J Pain Symptom Manage* 1991; **6**(7): 411–22.

40 Lucas LA, McMillen BA. Differences in brain area concentrations of dopamine and serotonin in Myers' high ethanol preferring (mHEP) and outbred rats. *J Neural Transm* 2002; **109**(3): 279–92.

41 Francesca F, Bader P, Echtle D, Giunta F, Williams J, Fall M *et al.* European Association of Urology Guidelines on Pain Management. 2003.

42 Portenoy RK, McCaffery M. Adjuvant analgesics. In: McCaffery M, Pasero C, eds. *Pain: Clinical Manual*, 2nd edn. St. Louis: Mosby, 1999.

43 Eaton CL, Coleman RE. Pathophysiology of bone metastases from prostate cancer and the role of bisphosphonates in treatment. *Cancer Treat Rev* 2003; **29**(3): 189–98.

44 Saad F, Gleason DM, Murray R, Tchekmedyian S, Venner P, Lacombe L *et al.* A randomized, placebo-controlled trial of zoledronic acid in patients with hormone-refractory metastatic prostate carcinoma. *J Natl Cancer Inst* 2002; **94**(19): 1458–68.

45 Ernst DS, Tannock IF, Winquist EW, Venner PM, Reyno L, Moore MJ *et al.* Randomized, double-blind, controlled trial of mitoxantrone/prednisone and clodronate versus mitoxantrone/prednisone and placebo in patients with hormone-refractory prostate cancer and pain. *J Clin Oncol* 2003; **21**(17): 3335–42.

46 Smith JA Jr. Palliation of painful bone metastases from prostate cancer using sodium etidronate: results of a randomized, prospective, double-blind, placebo-controlled study. *J Urol* 1989; **141**(1): 85–7.

47 Bouchelouche K, Nordling J. Recent developments in the management of interstitial cystitis. *Curr Opin Urol* 2003; **13**(4): 309–13.

48 Peters K, Diokno A, Steinert B, Yuhico M, Mitchell B, Krohta S *et al.* The efficacy of intravesical Tice strain bacillus Calmette–Guérin in the treatment of interstitial cystitis: a double-blind, prospective, placebo controlled trial. *J Urol* 1997; **157**(6): 2090–94.

49 Peters KM, Diokno AC, Steinert BW, Gonzalez JA. The efficacy of intravesical bacillus CalmetteGuérin in the treatment of interstitial cystitis: long-term followup. *J Urol* 1998; **159**(5): 1483–6; discussion 1486–7.

50 Peeker R, Haghsheno MA, Holmang S, Fall M. Intravesical bacillus Calmette–Guérin and dimethyl sulfoxide for treatment of classic and nonulcer interstitial cystitis: a prospective, randomized double-blind study. *J Urol* 2000; **164**(6): 1912–15; discussion 1915–16.

51 Hwang P, Auclair B, Beechinor D, Diment M, Einarson TR. Efficacy of pentosan polysulfate in the treatment of interstitial cystitis: a meta-analysis. *Urology* 1997; **50**(1): 39–43.

52 Sant GR, Propert KJ, Hanno PM, Burks D, Culkin D, Diokno AC *et al.* A pilot clinical trial of oral pentosan polysulfate and oral hydroxyzine in patients with interstitial cystitis. *J Urol* 2003; **170**(3): 810–15.

Index

Note: page numbers in *italics* refer to figures, those in **bold** refer to tables.

ABR-214936 mAb 250
ABX-EGF mAb 250
acetaminophen *see* paracetamol
N-acetyl cysteine 202
acetyl salicylic acid (ASA) 265
acetylcholine 39
acylaminopenicillins 142, 143
Aδ fibres 257, 275
  neurotransmission 276
  nociceptive impulses 275
adaptive resistance 99
adjuvant therapy
  analgesics 276, **281–2**, 289–91
  bladder cancer 199–201
  chemotherapy 165,
    199–201, 217, 238
  prostate cancer
    bicalutamide after radical
      prostatectomy 167–8
    hormone therapy 164–5
  renal cancer 238
  testicular cancer 217, 219
α-adrenergic antagonists 23–4, **25**
  benign prostatic hyperplasia 23–4, **25**
    combination therapy 26–30
  erectile dysfunction 51–2
  pelvic pain 286
    chronic 133
  renal colic 283–5
  sildenafil co-administration 45
  tadalafil contraindication 47
  vardenafil contraindication 49
α-adrenoceptor agonists 11
α_1-adrenoceptor antagonists 124
α_2-adrenoceptor antagonists 42, 52
β_2-adrenoceptor agonists 11
Adriamycin *see* doxorubicin
AIDS 149
alfuzosin 24, 286
alprostadil 41
  intracavernosal 53–4
  intraurethral 54–5
  topical 57
amethocaine 269
amifostine 202
amikacin 122

5-amino levulinic acid (ALA) photodynamic
  therapy 182–3
γ-aminobutyric acid (GABA) 276
aminoglycosides
  complicated urinary tract infection 96,
    97–106
  dosing 104–5
  monitoring 105–6
  nephrotoxicity 100, **101**, 105–6
  once-daily dosing 97–8
  ototoxicity 101–2
  single daily dosing 96, 97–106
    β-lactam combination 103
  switch therapy 96, 106–10
aminopenicillins
  perioperative prophylaxis 145, 146
  surgery without bowel segments 145
amitriptyline 65, **66**, 68, 276, **281**
amoxycillin, quinolone combination 110
amphoterocin B
  Candida cystitis 155–6
  candidiasis 157
  candiduria 153, 154
  fungal bezoars 157
  pyelonephritis 156
ampicillin
  resistance 80
  switch therapy in pregnancy 110
anaesthesia, local 262, 263, 269–71
analgesia/analgesics 276, **277–82**
  adjuvant 276, **281–2**, 289–91
  administration route 262–4
  antidepressants 65, 276
  cancer pain 287–8
  equivalent doses **280**
  individualizing doses 287–8
  interstitial cystitis 291–2
  ladder 287, 288–91
  minimum effective concentrations 263
  multimodal 271
  nonopioid 276, **277–8**
  oral 262, 264–6
  patient-controlled systems 262, 263–4,
    268, 271
  postoperative 257–72
    future 271–2
    stepwise planned approach 261
  simple 261
  WHO ladder 287, 288–91
  see also opioids

anaphylactic reactions, paclitaxel 194–5
androgen ablation in prostate cancer 161,
    162–4
  after radical surgery 167–8
  delayed treatment 168
  early treatment 168
  intermittent *versus* delayed 168–9
  locally advanced disease 167–9
  with radiotherapy 165, 167
  unwanted effects 163–4
androgen blockade, maximum 169
angiogenesis inhibition 239, 246–7
anti-adhesin-based vaccines 92
anti-androgens
  nonsteroidal 163
  prostate cancer 161, 163
    metastatic 169
  steroidal 163
anti-angiogenesis 239, 246–7
antibiotics, candiduria predisposition 151
anticholinergics in detrusor overactivity 4–8
  mixed action 8–10
anticonvulsants **282**
antidepressants
  analgesia 65, 276
  tricyclic 276, **281**
antidiuretic hormone (ADH) 285
anti-emetics 264
  regimens 189
antifungal agents, candiduria 155
antigen presenting cells 236, 248
antigens, tumour 236–7
antimicrobials
  acute bacterial prostatitis 127, 128
  bacterial prostatitis 120–2
  chronic pelvic pain syndrome 123, 132–3
  efficacy 89–91
  intraoperative administration 140–1
  minimum inhibitory concentration 79, 82
  perioperative prophylaxis 138–47
    administration route 142
    choice 142
    duration 141–2
    goals 139–40
    indications 140–1
    pharmacoeconomics 146–7
    timing 141–2
    urological interventions 143, **144**, 145–7
  pharmacokinetics/
    pharmacodynamics 81–2
  resistance 79–81, 91
    single daily dosing 99–100
  urinary tract infection
    complicated 96–111
    simple 78–91
apomorphine 50–1
apoptosis induction 35
L-arginine **67**, 68–9
arginine vasopressin 12
aspergillosis 149
  fungal bezoars 152
aspirin 265

autonomic neuropathy 150
Avastatin *see* bevacizumab
aztreonam, switch therapy in pregnancy 110
Azuprostat 35

bacille Calmette–Guérin (BCG),
    intravesical 69
  bladder cancer 178
  immunotherapy 180–1
  interstitial cystitis 291
bacterial killing, single daily dosing
    99–100
basic fibroblast growth factor 246
bedwetting 12
benign prostatic hyperplasia 21–36
  α-adrenergic antagonists 23–4, **25**
  combination therapy 26–30
  complementary therapy 32
  epidemiology 21
  management 21–2
  natural history 22–3
  pharmacotherapy guidelines *31*
  5α-reductase inhibitors 24–6
BEP combination chemotherapy
  plus paclitaxel 223
  testicular cancer 215, **216**, 217, 219, 221,
    222
  toxicity 227
bevacizumab 247
bicalutamide 163, 166–7
  after radical surgery 167–8
biochemotherapy, renal cancer 242, *243–5*,
    246
bioflavonoids 125
bisphosphonates
  adjuvant analgesia 289–91
  prostate cancer 161
    hormone-relapsed disease 172
bladder
  emptying failure 13
  neck dysfunction 123, 124
  outlet
    obstruction 123
    resistance 12–13
  overactive 3–10
    botulinum toxin 15
  pain 70
  pressure 3
  storage failure 13–15
  voiding disturbances 123
bladder cancer 176–84
  adjuvant therapy 199–201
  carcinoma *in situ* 176, 177, 181, 182
  chemoradiotherapy 205
  chemotherapy
    combination regimens 195–202
    doublet combinations 196–7
    future development 204–5
    intravesical 178–80, 183
    metastatic disease 198–202
    oral 177
    renal obstruction 203–4

sequential therapy 197–8
single-agent 195
systemic 188–207
triplet combinations 196–7
cystectomy 200
disease progression 176–7
gene therapy 206
immunotherapy 180–2, 183
intravesical therapy 176–82, 183–4
metastatic disease
  occult micro-metastatic 198–9
  systemic chemotherapy 198–202
monoclonal antibodies 205–6
neoadjuvant therapy 199, 201–2
novel therapies 183–4
organ-confined disease 198–9
patient selection for systemic
  chemotherapy 202–3
photodynamic therapy 182–3
radical local therapy 198
radical radiotherapy 200
recurrence rate 178, 183
renal tract obstruction 203–4
small cell 203
systemic therapy 188–207
targeted therapies 205–6
transitional cell carcinoma 188, 203
variant histology 203
virus vectors 184
bleomycin
  combination chemotherapy 215, **216**, 217,
    220, 221, 223
  toxicity 221, 227
bombesin 259
bone
  pain palliation 169–70
  prostate cancer metastases 172
BOP/VIP-B induction-sequential
  chemotherapy 223
botulinum toxin 13
  cystoscopic injection 15
  interstitial cystitis 71
bowel segments, surgical procedures 140,
  143, **144**, 145
bradykinin 258–9
brain metastases in testicular cancer 226
bupivacaine 269, 270
buprenorphine 268
buserelin 163

C fibres 70, 258, 275
  neurotransmission 276
  nociceptive impulses 275
  overactivity 13
  unmyelinated 13, 14
C225 206
calcitonin gene-related peptide (CGRP) 259
calcium channel blockers 285
  detrusor overactivity 10
cancer pain 287–8
  bone pain palliation 169–70
Candida 149–50

ascending infection 152
colonization 153
contamination 152–3
cystitis 152, 155–6
infection 153
isolation 152, 153
microbiology 150
pathogenesis 150–1
urosepsis 156–7
candidemia 152
  transient 151
  treatment 156
candidiasis
  disseminated 151, 152, 157
  nosocomial 150
  renal 152, 153, **154**, 157
candiduria 149–57
  asymptomatic 154–5
  clinical features 151–2
  diagnosis 152–3
  epidemiology 149–50
  localization 153
  pathogenesis 150–1
  risk factors 151
  treatment 154–6
capsaicin 13–14, 70
  interstitial cystitis 70
carbapenems
  prophylactic 142
  resistance 81
carbohydrates, topically applied 92
carboplatin
  cisplatin comparison 197
  renal function 204
  systemic in bladder cancer 193, 202
  testicular cancer 214, 221
cardiovascular risk factors of cisplatin 228
catheterization
  candiduria 150, 151, 153, 154
  clean intermittent 13
  indwelling 145
    Candida 151
  short-term 146
CD4 T cell response
  proliferative in chronic pelvic pain
    syndrome 125
CEB combination chemotherapy 221
cefotaxime 127
ceftriaxone 127
cefuroxime 127
celecoxib 266
cephalexin switch therapy in pregnancy 110
cephalosporins
  acute bacterial prostatitis 127
  resistance 81
  second generation 145, 146
  third generation 142, 143
cephalothin resistance 80
Cetuximab 206
chemoradiotherapy, bladder cancer 205
chemotherapy
  adjuvant therapy 199–201, 217, 238

chemotherapy (*contd*)
  combination regimens 195–202, 215–16, 217
    adjuvant 238
    doublet combinations 196–7
    infertility 227–8
    neoadjuvant 165, 199, 201–2
    renal cancer 235–6
    single-agent 195
    testicular cancer 214–29
      advanced disease 217
      side-effects 227–9
    triplet combinations 196–7, 238
    see also bladder cancer, chemotherapy
children, aminoglycoside single daily
    dosing 103
Chlamydia trachomatis, chronic bacterial
    prostatitis 122, 127
chloroprocaine 269
cholecystokinin 259
cimetidine **66,** 68
ciprofloxacin 87, 89
  acute bacterial prostatitis 127
  efficacy 91
  side-effects 108
  switch therapy 108, 109–10
CISCA chemotherapy regimen 196
cisplatin
  carboplatin comparison 197
  cardiovascular risk factors 228
  chemoradiotherapy 205
  combination chemotherapy
    salvage regimens 225
    testicular cancer 223, 227, 228
    toxicity 227, 228
  combination regimen 195–6, 202, 215, **216,** 217
    adjuvant 217
  gemcitabine combination 196
  nephrotoxicity 202, 204
  rechallenge in metastatic disease 198
  side-effects 189–90
  systemic in bladder cancer 188–90, 202
  testicular cancer 214, 220, 221, 223
  vascular complications 228
clavulanic acid switch therapy in
    pregnancy 110
clean intermittent catheterization (CIC) 13
clear cell carcinoma *see* renal cell carcinoma
clenbuterol 11
clindamycin, quinolone combination 110
clonidine 263, 264
CMV chemotherapy regimen 195–6
  neoadjuvant 201
cocaine 269
co-codamol 289
codeine phosphate 267
complementary therapy, benign prostatic
    hyperplasia 32
costs of switch therapy 108
cotrimoxazole, perioperative
    prophylaxis 146

COX-1 264
  inhibition 265
COX-2 inhibitors
  chronic pelvic pain syndrome 125–6
  postoperative pain 264, 266
  prostatitis 286
  renal colic 284
cranberry products 91–2
creatinine serum levels 105–6
cryptococcosis 149
cyclizine 264
cyclo-oxygenase (COX) inhibitors 264, 275, **278**
  see also COX-1; COX-2 inhibitors
cyclophosphamide combination regimen
    196
cyclosporin 64, 69
CYP3A4 system inhibitors 48
cyproterone acetate 163, 169
cystitis, acute 77
  clinical trials of therapy 87–91
  cranberry products 91–2
  fosfomycin 86
  treatment duration 88–9
  trimethoprim–sulphamethoxazole 83
cystitis, *Candida* 152, 155–6
cystitis, interstitial 62–71, 287
  diagnostic criteria 62–3
  drug treatment 65, **66–7,** 67–70
  pain management 291–2
  therapy 63–5
cytokines
  chronic pelvic pain syndrome 125
  inhibitors 125–6
  renal cancer 237
cytotoxic T cells 237

darifenacin 10
dendritic cell vaccines 247–8
dendritic cells 236, 248
desmopressin 12, 285
detrusor areflexia 15
detrusor hypocontractility 12–13
detrusor overactivity 3–10
  neurogenic 10, 13, 15
detrusor sphincter dyssynergia 12–13
dextropropoxyphene 267
dhfr gene 82, 83
dhps gene 82, 83
diabetes mellitus, candiduria 150, 155
diclofenac 266
dihydrocodeine 267
dihydrofolate reductase 82
  inhibition 190, 191
dihydropteroate synthase 82
dihydrotestosterone 25
dimethyl sulphoxide **66,** 68
docetaxel 165, 170
  plus prednisolone 170–1
doxazosin 24
  finasteride combination
    26–30

doxorubicin
  combination regimen 195–6
  intravesical for bladder cancer 178–9
  side-effects 192–3
  systemic in bladder cancer 192–3
duloxetine 11
dutasteride 25–6
  prostate cancer prevention 162
  tamsulosin combination 30

EMLA cream 270
Enterobacter aerogenes 120
enterococci 78
  surgery without bowel segments 145
Enterococcus faecalis 120
Entonox 263
enuresis, nocturnal 12
EP combination chemotherapy 215, **216,**
    217, 221
  testicular cancer 222
epidermal growth factor receptor
    (EGFR) 205, 250
epidural analgesia 263, 271
epirubicin, bladder cancer
  intravesical 179
  systemic 202
erectile dysfunction 40–58
  causes 40, **41**
  centrally acting agents 50–1
  drug-induced 40, *41*
  locally active agents 53–5
  melanocortin analogues 56–7
  orally active agents 42–53
  testosterone 55–6
  therapy principles 41–2
erection, physiology 39–40
erythromycin 127
Escherichia coli 78
  nitrofurantoin 85
  prostatitis 120
  surgery without bowel segments 145
  urinary tract infection 82
estramustine 165, 170, 171
etidocaine 271
etoposide
  combination chemotherapy 215, **216,** 217
    salvage regimens 225
    testicular cancer 223
  testicular cancer 221
extracorporeal shock wave lithotripsy
    (ESWL) 143, 146

farnesyl transferase inhibitors 206
fentanyl 264
finasteride 24–5, 26
  doxazosin combination 26–30
  pelvic pain 286
  prostate cancer prevention 162
  tamsulosin combination 29
  terazosin combination 26–30
fleroxacin 87, 89
fluconazole

Candida cystitis 155
candidiasis 157
candiduria 154, 155, 156
fungal bezoars 157
pyelonephritis 156
flucytosine 155, 156
fluoroquinolones 82, 86–7
  efficacy 90–1
  perioperative prophylaxis 142,
    145, 146
  resistance 81
  surgery without bowel segments 145
  treatment duration 89
5-fluorouracil
  chemoradiotherapy 205
  renal cancer 235, 238
    biochemotherapy 242, *243–5,* 246
flutamide 163, 164–5
folinic acid 'rescue' 191
fosfomycin 78, 79, **80,** 86
  efficacy 90
fungal bezoars 152, 156–7

G250 mAb 249
gabapentin 65, **282**
gatifloxacin 87, 91
gemcitabine
  chemoradiotherapy 205
  cisplatin combination 196
  combination regimen 196
  farnesyl transferase inhibitor
    combination 206
  systemic in bladder cancer 193–4
  toxicity 194
gene therapy in interstitial cystitis 71
genitourinary system
  cancer pain 287–8
  infection prevention 139–40
gentamicin
  acute bacterial prostatitis 127
  complicated urinary tract infection 97–8
  single daily dosing 98–106
    benefits **99**
    contraindications 103
    convenience 102
    cost 102
    efficacy 102–3
    monitoring 105–6
    procedure 104–5
    toxicity decrease 100–2
germ cell tumours, non-seminomatous 218
  metastatic 221–3, 227
  stage I 217–19
  stage II–IV 219–23
  see also seminoma
glomerular filtration rate 81–2, 204
glucose-6-phosphage dehydrogenase (G6PD)
    deficiency 83, 85
goserelin 163
graft-*versus*-tumour response 248
guanosine monophosphate (GMP) 39, *40*
guanosine triphosphate (GTP) 39, *40*

heparin 69
Herceptin 206, 249
histamine release inhibition 64
histoplasmosis 149
hospital stay, length 108
hospitalization in acute bacterial
    prostatitis 132
human chorionic gonadotrophin (hCG) 212
human leukocyte antigens (HLA) 236
hyaluronic acid **66,** 67–8
hydrocortisone with/without
    mitoxantrone 170
hydronephrosis 157
5-hydroxytryptamine
    (5-HT) 258–9, 276
hydroxyzine **66,** 68
hypernephroma *see* renal cell carcinoma
hypersensitivity reactions, paclitaxel 194–5
hypertension, cisplatin 228
hypothalamus dopaminergic transmission 42
Hypoxis rooperi (star grass) 34–5

ibandronate 289–91
ibuprofen 265
ifosfamide combination chemotherapy 215,
    216, 217, 222, 223
    salvage regimens 225
imipramine 276
immune modulators, chronic pelvic pain
    syndrome 125–6
immunocompromised patients
    candiduria 150, 155
    urinary tract infection 103
immunogenic response modulation 64
immunoglobulin E (IgE) 258–9
immunotherapy
    bladder cancer 180–2, 183
    renal cancer 235, 236–8
    combined 242
indomethacin 266
infertility with chemotherapy 227–8
inflammatory response mediators 258–9
instrumentation 150
interferon α (IFN-α)
    IL-2 combination 242
    intravesical immunotherapy 181
    renal cancer 235, 237–8, 238–40
    biochemotherapy 242, *243–5,* 246
    toxicity 240
interferons 238–40
interleukin 2 (IL-2) 237
    continuous infusional 241
    IFN-α combination 242
    renal cancer 235, 240–1
    biochemotherapy 242, *243–5,* 246
    self-administered
        subcutaneous 241
    side-effects 241
interleukin 8 (IL-8) 246
intestinal segment, colonized 145
intracavernosal therapy 53–4
intrathecal analgesia 263

intravesical therapy 176–82, 183–4
Iressa 206
isosorbide dinitrite 285

ketamine 264
ketoprofen 265
ketorolac 266
keyhole limpet
    haemocyanin 181–2
Klebsiella 78
    prostatitis 120
    surgery without bowel segments 145
Klebsiella pneumoniae 82

β-lactamase inhibitors 142
    perioperative prophylaxis 146
    surgery without bowel segments 145
β-lactams 82, 84
    aminoglycoside single daily dose
        combination 103
    efficacy 90
    quinolone combination 110
    treatment duration 89
lactobacillus probiotic 92
leucovorin 'rescue' 191
leukotriene D receptor 65
leuprorelin 163, 164–5
levofloxacin 87
    efficacy 91
    switch therapy 109–10
lignocaine 269, 270
lipid abnormalities with cisplatin 228
lomefloxacin 87
lower urinary tract symptoms (LUTS) 21, 22
    sexual function 22–3
luteinizing hormone-releasing hormone (LH-
    RH) 161
luteinizing hormone-releasing hormone (LH-
    RH) agonists 163
    metastatic prostate cancer 169
luteinizing hormone-releasing hormone (LH-
    RH) analogues 162–3
luteinizing hormone-releasing hormone (LH-
    RH) antagonists 169

major histocompatibility complex
    (MHC) 236
mast cell inhibition 64
MCAVI chemotherapy regimen 196
MDR-1 gene 236
medroxyprogesterone acetate 235, 246
melanocortin analogues 42, 56–7
melanocortin receptors 57
meloxicam 266
mepivacaine 269
meptazinol 268
metabolic syndrome, testicular cancer 228
metastases
    bladder cancer 198–202
    prostate cancer 169, 172
    renal cancer 234
    testicular cancer 221–3, 226, 227

methicillin-resistant *Staphylococcus aureus* (MRSA) 145
methotrexate
    combination regimen 195–6
    side-effects 191
    systemic in bladder cancer 190–1, 202
metronidazole, quinolone combination 110
MIB-1 monoclonal antibody 218
micturition reflex 13
midazolam 264
Mishima regimen 180
misoprostol 65, 69
mitomycin C
    intravesical in bladder cancer 179–80
    side-effects 180
mitoxantrone 170–1
    intravesical in bladder cancer 180
monoclonal antibodies (mAbs) 205–6, 218, 249
    renal cancer 247, 249–50
montelukast 65, 69
morphine **279–80**
    oral 267
    PCAS delivery 263
    postoperative pain 262–3
moxifloxacin 87
multi-drug resistance, renal cancer 236
muscarinic (M) receptors 4, 5
    detrusor muscle activation 10
MUSE system 54–5
MVAC chemotherapy regimen 195–6
    neoadjuvant 201
    outcome 203
MVEC chemotherapy regiment 202
MVECA chemotherapy regiment 202

nalbuphine 268
naloxone 268
naproxen 265
neobladder 145
nephrectomy 156
    radical 234, 237–8
        relapse *243–5*
nephro-protective agents 202
nephrostomy tubes, percutaneous 150, 157
nephrotoxicity
    aminoglycosides 100, **101**, 105–6
    single daily dosing 100, **101**
neuraxial blockade 263
neuroanatomy 257–8
neurogenic inflammation modulation 64–5
neurokinins A and B 259
neurones, wide dynamic range 259
neuropharmacology 258–9
neurophysiology 258–9
neurotensin 276
neurotransmitters 259
    inhibition 276
nifedipine 285
nitric oxide 39, *40*

erectile function 42–3
    interstitial cystitis 64–5
nitrofurantoin 78, 79, **80**, 84–5
    adverse events 85
    efficacy 90, 91
    resistance 81
    treatment duration 88–9
nitrous oxide 263
nociception modulation 65
nociceptors 258, 259, 275
non-steroidal anti-inflammatory drugs (NSAIDs) 264, 271, 276, **277–8**
    administration route 262
    adverse effects 271
    analgesic effects 274–5
    cancer pain 288–9
    chronic pelvic pain syndrome 125
    interstitial cystitis 65
    opioid supplementation 289
    postoperative pain 261, 262, 264, 265, 266
    renal colic 283, 285
norephedrine 11
norepinephrine 276
norfloxacin 89

oestrogens, vaginally administered 11
ofloxacin 87
    acute bacterial prostatitis 127
    efficacy 90–1
ondansetron 264
opioids 276, **278–80**
    endogenous 276
    epidural 271
    interstitial cystitis 65
    NSAID supplementation 289
    patient response 289
    postoperative analgesia 262, 263, 264, 266–8
    precursors 71
    renal colic 283
orchiectomy
    non-seminoma stage II–IV 219
    radical inguinal 214, 217
        non-seminomatous cancer 222, 223
        retroperitoneal lymph node dissection 219
        without retroperitoneal node dissection 218
ototoxicity
    aminoglycosides 101–2
    single daily dosing 101–2
    switch therapy 108
oxaliplatin 204–5
oxybutinin 8–9
    tolterodine comparative trials 6–7
    trospium chloride comparative trials 7–8
oxycodone 268

p53 mutations 205, 206
p53-selective oncolytic adenovirus dl1520 (ONYX-015) 206

paclitaxel
  side-effects 194–5
  systemic in bladder cancer 194–5
  testicular cancer 223
pain
  ascending impulses 275–6
  assessment 282–3
    postoperative 259–61
  bladder 70
  cancer 287–8
    bone pain palliation 169–70
  classification 274–6
  gate theory 259
  intensity 283
  interstitial cystitis 291–2
  management 283–8
  measurement 282–3
  modulation 259
  neuropathic 65, 276
    adjuvant analgesics 289, **290**
  nociceptive 275
  physiological entity 257–9
  physiology 274–6
  postoperative
    assessment 259–61
    drugs used 264–71
    treatment 261–2
  questionnaires 261
  rating scales 282–3
  sensations 258
  somatic 257–8
  transmission 259
  underestimation 260–1
  urological 274, 282–92
  visceral 258
    adjuvant analgesics 289, **290**
papaverine 41
para-amino benzoic acid (PABA) 269
paracetamol 264, 265, 271, 276, **277**
  cancer pain 288–9
  postoperative pain 261
parecoxib 266
pelvic floor exercises 3–4
pelvic pain syndrome, chronic 121, 123–6
  analgesia 285–7
  clinical trials 132–3
  developments 133–4
  drugs 127–8, **129–30**
  therapeutic strategies 123–4
penicillin resistance 81
Penicillium, fungal bezoars 152
penile erection 39–40
  see also erectile dysfunction
pentazocine 268
pentosan polysulphate **66**, 67
  chronic pelvic pain syndrome 124, 287
  interstitial cystitis 291–2
perfloxacin 91
Permixon 33, 34
pethidine 264, 268
  postoperative pain 262

P-glycoprotein 236
pharmacoeconomics of perioperative
    prophylaxis 146–7
phenoxybenzamine 23
phentolamine 41–2
  erectile dysfunction 51–2
  vasoactive intestinal peptide
    combination 57
phenylpropanolamine 11
phosphodiesterase type 5 39, *40*, 42–3
phosphodiesterase type 5 inhibitors 42–50
  apomorphine comparison 51
  comparison 49–50
  contraindications 44, 50
phosphodiesterase type 6 43, 45
phosphodiesterase type 11 43
phospholipase inhibition 275
photodynamic therapy, bladder
    cancer 182–3
phytotherapeutic agents 30, 32–5
  benign prostatic hyperplasia 22
  chronic pelvic pain syndrome 125
  mechanism of action 32
piperacillin resistance 81
piroxicam 266
post-antibiotic effect 99–100
potassium channel openers (KCOs), detrusor
    overactivity 10
pRB mutations 205, 206
prednisolone 170–1
pregnancy, urinary tract infection 110
preproencephalin 71
prilocaine 269, 270
probiotics 92
procaine 269
prochlorperazine 264
propiverine 9–10
prostaglandin E1 41, 53
  analogues 65
  gel 57
prostaglandins 258–9
prostate
  immune responses 125
  transrectal biopsy 140, 146
  see also benign prostatic hyperplasia
prostate cancer
  androgen ablation 161, 162–4
    after radical surgery 167–8
    delayed treatment 168
    early treatment 168
    intermittent *versus* delayed 168–9
    locally advanced disease 167–9
    with radiotherapy 165, 167
    unwanted effects 163–4
  androgen maximum blockade 169
  bisphosphonates 161
    hormone-relapsed disease 172
  chemoprevention 161–2
  chemotherapy
    hormone-relapsed
      disease 170–1

neoadjuvant 165
diagnosis 161
hormone therapy 162–4
  locally advanced disease 166–9
  neoadjuvant 164–5
hormone-relapsed 169–72
localized 164–5
locally advanced 166–9
metastatic 169
  bone 172
palliative treatment 169–70
pharmacotherapy 161–73
radical prostatectomy
  adjuvant bicalutamide 167–8
  and neoadjuvant chemotherapy 165
  preceded by hormone therapy 164–5
radiotherapy plus androgen ablation 165,
  167
skeletal fractures 172
surgery 161
tumour flare 163
watchful waiting 164
prostatectomy, radical
  adjuvant bicalutamide 167–8
  and neoadjuvant chemotherapy 165
  preceded by hormone therapy 164–5
prostate-specific antigen (PSA) 22
  asymptomatic prostatitis 126–7, 128,
    131
  bicalutamide effects 167
  proliferative CD4 T cell response 125
  raised 134
  testosterone therapy 56
prostatic massage 123
prostatitis 120–34
  acute bacterial 120–1, 128, 132
    developments 133
    treatment 127
  asymptomatic 126–7, 128, **131**, 133, 134
  chronic bacterial 121–2, 127–8
    clinical trials 132
    developments 133
  chronic nonbacterial 285–7
  classification 120, **121**
Proteus, surgery without bowel
    segments 145
Proteus mirabilis 78
Provera *see* medroxyprogesterone acetate
Pseudomonas aeruginosa
  minimum inhibitory concentration 104
  prostatitis 120
PVB combination chemotherapy 220
pVHL 249
pyelonephritis
  Candida 151, 152, **154**
    ascending 156–7
  in pregnancy 110
  switch therapy 106, 107–8
Pygmeum africanum (African plum) 34

quinolones
  acute bacterial prostatitis 127

chronic bacterial prostatitis 132
contraindication in pregnancy 110
resistance 110
side-effects 108
switch therapy 109–10

radiation recall phenomenon 192–3
radiotherapy
  with androgen ablation 165
  dog-leg field 213–14
  doxorubicin toxicity 192–3
  renal cancer 234–5
  seminoma
    stage I 213–14
    stage IIA/B 214, 215
    stage IIC advanced disease 215, 216
  whole-brain irradiation 226
Raynaud's phenomenon 227, 228
receptor tyrosine kinase inhibitors 206, 250
5α-reductase inhibitors 24–6, 162
  benign prostatic hyperplasia combination
    therapy 26–30
  chronic pelvic pain syndrome 124
renal cancer 234–50
  anti-angiogenesis agents 239, 246–7
  biochemotherapy 242, *243–5*, 246
  chemotherapy 235–6
    adjuvant 238
  dendritic cell vaccines 247–8
  5-fluorouracil biochemotherapy 242,
    243–5, 246
  hormone therapy 235
  IFN-α 235, 237–8, 238–40
    biochemotherapy 242, *243–5*, 246
  IL-2 235, 237, 240–1
    biochemotherapy 242, *243–5*, 246
  immunotherapy 235, 236–8
    combined 242
  medroxyprogesterone acetate 235, 246
  metastatic disease 234
  monoclonal antibodies 247, 249–50
  multi-drug resistance 236
  palliation 235
  risk factors 234
  staging 234
  stem cell transplantation 248–9
  surgery 237–8
    adjuvant therapy 238
  tamoxifen 235, 242
  thalidomide 246–7
  triple therapy 242, *243–5*, 246
  vinblastine 235, 239
renal cell carcinoma 234
renal colic 283–5
renal function, impaired 204
renal transplantation, candiduria 155
resiniferatoxin 14–15
  interstitial cystitis 70
resistance
  adaptive 99
  antimicrobials 79–81, 91
    single daily dosing 99–100

resistance (*contd*)
  multi-drug in renal cancer 236
  vancomycin 142
retroperitoneal lymph node nerve-sparing
      dissection 217–18, 219
Rexed's laminae 257, 258, 259
Reye's syndrome 265
Rituximab 249
rofecoxib 266, 286
ropivacaine 269, 271
rufloxacin 91

Sabal serrulatum (saw palmetto) 33
saw palmetto 32, 33–4
selenium, prostate cancer prevention 162
seminoma
  carboplatin chemotherapy 215–16
  residual abnormalities 216
  stage I 213–14
  stage IIA/B 214–15
  stage IIC advanced disease 215–17
Serenoa repens (saw palmetto) 33–4
Serratia, prostatitis 120
sexual function, LUTS 22–3
sildenafil 41–2, 43, 44–6
  apomorphine comparison 51
  contraindications 45
  pharmacokinetics 43–4
  safety 46
  side-effects 45
single daily dosing of aminoglycosides 96,
      98–106
  antimicrobial resistance reduction
      99–100
  contraindications 103
  dosing 104–5
  gentamicin
    contraindications 103
    convenience 102
    cost 102
    efficacy 102–3
    monitoring 105–6
    procedure 104–5
  nephrotoxicity 100, **101**
  ototoxicity 101–2
  toxicity decrease 100–2
beta-sitosterol 35
skeletal fractures in prostate cancer 172
smoking
  bladder cancer 202
  renal cancer risk 234
sodium hyaluronate **66**, 67–8
soft enhancer of percutaneous absorption
      (SEPA) 57
solifenacin 10
sphincterotomy, surgical 13
spinal cord, dorsal horn 274, 275–6
staphylococcal infection prophylaxis 145
Staphylococcus aureus, methicillin-
      resistant 145
Staphylococcus saprophyticus 78, 82
star grass 34–5

stem cell transplantation
  mini allogenic 248–9
  testicular cancer 223, 226
stents
  candiduria 150
  ureteral 157
steroids
  analgesic effects 274–5
  hydrocortisone with/without
      mitoxantrone 170
  prednisolone 170–1
substance P 258–9
sulphamethoxazole *see*
      trimethoprim–sulphamethoxazole
sulphonamides 81
suplatast tosilate 70
surgery
  diagnostic urological interventions 146
  endourological 146
  erectile dysfunction 40, *41*
  including bowel segments 143, 145
  outside urinary tract 145
  perioperative antimicrobial
      prophylaxis 138–47
  prostate cancer 161
  refractory candiduria 156
  renal cancer 237–8
  sphincterotomy 13
  testicular cancer 214, 217–18, 219, 222,
      223
    after chemotherapy 224
    salvage 225, 226
switch therapy
  acute bacterial prostatitis 127
  aminoglycosides 96, 106–10
  contraindications 109
  definition 106
  dosing 109–10
  efficacy 107–8
  patient selection 109
  pregnancy 110
  rationale 107–8
  underutilization 107
syndrome X, testicular cancer 228

T cell receptor (TCR) 236
T cells
  activation 236–7
  proliferative response in chronic pelvic pain
      syndrome 125
tadalafil 41, **42**, 43, 46–7
  pharmacokinetics 43–4
  safety 47
  side-effects 46–7
tamoxifen, renal cancer 235, 242
tamsulosin 24
  dutasteride combination 30
  finasteride combination 29
  renal colic 284–5
  saw palmetto combination/comparison 34
Tarceva 206

taxanes
  bladder cancer 194–5
  platinum doublets 197
tazobactam resistance 81
tenoxicam 266, 285
terazosin 24
  finasteride combination 26–30
testicular cancer 212–29
  adjuvant therapy 217, 219
  brain metastases 226
  chemotherapy 214–28
    high-dose 225, 226
    with peripheral stem cell
      transplantation 223
    recurrent disease 225–6
    salvage regimens 225
    side-effects 227–9
    toxicity 227–9
  classification 212, **213**
  diagnosis 212
  disseminated 219–23
  follow-up 226–7
  germ cell tumours 220
  metabolic syndrome 228
  monoclonal antibodies 218
  non-seminomatous germ cell tumours
    218
    metastatic 221–3, 227
    stage I 217–19
    stage II–IV 219–23
  prognosis 220
  relapse 225–6
    rates 219, 227
  retroperitoneal lymph node nerve-sparing
    dissection 217–18, 219
  seminoma
    stage I 213–14
    stage IIA/B 214–15
    stage IIC advanced disease 215–17
  staging 212, **213**
  stem cell transplantation 223, 226
  surgery 214, 217–18, 219, 222, 223
    after chemotherapy 224
  surveillance 218–19, 219
  syndrome X 228
testosterone
  administration 55
  bicalutamide effects 166
  erectile dysfunction 40, 55–6
  preparations **56**
tetracaine 269, 271
tetracycline 127
thalidomide, renal cancer 246–7
thiotepa, intravesical in bladder cancer 178
thymidine synthase 190
tolterodine 5–7
  trospium chloride comparative trials 8
tramadol 264, 268, **278–9**
transforming growth factor β$_1$ (TGF-
  β$_1$) 34–5
transurethral resection of prostate
  (TURP) 21

perioperative prophylaxis 140
Trastuzumab 206
trazodone 42, 52–3
triethylene thiophosphoramide *see* thiotepa
Trilene 263
trimethoprim 83–4
trimethoprim–sulphamethoxazole 78, 79,
  80, 82–3
  acute bacterial prostatitis 127
  efficacy 89–91
  pharmacokinetics 83
  resistance 80
  switch therapy in pregnancy 110
  treatment duration 88
triptorelin 163
tromethamine 86
trospium chloride 7–8
trovafloxacin 87
tumour antigens 236–7
tumour necrosis factor
  α (TNF-α) 246
tumour-associated
  antigens (TAAs) 239, 247–8
tunica albuginea 40
tyrosine kinase inhibitors
  206, 250

Ureaplasma urealyticum, bacterial
  prostatitis 122, 127
ureteric obstruction 284
urethral closure pressure
  maximum (MUCP) 10–11
    chronic pelvic pain syndrome 123
  reduction 124
urge incontinence 3
urgency 3
urinary drainage
  acute bacterial prostatitis 128
  bacterial contamination 140
  postoperative 146
urinary incontinence 3–15
  neurogenic 12–15
  overactive bladder 3–10
  stress 3, 10–12
urinary retention, acute
  benign prostatic hypertension 22
  combination therapy 27–9
urinary stasis 150
urinary tract
  obstruction 140, 150
  see also lower urinary
    tract symptoms (LUTS)
urinary tract infection 77–92
  complicated 96–111
    duration of treatment 110
    immunocompromised patients 103
  fungal 149
  pathogens 78
  postoperative complication 146
  pregnancy 110
  recurrent in prostatitis 122
  therapy principles 78–82

urological interventions,
        diagnostic 146
urothelial protection 64

valrubicin, intravesical in bladder cancer
        180
vancomycin resistance 142
vanilloid receptor antagonists 70
vanilloid receptors 13–14
vardenafil 41, **42**, 43, 47–9
    pharmacokinetics 43–4
    safety 49
    side-effects 48–9
vascular endothelial growth factors (VEGF)
    monoclonal antibodies 247
    renal cancer 246
vasoactive intestinal peptide (VIP) 39, 259
    phentolamine combination 57
verapamil 10
VHL gene 249
vinblastine
    combination chemotherapy 195–6
        salvage regimens 225
    renal cancer 235, 239
    systemic in bladder cancer 191–2, 202

testicular cancer 220
vincristine 191, 192
    combination chemotherapy in testicular
        cancer 223
vinflunine 205
VIP combination chemotherapy 215, **216**,
        217, 222, 223, 226
virus vectors 184
vitamin E, prostate cancer
        prevention 162
von Hippel–Lindau (VHL)
        syndrome 234

whole-brain irradiation 226
World Health Organization (WHO) analgesic
        ladder 288–91
wound infections, postoperative
        complication 145, 146

yohimbine 42, 52

Zoladex 169
zoledronic acid 172, *173*
    adjuvant analgesia 289–91
zygomycetes, fungal bezoars 152